CRITICAL CARE MANAGEMENT
Case Studies:
Tricks and Traps

Editors

G. R. Park MD, MA, BSc, MBChB, FRCA
Director
The John Farman Intensive Care Unit
Addenbrooke's Hospital
Cambridge, UK

and

M R Pinsky MD
Professor of Anesthesiology, Critical Care Medicine and Medicine
Director of Research
Division of Critical Care Medicine
University of Pittsburgh Medical Center
Pittsburgh, USA

W B Saunders Company Ltd
London   Philadelphia   Toronto   Sydney   Tokyo

W.B. Saunders Company Ltd   24–28 Oval Road
London NW1 7DX, UK

The Curtis Center
Independence Square West
Philadelphia, PA 19106-3399, USA

Harcourt Brace & Company
55 Horner Avenue
Toronto, Ontario M8Z 4X6, Canada

Harcourt Brace & Company, Australia
30–52 Smidmore Street
Marrickville, NSW 2204, Australia

Harcourt Brace & Company, Japan
Ichibancho Central Building, 22–1 Ichibancho
Chiyoda-ku, Tokyo 102, Japan

© 1997 W.B. Saunders Company Ltd

A catalogue record for this book is available from the British Library

ISBN 0–7020–1909–7

Typeset by LaserScript, Mitcham, Surrey
Printed and bound in Great Britain by The University Press, Cambridge

Contents

[†] Deceased

List of Contributors

Graeme J M Alexander, MA, MD, FRCP, Lecturer in Medicine and Honorary Consultant Physician, Department of Medicine, Clinical School of Medicine, University of Cambridge, Addenbrooke's NHS Trust, Cambridge, UK

Derek C Angus, MPH, FCCP, Assistant Professor, Critical Care Medicine Division, Department of Anesthesiology/Critical Care Medicine, University of Pittsburgh School of Medicine, Pittsburgh, USA

Trevor Baglin, MA, PhD, FRCP, MRCPath, Consultant Haematologist, Department of Clinical Haematology, Addenbrooke's NHS Trust, Cambridge, UK

Sarah E Bakewell, FRCA, The John Farman Intensive Care Unit, Addenbrooke's NHS Trust, Cambridge, UK

Rinaldo Bellomo, MD, Intensive Care Unit, Austin Hospital, Victoria 3084, Australia

Morris I Bierman[†], MD, Assistant Professor, Division of Critical Care Medicine, University of Pittsburgh Medical Center, Pittsburgh, USA

Stephen A Bowles, MD, Assistant Professor, Division of Critical Care Medicine, Presbyterian University Hospital, University of Pittsburgh Medical Center, Pittsburgh, USA

P H Carroll, MA, DA, FRCA, The John Farman Intensive Care Unit, Addenbrooke's NHS Trust, Cambridge, UK

Victor M Chavez, MD, Division of Pulmonology, Saint Louis University Medical Center, St Louis, USA

Tarek A Chidiac, MD[a], Department of Critical Care Medicine, St John's Mercy Medical Center, St Louis, USA

John G Cunniffe, MSC, MRCPath, The Department of Medical Microbiology, Addenbrooke's NHS Trust, Cambridge, UK

Robert E Cunnion, MD, Senior Investigator, Critical Care Medicine Department, National Institutes of Health, Bethesda, USA

[†] Deceased
[a] Present address: Department of Hematology and Medical Oncology, Cleveland Clinic Foundation, Cleveland, USA

P Diesel, DPharm, Research Pharmacist, The John Farman Intensive Care Unit, Addenbrooke's NHS Trust, Cambridge, UK

Geoff Dobb, BSc, MRCP, FRCA, FANZCA, FFICANZCA, MD, Specialist in Intensive Care, Intensive Care Unit, Royal Perth Hospital, Perth, Australia

J C Farmer MD, Director, Critical Care Medicine, Wilford Hall, USAF Medical Center, Lackland, USA

D G Greig, FRCA, Senior Registrar in Anaesthetics, Department of Anaesthesia, Withington Hospital, Manchester, UK

John A Kellum, MD, Assistant Professor of Medicine, Division of Critical Care Medicine, University of Pittsburgh Medical Center, Pittsburgh, USA

Lisa L Kirkland, MD, University of Tennessee Medical Center, Knoxville, USA

David J Kramer, MD, Co-Director, Liver Transplant Unit, Associate Professor, Division of Critical Care Medicine, Pittsburgh, USA

G Daniel Martich, MD, Assistant Professor, Division of Critical Care Medicine, University of Pittsburgh Medical Center, Pittsburgh, USA

B F Matta, BA, DA, FRCA, Senior Registrar, The John Farman Intensive Care Unit, Addenbrooke's NHS Trust, Cambridge, UK

George M Matuschak, MD, Professor of Internal Medicine, Co-Director, MICU, Division of Pulmonology, Saint Louis University Medical Center, St Louis, USA

Adelaida M Miro, MD, Associate Professor of Anesthesiology, Division of Critical Care Medicine, University of Pittsburgh Medical Center, Pittsburgh, USA

N D Murphy, BS, FRCA[a], The John Farman Intensive Care Unit, Addenbrooke's NHS Trust, Cambridge, UK

Gilbert R Park, MD, MA, BSc, MBChB, FRCA, Director of Intensive Care & Consultant in Anaesthesia, The John Farman Intensive Care Unit, Addenbrooke's NHS Trust, Cambridge, UK

Michael R Pinsky, MD, CM, Professor of Anesthesiology, Critical Care Medicine and Medicine, Director of Research, Division of Critical Care Medicine, University of Pittsburgh Medical Center, Pittsburgh, USA

Philippe Rico, MD[b], Critical Care Medicine Division, Department of Anesthesiology/Critical Care Medicine, University of Pittsburgh School of Medicine, Pittsburgh, USA

---

[a] Present address: Kings College Hospital, Denmark Hill, London, UK
[b] Present address: Hopital du Sacré-Coeur de Montreal, Montreal, Canada

Hamid R Sadaghar, MD, Assistant Professor, Division of Critical Care Medicine, University of Pittsburgh Medical Center, Pittsburgh, USA

Jeffrey E Salon, MD[a], Department of Critical Care Medicine, St John's Mercy Medical Center, St Louis, USA

Steven M Scharf, MD, PhD, Division of Pulmonary and Critical Care Medicine, Long Island Jewish Medical Center, New York, USA

Maire P Shelly, FRCA, Consultant in Anaesthesia and Intensive Care, Withington Hospital, West Didsbury, Manchester, UK

Subhash Todi, MD, Department of Critical Care Medicine, St Johns Mercy Medical Center, St Louis, USA

R William Vandivier, MD, Senior Staff Fellow, Critical Care Medicine Department, National Institutes of Health, Bethesda, USA

Christopher Veremakis, MD, Chairman, Department of Critical Care Medicine, St John's Mercy Medical Center, Associate Clinical Professor of Medicine, Saint Louis University, St Louis, USA

Neil Watkins, MBBS, FRACP, NH and MRC Scholar, Department of Medicine, University of Western Australia, QEII Medical Centre, Nedlands, Australia

---

[a] Present address: Director, Buckeye Critical Care Institute, Mount Carmel Medical Center, Columbus, Ohio

Preface

Effectively treating the critically ill and unstable patient is a difficult and demanding task. Complex and often life threatening changes occur to the patient which need immediate decisions and treatment. Even appropriate treatment, if delayed, is often associated with a poor outcome. In these circumstances of rapid change in the patient's status, and the urgent demands associated with such change, the clinician's knowledge and skill will be tested to the full. Every physician has had patients in whom care was suboptimal because they fell into a trap of incorrect logic: while this logic would have been reasonable under other circumstances, it was not correct in this case. This book attempts to highlight some of the common traps encountered in every day intensive care. Reading this most clinicians will feel 'there but for the grace of God go I' and try not to fall for this trap. Just reporting the specific trap, however, is not enough. Thus, we asked the authors not only to describe these specific traps, but also to detail how they could have been recognized earlier, which additional tests could have been done to prevent the trap, and also how they would have extricated themselves from the trap once 'sprung'. Finally, supplemental references on each subject are included for additional reading.

In writing an international textbook several obstacles had to be cleared. Regrettably there are still no standard units for all laboratory measurements. The Europeans favouring System Internationale, while the Americans continue with Imperial or conventional units. Chapters in this book give as the primary units those used by the author, and in the square brackets next to it we give the value in the alternative units. Where the numbers are identical in both systems the change in units is ignored. For example, a serum potassium of 4.5 mEq L^{-1} would not be changed to 4.5 mmol L^{-1}. A similar problem existed with the generic names of some drugs. Again we have left these as the author wrote them, but on their first mention in each chapter we have given the alternative name.

We hope that this book will serve the reader well in the bedside practice of critical care medicine. As novel and advanced therapies continue to develop and more unstable patients are presented to the intensive care unit one thing remains clear, there is no substitute for an experienced bedside health care team dedicated to excellence in patient care and willing to learn both from their own mistakes and from those of others.

GR Park
Cambridge, UK
MR Pinsky
Pittsburg, USA

1 Cardiac Instability

1.1 Hypotension in a Cancer Patient
R.W. Vandivier and R.E. Cunnion

History

A 61-year-old man was admitted for management of hypotension. A former shipyard worker, he had been found 11 months earlier to have a locally invasive, pleural-based, mass lesion (Figure 1.1.1), which was biopsied and found to be a malignant mesothelioma. Despite palliative irradiation, as well as chemotherapy, including adriamycin (total dose 400 mg m^{-2}), his disease had metastasized to the mediastinum, the contralateral lung and the liver. The most recent cycle of chemotherapy had been nine days before admission.

On initial examination he was alert but uncomfortable, complaining of dyspnea and right-sided chest discomfort, which had developed over the preceding day or two. He denied cough, hemoptysis, fever, chills, abdominal discomfort, bleeding or dysuria. His blood pressure was 88/68 mmHg, his pulse rate 115/minute, his temperature 38.3°C and his respiratory rate 24/minute. His ears, nose and throat were unremarkable. His fingernails were clubbed and cyanotic. Elevated jugular veins and indurated supraclavicular lymph nodes were present bilaterally. There was dullness to percussion and absence of breath sounds at both lung bases. Heart sounds were soft; no murmurs were heard. His abdomen was protuberant but not tender, with active bowel sounds, and his liver edge was palpable 4 cm below the right costal margin. Both legs were edematous, but no cords were appreciable and Homans' sign was absent.

His routine serum chemistries were within normal limits except for mildly elevated BUN (28 mg dL^{-1} [10 mmol L^{-1}]), creatinine (1.9 mg dL^{-1} [168 µmol L^{-1}]) and bilirubin (2.0 mg dL^{-1} [34 µmol L^{-1}]). Arterial gases, obtained on supplemental oxygen at 4 L min^{-1} by nasal cannula, showed pH 7.45 [H$^+$ 36 nmol L^{-1}], $P_a\text{CO}_2$ 33 mmHg [4.4 kPa] and $P_a\text{CO}_2$ 62 mmHg [8.3 kPa]. Total white blood cell count was 0.9×10^9 L^{-1} (900 mm^{-3}), hemoglobin and hematocrit were 9.8 g dL^{-1} and 29.9%, respectively, and platelet count was 60×10^9 L^{-1} (60 000 mm^{-3}). Urine specific gravity was 1.021 and urine dipstick tests were negative. Urine and blood cultures were sent. His chest radiograph is shown in Figure 1.1.2 and his electrocardiogram in Figure 1.1.3.

0.9% Saline was started intravenously at 500 mL h^{-1} and empiric broad-spectrum antibiotic therapy was ordered. Four hours later, his blood pressure was 84/62 mmHg, his pulse rate 130/minute, his respiratory rate 28/minute and his urine output less than 20 mL h^{-1}.

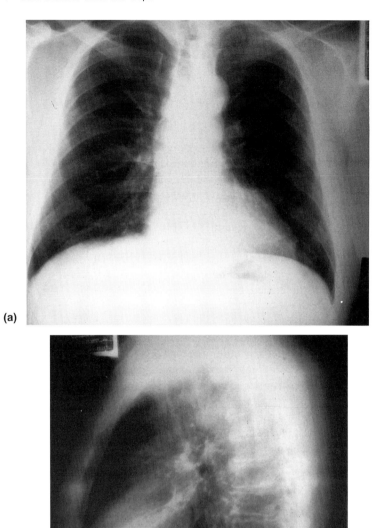

(a)

(b)

Figure 1.1.1. (*a*) Posteroanterior and (*b*) Lateral Chest radiographs obtained 11 months earlier. The primary mesothelioma, located posteriorly above the left hemidiaphragm, is best seen on the lateral film. The cardiac silhouette is normal.

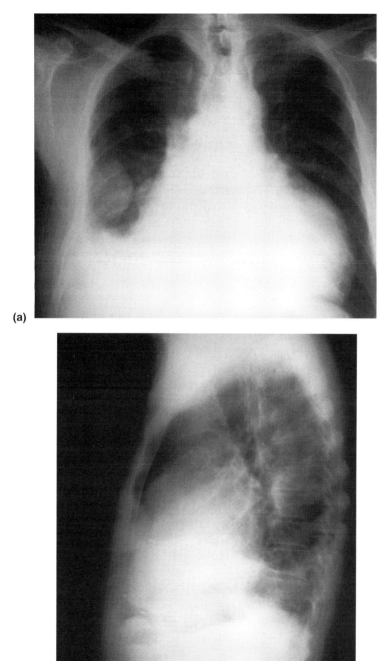

(a)

(b)

Figure 1.1.2. (*a*) Posteroanterior and (*b*) lateral chest radiographs obtained on admission, showing nodular lung densities, a large right pleural effusion, and an enlarged, globular, cardiac silhouette.

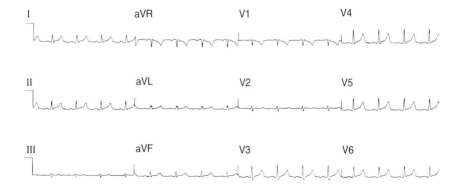

Figure 1.1.3. A 12-lead electrocardiogram obtained on admission, notable for the absence of Q waves or ischemic ST segment or T wave abnormalities, and for the presence of low QRS voltage (<0.5 mV) in the limb leads.

Traps

- When admitting a complex medical patient to a busy intensive care unit, it is tempting to treat hypotension based on the initial diagnostic impression (in this case, sepsis) without adequately considering other potential causes (such as hemorrhage, dehydration, heart failure, pulmonary embolism or tamponade) that have specific therapeutic implications.
- Rapid infusion of crystalloid or colloid solutions is central in the initial resuscitation of any hypotensive patient. However, if blood pressure does not respond quickly, it is important to consider administering fluid even more aggressively, starting inotropic or vasopressor agents, and implementing invasive hemodynamic monitoring. The longer hypotension persists, the more likely the patient will develop multiorgan dysfunction.

Tricks

Confronted with a hypotensive patient, the clinician can discern the elements of the differential diagnosis quickly using the history, physical findings and routine ancillary tests. Then, while initial resuscitative measures are underway, an orderly sequence of further diagnostic and therapeutic steps can be established.

In this patient, who presented with hypotension and low-grade fever in the setting of chemotherapy-induced leukopenia, it was important and entirely appropriate to obtain cultures and start empiric antibiotics for the possibility of *sepsis*, even in the absence of an identifiable site of infection.[1]

Nothing in his clinical presentation indicated *dehydration*; in fact, his elevated neck veins and edematous legs were suggestive of fluid overload.

Similarly, there was no overt evidence of *hemorrhage*. However, because of his leukopenia, no rectal examination was performed to see if there was any fresh or old blood in his stool, and his combination of anemia and thrombocytopenia warranted ongoing vigilance for any signs of bleeding.

At first glance, *heart failure* would seem unlikely, given his relatively acute onset of symptoms and the absence of Q waves or ischemic ST segment and T wave abnormalities on his electrocardiogram. Nonetheless, he had received adriamycin, which can cause biventricular heart failure.[2] Adriamycin cardiotoxicity usually is seen when cumulative total doses have exceeded $550\,mg\,m^{-2}$, but it can be seen at lower cumulative doses. Syndromes of acute adriamycin cardiotoxicity, unrelated to cumulative dose, have also been described. In this patient, heart failure could not be excluded without further measures, such as echocardiography, radionuclide heart scanning or pulmonary artery catheterization.

This patient had a number of features consistent with acute *pulmonary embolism*, particularly hypoxemia, tachycardia and chest pain. Ordinarily, hypotension is a feature of pulmonary embolism only when more than 50% of the pulmonary vascular cross-sectional area is occluded. Patients with malignancies are at increased risk of thromboembolic complications, and pulmonary embolism certainly can occur in cancer patients despite thrombocytopenia or other coagulopathies.[3] Excluding pulmonary emboli in critically ill patients is often problematic. If the chest radiograph is markedly abnormal, as in this patient, the sensitivity and specificity of ventilation–perfusion lung scanning are diminished. Transportation and proper positioning of hemodynamically unstable patients are difficult. Pulmonary arteriography has enough potential morbidity to inhibit its use when the suspicion of pulmonary embolism is low. Less invasive tests, such as impedance plethysmography or Doppler sonography of lower extremity veins, are sometimes useful. Even when the diagnosis has been established, critically ill patients often have absolute or relative contraindications to therapy with heparin or thrombolytic agents, such that therapeutic intervention is limited to placement of an inferior vena caval filter. In this particular patient, pulmonary embolism was considered an improbable cause for hypotension, and a judgement was made that other diagnostic considerations should assume priority.

Pericardial tamponade, defined as an accumulation of fluid in the pericardial space sufficient to compress the heart and impair diastolic filling, occurs in a wide variety of settings, ranging from chest trauma to uremia to collagen vascular diseases to idiopathic pericarditis.[4] Among cancer patients, tamponade most commonly occurs with neoplasms that invade the pericardium and give rise to malignant pericardial effusions, namely breast and lung carcinomas, melanomas, Hodgkin's and non-Hodgkin's lymphomas, and mesotheliomas.

Tamponade, irrespective of course, classically presents with many of the features found in this case: dyspnea, tachycardia, distended neck veins, distant heart sounds, an enlarged cardiac silhouette on the chest radiograph and decreased electrocardiographic QRS voltage.[5] Pulsus paradoxus, defined as $>10\,mmHg$ decrease in systolic blood pressure with inspiration, is often present, but can be quite difficult to measure accurately in a patient who has already become hypotensive and who has a narrow pulse pressure. Unfortunately, even when pulsus paradoxus is appreciated, the finding is not specific for tamponade; pulsus paradoxus may also be found in hypovolemia, cor pulmonale and other conditions.

Two tests are highly useful in diagnosing pericardial tamponade: echocardiography and pulmonary artery catheterization. Echocardiography will demonstrate the presence or absence of a pericardial effusion. If an effusion is present, the presence of diastolic collapse of the right atrium and the right ventricular free wall are pathognomonic of tamponade.[6] Concomitantly, echocardiography permits assessment of the heart itself for any abnormalities of myocardial or valvular function.[7] Pulmonary artery catheterization in tamponade will demonstrate that right-sided pressures – right atrial, right ventricular end-diastolic, pulmonary artery diastolic and pulmonary artery occlusion – all are elevated and equalized (i.e. within 5 mmHg of one another).

It is important to recognize that hypotension is a late finding in tamponade. As pericardial pressure increases, the cardiovascular system compensates, maintaining diastolic filling by intravascular volume expansion, maintaining stroke volume by catecholamine-mediated increases in contractility, maintaining cardiac output through increases in heart rate, and maintaining blood pressure by augmenting systemic vascular resistance.[8] Only when these compensatory mechanisms are overcome does frank hypotension develop.

Follow-up

This patient's physicians did suspect tamponade, given his underlying malignancy, the enlarged cardiac silhouette on chest radiography, and the low QRS voltage on the ECG. They requested a portable echocardiogram, which showed a large anterior and posterior pericardial effusion, with diastolic right atrial and right ventricular free wall collapse. Further, the echocardiogram showed vigorous systolic contraction of both ventricles, thus effectively excluding adriamycin cardiomyopathy. As arrangements were being made for percutaneous pericardiocentesis, a pulmonary artery catheter was placed (Table 1.1.1).

Table 1.1.1. Hemodynamic measurements before pericardiocentesis

Arterial pressure	80/58 mmHg
Heart rate	135/minute
Right atrial pressure	20 mmHg
Right ventricular pressure	35/10 mmHg
Right ventricular end-diastolic pressure	18 mmHg
Pulmonary artery pressure	34/22 mmHg
Pulmonary artery occlusion pressure	19 mmHg
Cardiac output	$3.0 \, L \, min^{-1}$
Cardiac index	$1.7 \, L \, min^{-1} \, m^{-2}$
Systemic vascular resistance	$1209 \, dyn\text{-}sec \, cm^{-5}$
Systemic vascular resistance index	$2133 \, dyn\text{-}sec \, cm^{-5} \, m^{-2}$

A pericardial needle was inserted from the subxiphoid approach. Serosanguinous fluid was obtained and sent for cytology, cultures, counts and chemistries. As soon as the first 100 ml of fluid was removed, the patient's hypotension and tachycardia began to improve. It is common for pericardiocentesis to produce this sort of immediate physiologic response. Removal of just the first 50 or 100 mL of fluid dramatically reduces the intrapericardial pressure, facilitating ventricular filling and augmenting stroke volume. In this patient, a pigtail catheter was advanced into the pericardium, a total of 810 mL was removed, and hemodynamic determinations were repeated (Table 1.1.2).

Table 1.1.2. Hemodynamic measurements after pericardiocentesis

Arterial pressure	136/80 mmHg
Heart rate	90/minute
Right atrial pressure	4 mmHg
Right ventricular pressure	32/2 mmHg
Right ventricular end-diastolic pressure	5 mmHg
Pulmonary artery pressure	30/16 mmHg
Pulmonary artery occlusion pressure	11 mmHg
Cardiac output	$6.6\,\text{L min}^{-1}$
Cardiac index	$3.7\,\text{L min}^{-1}\,\text{m}^{-2}$
Systemic vascular resistance	$1196\,\text{dyn-sec cm}^{-5}$
Systemic vascular resistance index	$2111\,\text{dyn-sec cm}^{-5}\,\text{m}^{-2}$

These numbers were reassuringly normal, allaying any concern that the patient might have had septic shock, heart failure or pulmonary embolism concomitant with his tamponade. If sepsis were present, one would have expected the cardiac index to be higher and the systemic vascular resistance index to be lower. If heart failure were present, one would have expected the cardiac index to be lower and the pulmonary artery occlusion pressure to be higher. If extensive pulmonary embolism were present, one would have expected persistent elevation of pulmonary artery pressures following pericardiocentesis.

Sometimes pericardiocentesis fails to produce the expected improvement. When this occurs, other explanations should be sought. Pericardial effusions can be loculated, leading to incomplete drainage. Alternatively, some patients have effusive–constrictive pericarditis, in which the physiology may represent a composite of tamponade and of constriction caused by pericardial fibrosis.[9]

This patient had a brisk spontaneous diuresis over the next few hours, and his oxygenation improved markedly. Daily drainage from the pericardial catheter remained $> 200\,\text{mL}$. The patient was informed of the available therapeutic options.[10] Instead of sclerotherapy or balloon pericardiostomy, he elected to undergo surgical pericardiotomy, which was successfully accomplished four days after the pericardiocentesis.

References

1 Cunnion RE and Parrillo JE. Cardiovascular diseases. In: Parrillo JE, Masur H (eds) *The Critically Ill Immunosuppressed Patient.* Rockville, Aspen Publishers, pp 3–38, 1987.

2 Buzdar AU, Marcus C, Smith TL, and Blumenschein GR. Early and delayed clinical cardiotoxicity of doxorubicin. *Cancer* (1985) **55**: 2761–2765.

3 Moser KM. Venous thromboembolism. In: Shelhamer JH, Pizzo AA, Parrillo JE and Masur H. (eds) *Respiratory Disease in the Immunosuppressed Host.* Philadelphia, J.B. Lippincott, pp 530–534, 1991.

4 Ameli S and Shah PK. Cardiac tamponade: pathophysiology, diagnosis, and management. *Cardiology Clinics* (1991) **9**: 665–674.

5 Spodick DH. Pericarditis, pericardial effusion, cardiac tamponade, and constriction. *Critical Care Clinics* (1989) **5**: 455–476.

6 Singh S, Wann LS, Klopfenstein HS, Hartz A and Brooks HL. Usefulness of right ventricular diastolic collapse in diagnosing cardiac tamponade and comparison to pulsus paradoxus. *American Journal of Cardiology* (1986) **57**: 652–656.

7 Parker MM, Cunnion RE and Parrillo JE. Echocardiography and nuclear cardiac imaging in the critical care unit. *Journal of the American Medical Association* (1985) **254**: 2935–2939.

8 Reddy PS, Curtiss EI, O'Toole JD, and Shaver JA. Cardiac tamponade: hemodynamic observations in man. *Circulation* (1978) **58**: 265–272.

9 Brockington GM, Zebede J and Pandian NG. Constrictive pericarditis. *Cardiology Clinics* (1990) **8**: 645–661.

10 Hawkins JW and Vacek JL. What constitutes definitive therapy of malignant pericardial effusion? 'Medical' versus surgical treatment. *American Heart Journal* (1989) **118**: 428–432.

1.2 Acute Myocardial Infarction with Pulmonary Edema

R.W. Vandivier and R.E. Cunnion

History

A hypertensive 67-year-old man presented to the emergency room at 18.00 h with substernal pain of 6 hours' duration. His electrocardiogram showed ST segment elevations in the anterior precordial leads. He received 100 mg of recombinant tissue plasminogen activator, with resolution of his chest pain, and was brought to the coronary intensive care unit with a blood pressure of 110/60 mmHg and a pulse rate of 90/minute. On examination, he had no jugular venous distension or edema, but he did have rales at the left lung base and a subtle S3 gallop.

He was maintained overnight on heparin 1000 units h^{-1}, nitroglycerin 20 µg min^{-1} and oxygen 2 L min^{-1}. He slept fitfully but remained pain-free. At 06.00 h his creatine phosphokinase was 3942 IU mL^{-1} [66 µmol L^{-1}] and his electrocardiogram revealed Q waves in leads V1 to V4, consistent with a large transmural anterior wall infarction.

At 07.00 h he was noted to be sitting upright in bed coughing; his lips and nailbeds appeared somewhat bluish. On examination, his blood pressure was 118/64 mmHg, his pulse rate 114/minute and his respiratory rate 28/minute. Rales were audible to the apices bilaterally and a loud S3 gallop was evident.

Because of the obvious presence of pulmonary edema, intravenous furosemide [frusemide] 40 mg was given and supplemental oxygen increased to 50% by aerosol face mask. Within 45 minutes, the patient produced 550 mL of urine and his respiratory rate decreased to 24/minute. However, his blood pressure decreased to 96/66 mmHg and his heart rate increased to 122/minute. A pulmonary artery catheter was then placed (Table 1.2.1) and a chest radiograph was obtained (Figure 1.2.1).

Table 1.2.1. Hemodynamic measurements following furosemide

Arterial pressure	90/62 mmHg
Heart rate	126/minute
Right atrial pressure	2 mmHg
Right ventricular pressure	28/0 mmHg
Pulmonary artery pressure	27/14 mmHg
Pulmonary artery occlusion pressure	9 mmHg
Cardiac output	3.1 L min^{-1}
Cardiac index	1.9 L min^{-1} m^{-2}

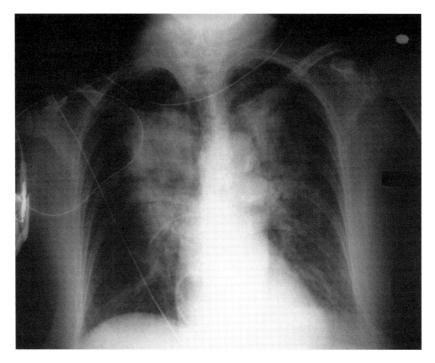

Figure 1.2.1. In this chest radiograph of a patient with severe, acute heart failure, the heart size is normal and there is alveolar pulmonary edema in a 'bat-wing' configuration. A femoral pulmonary artery catheter is seen, with its tip in the right pulmonary artery and a redundant loop coiled in the right atrium. In milder cases of heart failure, the typical radiographic changes are subtler: pulmonary vascular redistribution, perihilar haziness, Kerley B lines and perhaps pleural effusions.

Traps

- Sometimes, in patients with acute myocardia infarction, the judicious use of furosemide can be useful in relieving pulmonary congestion and hypoxemia.[1,2] Symptoms may improve significantly, even before diuresis occurs. This reflects a direct venodilating effect of furosemide, reducing central venous return and thus reducing pulmonary venous pressure.[3] In general, though, as this case illustrates, diuretics usually should not be used acutely in patients with a large myocardial infarction, because of the potential for reducing cardiac output and lowering blood pressure.

  The acutely infarcted ventricle has poor compliance, i.e. is stiff, so that the left ventricle fills well only when pulmonary venous pressure is relatively high. In this setting, small decreases in intravascular volume can substantially impair left ventricular filling, considerably reducing cardiac output and resulting in hypotension. Hypotension, in turn, can reduce coronary perfusion, worsening myocardial ischemia and creating a vicious cycle. After myocardial infarction, pulmonary edema does need to be treated aggressively, but it is important to use an approach that will improve hemodynamic performance without exacerbating ischemia.[2,4]

- Usually, when a patient with an anterior myocardial infarct develops pulmonary edema, the explanation is that the affected area of myocardium is large, leading to marked derangement of systolic and diastolic ventricular function. However, the possibility of a mechanical complication (such as acute mitral regurgitation or ventricular septal rupture) should always be considered.[4] Optimal treatment of these complications depends on their prompt recognition, usually by physical examination or echocardiography.

Tricks

For conceptual, therapeutic and prognostic purposes, the Killip classification offers a useful way of stratifying patients with acute myocardial infarction.[5] Patients in Killip class I have no clinical or radiographic signs of heart failure and have a favorable prognosis. Patients in Killip class II have mild failure, with bibasilar rales and S3 gallops. Dyspnea is usually mild, and radiographic abnormalities usually are confined to pulmonary vascular redistribution. Short-term mortality is 3–5 times higher in class II than in class I. Patients in Killip class III, like the patient in this case, develop frank pulmonary edema with dyspnea, orthopnea, diffuse rales, an S3 gallop and radiographic evidence of interstitial and alveolar edema. If pulmonary artery catheterization is performed, class III patients typically have moderately decreased cardiac outputs and high pulmonary artery occlusion pressures (usually exceeding 18 mmHg). Their mortality is 5–6 times higher than class I patients. Patients in Killip class IV have cardiogenic shock with hypotension and signs of hypoperfusion, such as oliguria, metabolic acidosis and confusion. These signs of hypoperfusion typically occur when the cardiac index falls below $2.0\,L\,min^{-1}\,m^{-2}$. With pharmacological therapy alone, the mortality of cardiogenic shock exceeds 90%.[6]

Almost all Killip class I and II patients, and some Killip class III patients, can be treated effectively without invasive hemodynamic monitoring. The use of oxygen and intravenous furosemide in small doses may be all that is required. However, as already mentioned, the salutary effects of diuretics after acute myocardial infarction are predicated on reduction of preload, and hence on reduction of cardiac output.[1,3] Clinical response to treatment can be gauged by relief of symptoms, improvement of oxygenation, and reduction of heart rate and respiratory rate. However, if tachycardia, oliguria or hypotension supervene, prompt pulmonary artery catheterization can be very helpful, not only to define filling pressures and cardiac performance (Figure 1.2.2) but also to guide titration of parenteral vasodilators and positive inotropic agents.[2,8] In class III and IV patients, the goals of aggressive pharmacological therapy are to improve myocardial oxygen delivery, minimize myocardial oxygen demand, reduce the work of breathing, and maintain levels of blood pressure and cardiac output sufficient to prevent or reverse the signs of hypoperfusion.

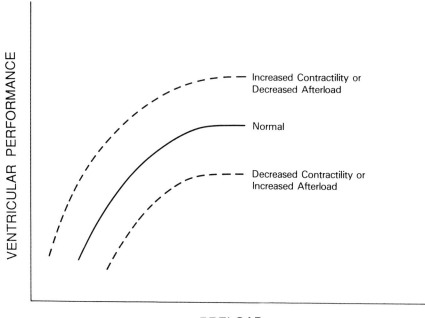

PRELOAD

Figure 1.2.2. A schematic representation of the Frank–Starling curve, which relates preload (*x*-axis) to ventricular performance (*y*-axis). Preload is the stretch on cardiac myofibrils at the beginning of systole, and hence is a function of ventricular end-diastolic volume. There are no clinically convenient methods for accurate serial assessment of ventricular volumes, so pulmonary artery occlusion pressure is widely used as an indirect measure of preload. Changes in ventricular performance probably are assessed most accurately by measuring ejection fraction or stroke work index, but for practical purposes stroke volume, cardiac output or blood pressure can be measured instead. As preload increases, ventricular performance increases in a curvilinear fashion until a plateau is reached. Preload is optimal in most patients at a pulmonary artery occlusion pressure of 14–18 mmHg, or perhaps slightly higher in acute infarction.[8] Diuretics can impair ventricular performance if preload is reduced excessively.[1,8] In patients with poor contractility, ventricular performance may be enhanced, at any given level of preload, by using positive inotropic agents or afterload reducing agents.[1,7]

All patients with heart failure should receive enough oxygen supplementation to keep arterial oxygen saturation above 90%. In patients who have severe pulmonary edema or cardiogenic shock, consideration should be given to tracheal intubation and mechanical ventilation, to improve oxygenation, permit heavy sedation for the relief of anxiety, reduce the work of breathing and allow respiratory compensation for the metabolic acidosis.[4]

Parenteral vasodilators such as nitroglycerin and sodium nitroprusside cause relaxation of smooth muscle in the arterial circulation, decreasing afterload (impedance to left ventricular emptying).[2] They also decrease preload, by increasing venous capacitance and reducing central venous return, thus serving to relieve pulmonary congestion. When vasodilators are titrated appropriately, arterial relaxation predominates and cardiac output improves despite the decreased preload. When this is accomplished, the beneficial effects of vasodilators will not be accompanied by marked changes in blood pressure or heart rate, because the increased cardiac output will compensate for the reduced systemic vascular resistance. At high doses, however, vasodilators may reduce afterload or preload excessively, resulting in tachycardia, hypotension, reduced cardiac output, reduced coronary perfusion, increased myocardial oxygen demand and myocardial ischemia.

Nitroglycerin is both a venous and an arterial vasodilator, but its effects on preload predominate over its effects on afterload. Sodium nitroprusside is a combined venous and arterial vasodilator, but its actions on afterload are more potent than those of nitroglycerin. Many clinicians prefer nitroglycerin over nitroprusside in acute myocardial infarction, because of its beneficial effects on coronary hemodynamics and its potential to reduce infarct size. Nitroprusside certainly is useful, particularly in severe heart failure or hypertension, but it has the potential to exacerbate ischemia. Treatment with either vasodilator should be started at low doses (e.g. nitroglycerin $20 \, \mu g \, min^{-1}$ or nitroprusside $0.5 \, \mu g \, kg^{-1} \, min^{-1}$) and then rapidly titrated upward. The end-points of titration are reduced pulmonary congestion, improved oxygenation and increased cardiac output, without increased heart rate or decreased blood pressure. In most studies of acute myocardial infarction, the optimal pulmonary artery occlusion pressure for these end-points has been in the range of 16–22 mmHg.[7]

Positive inotropic agents may be helpful, usually in combination with parenteral vasodilators, in treating heart failure in acute myocardial infarction.[8] These agents enhance myocardial contractility, increasing cardiac output. They are indicated for patients with severe heart failure, especially those with severely depressed cardiac output or hypotension. However, they can induce or worsen ischemia, so only the lowest dose that produces the desired physiological effects should be employed.

Dobutamine, in doses of $5-20 \, \mu g \, kg^{-1} \, min^{-1}$, is generally the inotropic agent of choice for acute severe heart failure.[8,9] Dobutamine, a beta adrenergic agonist, tends to decrease pulmonary venous pressure and relieve pulmonary congestion, whereas dopamine, possessing both alpha and beta adrenergic agonist effects, can exacerbate pulmonary congestion and has more of a tendency to cause tachycardia.[9] The hemodynamic effects of dobutamine resemble those of dopamine combined with a vasodilator. All positive inotropic agents increase myocardial oxygen demand, but with dobutamine the increased demand is balanced by increased coronary blood flow. Digoxin, while certainly useful for atrial arrhythmias and for long-term treatment of heart failure, is not potent enough to have a significant role in the treatment of acute heart failure after myocardial infarction.

In a great many Killip class III and IV patients, invasive hemodynamic monitoring and stabilization with parenteral vasodilators and inotropic agents serve as a prelude to more aggressive therapy, often including intra-aortic balloon counterpulsation[10] and coronary arteriography to assess the prospects for revascularization.[6]

Follow-up

Once the initial results of pulmonary artery catheterization were obtained, showing a pulmonary artery occlusion pressure of only 9 mmHg and a cardiac index of only $1.9\,L\,min^{-1}\,m^{-2}$, the patient was given a bolus of 500 mL of 0.9% saline. It was felt that he could benefit from both a positive inotropic agent and a vasodilator, so dobutamine and nitroprusside were started and titrated upward, while observing blood pressure, heart rate, urine output and arterial oxygen saturation. Within an hour, marked clinical improvement was noted, and repeat hemodynamic measurements were obtained (Table 1.2.2).

Table 1.2.2. Repeat hemodynamic measurements after administration of saline, nitroprusside and dobutamine

Arterial pressure	108/70 mmHg
Heart rate	96/minute
Right atrial pressure	3 mmHg
Right ventricular pressure	32/2 mmHg
Pulmonary artery pressure	31/20 mmHg
Pulmonary artery occlusion pressure	17 mmHg
Cardiac output	$4.2\,L\,min^{-1}$
Cardiac index	$2.6\,L\,min^{-1}\,m^{-2}$

Comcomitant with these therapeutic maneuvers, a diagnostic bedside echocardiogram was performed. Mild concentric left ventricular hypertrophy was noted. Left ventricular wall motion was abnormal, with anteroseptal akinesis and anterolateral hypokinesis. There was no echocardiographic evidence of significant mitral regurgitation, ventricular septal rupture or fluid in the pericardium.

The patient was deemed sufficiently stable on this pharmacological regimen that tracheal intubation and intra-aortic balloon counterpulsation were felt to be unnecessary. He was taken for coronary arteriography, which revealed one-vessel coronary disease. The right and circumflex coronary arteries had only minor luminal irregularities, while the left anterior descending coronary artery had a complete proximal occlusion. Attempts at percutaneous transluminal coronary angioplasty were unsuccessful, and the patient was returned to the coronary intensive care unit.

Subsequently, the patient's parenteral therapy was tapered off and he was started on an oral regimen of digoxin, nitrates, furosemide, enalapril and aspirin.[2] He was able to leave intensive care on the fifth hospital day and thereafter entered a cardiac rehabilitation program.

References

1 Sica DA and Gehr T. Diuretics in congestive heart failure. *Cardiology Clinics* (1989) **7**: 87–97.

2 Jain P and Vlay SC. Pharmacological management of acute myocardial infarction. *Clinical Cardiology* (1992) **15**: 795–803.

3 Biddle TL and Yu PN. Effects of furosemide on hemodynamics and lung water in acute pulmonary edema secondary to myocardial infarction. *American Journal of Cardiology* (1979) **43**: 86–90.

4 The American College of Cardiology/American Heart Association Task Force. Guidelines for the early management of patients with acute myocardial infarction. *Circulation* (1990) **82**: 664–707.

5 Killip T and Kimball JT. Treatment of myocardial infarction in a coronary care unit. *American Journal of Cardiology* (1967) **20**: 457–464.

6 Schreiber TL, Miller DH and Zola B. Management of myocardial infarction shock: current status. *American Heart Journal* (1989) **117**: 435–443.

7 Crexells C, Chatterjee K, Forrester JS, Dikshit K and Swan HJC, Optimal level of filling pressure in the left side of the heart in acute myocardial infarction. *New England Journal of Medicine* (1973) **289**: 1263–1266.

8 Om A and Hess ML. Inotropic therapy of the failing myocardium. *Clinical Cardiology* (1992) **16**: 5–14.

9 Maekawa K, Liang C-S and Hood WB. Comparison of dobutamine and dopamine in acute myocardial infarction. *Circulation* (1983) **67**: 750–759.

10 O'Rourke MF, Norris RM, Campbell TJ, Chang VP and Sammel NL, Ramdomized controlled trial of intraaortic balloon counterpulsation in early myocardial infarction with acute heart failure. *American Journal of Cardiology* (1981) **47**: 815–820.

1.3 Recurrent Chest Discomfort and Hypotension Three Days after Acute Myocardial Infarction

R.W. Vandivier and R.E. Cunnion

History

A 70-year-old man was admitted with new onset of anterior chest pain. Although he had not experienced chest pain before, he had multiple risk factors for atherosclerosis including heavy tobacco use, hypercholesterolemia and hypertension. On examination he was obese and barrel-chested. His blood pressure was 150/90 mmHg, his pulse rate 90/minute and his respiratory rate 24/minute. His chest was hyperresonant to percussion, with scattered expiratory wheezes, but no rales. No murmurs or gallops were heard. The admission chest radiograph was interpreted as consistent with chronic obstructive pulmonary disease and the electrocardiogram revealed a right bundle branch block without obvious ischemic changes.

After administration of sublingual nitroglycerin, his chest pain quickly disappeared. Additional treatment consisted of aspirin 325 mg orally, nasal oxygen $2\,L\,min^{-1}$ and intravenous nitroglycerin $50\,\mu g\,min^{-1}$. Serial creatine phosphokinase levels peaked 18 hours after admission at $766\,IU\,m\,L^{-1}$ [$13\,\mu mol\,L^{-1}$] with an elevated MB fraction.

On the second day, oral nitrates were started and intravenous nitroglycerin was stopped. His chest pain did not recur but, since his blood pressure remained mildly elevated, oral diltiazem was started. Aspirin and oxygen were continued, and he was permitted out of bed in a chair for brief periods.

On the third day, while sitting in a chair, he suddenly became light-headed and asked to get back into bed. On questioning, he admitted to feeling short of breath and also to having an ill-defined sensation of anterior chest tightness. His blood pressure was 85/50 mmHg, his pulse rate 116/minute and his respiratory rate 30/minute. Auscultation of his lungs again revealed scattered wheezes, without rales, rubs or signs of consolidation. Cardiac examination again revealed no murmurs, but a right ventricular S3 gallop was heard. On the electrocardiogram (Figure 1.3.1), new abnormalities were present and the right bundle branch block had disappeared. His chest radiograph was unchanged.

The house officer felt that this acute onset of hypotension and chest discomfort were probably caused by recurrent ischemia and infarct extension. To exclude acute mechanical complications of myocardial infarction (e.g. papillary muscle rupture, ventricular septal rupture or ventricular free wall rupture), he contacted the cardiology fellow to obtain an echocardiogram and to consider right-sided heart catheterization. He continued the nitrates and diltiazem at an unchanged rate and increased the supplemental oxygen to $4\,L\,min^{-1}$.

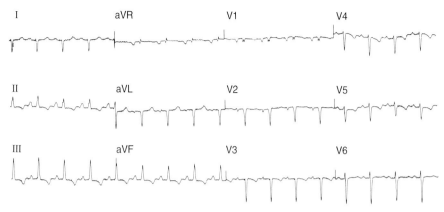

Figure 1.3.1. In this abnormal 12-lead electrocardiogram, the Q waves in leads V1 through V3 are due to anteroseptal myocardial infarction. The large R waves in leads 2, 3, and aVF, the deepening rS pattern across the lateral precordium, the right axis deviation and the ST segment depression and T wave inversion in leads 2, 3, and aVF result from right ventricular hypertrophy and strain. The prominent P waves in leads 2, 3, and aVF reflect enlargement of the right atrium.

Traps

- In evaluating hypotension and chest discomfort in the immediate post-infarct period, it is not merely appropriate, but imperative to carefully evaluate the possibility of infarct extension or of a mechanical complication. Nonetheless, in a patient with potentially life-threatening instability, it is also crucial to consider other possibilities – in this case, acute pulmonary embolism. In one published consecutive series of pulmonary emboli, 12% occurred after acute myocardial infarction.[1]
- The physical findings in this case were not those typically seen in acute infarct extension or in an acute mechanical complication. Usually, if a patient has enough acute left ventricular dysfunction to cause hypotension, some degree of pulmonary edema will be present. Similarly, hypotension from papillary muscle rupture or ventricular septal rupture will almost always be accompanied by pulmonary edema. Ventricular free wall rupture most often causes pericardial tamponade and electromechanical dissociation.
- Since the physical findings and electrocardiographic findings in this case pointed predominantly to dysfunction of the right ventricle, another potential consideration in the differential diagnosis of hypotension here was right ventricular infarction. However, right ventricular infarction ordinarily arises from occlusion of the right coronary artery in association with inferior or inferoposterior infarction. Nothing about this patient's electrocardiogram was suggestive of such an event.
- Diagnosis and management of this patient were difficult because the signs

and symptoms of two acute processes (myocardial infarction and pulmonary embolism) had to be distinguished from each other, as well as from his underlying chronic lung disease.

Tricks

Clinical findings are notoriously unreliable in diagnosing pulmonary emboli.[2,3] Significant emboli almost always produce dyspnea, but chest pain and hemoptysis are usually absent. When pain does occur, it is most often located laterally in the chest and it is often pleuritic (sharp, knife-like and aggravated by each breath), especially if pulmonary infarction has occurred. This contrasts with the deep, dull, steady pain characteristic of myocardial infarction.

The most common electrocardiographic abnormalities in acute pulmonary embolism are sinus tachycardia and non-specific ST segment and T wave changes. The more classically described changes (right bundle branch block, right axis deviation, P pulmonale, right ventricular hypertrophy) are less commonly seen.[3,4] The electrocardiographic changes are probably due to acute pulmonary hypertension with right atrial and ventricular dilatation, hypoxia and perhaps myocardial ischemia. The changes are often transient and non-specific, so that serial tracings are helpful. The electrocardiographic manifestations of acute pulmonary embolism and of acute myocardial infarction may be particularly difficult to discern in patients with pre-existing chronic obstructive lung disease and cor pulmonale.

In electrocardiograms such as that in Figure 1.3.1, it is difficult to discern whether the Q waves in the anterior precordial leads represent an anteroseptal infarction or whether they merely represent clockwise rotation of the QRS vector. Similarly, without serial tracings it is difficult to know whether the manifestations of right ventricular strain are chronic (reflecting the underlying lung disease) or acute (reflecting acute pulmonary embolism).

In patients who do not have pre-existing cardiopulmonary disease, right ventricular afterload begins to increase sharply once thrombotic obstruction reduces the cross-sectional area of the pulmonary vascular bed by 25% or more. To compensate for this impairment, pulmonary artery pressures and right ventricular pressures increase (which can be demonstrated by pulmonary artery catheterization), and the right ventricle dilates and becomes hypokinetic (which can be observed echocardiographically). As the right ventricle fails, right atrial pressure increases and cardiac output decreases. Such patients are said to have *massive* pulmonary embolism, which usually is manifested clinically by some combination of profound dyspnea, syncope and incipient cardiogenic shock, which may culminate in electromechanical dissociation and cardiac arrest.

In a patient such as this it is important to establish the diagnosis of pulmonary embolism both quickly and definitively so that therapy may proceed. Therapeutic doses of heparin should be given immediately rather than waiting for diagnostic tests to be completed. The sensitivity and specificity of ventilation–perfusion lung scanning are limited in patients with chronic obstructive pulmonary disease; accordingly, in the face of hemodynamic instability and a high index of clinical suspicion, many clinicians would go directly to pulmonary arteriography.

Therapy for massive pulmonary embolism consists of administration of a thrombolytic agent, such as recombinant tissue plasminogen activator, to accelerate dissolution of emboli, improve pulmonary perfusion and reverse right ventricular failure.[5-7] If the thrombus arose from the lower extremities, and the hemodynamic status of the patient was so marginal that further emboli might prove fatal, consideration might be given to placement of an inferior vena caval filter, weighing the potential benefit against the risk of hemorrhagic complications.[8] Surgical thromboembolectomy, which involves thoracotomy and exploration of the pulmonary arteries under cardiopulmonary bypass, is associated with a high mortality and normally is reserved for patients *in extremis* in whom thrombolytic therapy is contraindicated or is failing.[9] Transvenous pulmonary embolectomy, using a specialized suction catheter, is another therapeutic option available in some hospitals.

Follow-up

The echocardiogram in this patient showed an area of akinesis in the anteroseptal left ventricular wall, without evidence of mitral regurgitation, ventricular septal rupture, or ventricular free wall rupture. The right ventricle was markedly dilated and diffusely hypokinetic.[10] A presumptive diagnosis of massive pulmonary embolism was made, and heparin was given intravenously (5000 U bolus and 1200 U h^{-1} infusion). As the house officer was arranging for urgent pulmonary arteriography, the cardiology fellow inserted a pulmonary artery catheter from a femoral vein. The findings, shown in Table 1.3.1, showed that the pulmonary capillary wedge pressure was normal, but with markedly elevated pulmonary arterial and right ventricular pressures and a markedly diminished cardiac index. Dobutamine was started (at 10 µg kg^{-1} min^{-1}) with the goal of enhancing right ventricular function, with cognizance of the potential for dobutamine to induce ischemia.

Pulmonary arteriography was performed using the same sheath that had been used for the pulmonary artery catheter. In view of the high pulmonary artery

Table 1.3.1. Hemodynamic measurements

Arterial pressure	85/50 mmHg
Heart rate	116/minute
Right atrial pressure	19 mmHg
Right ventricular pressure	62/12 mmHg
Pulmonary artery pressure	60/35 mmHg
Pulmonary artery occlusion pressure	10 mmHg
Cardiac output	2.9 L min^{-1}
Cardiac index	1.7 L min^{-1} m^{-2}

pressures and the attendant risk, the study was done selectively and with digital subtraction technique, injecting contrast material only into one branch of the right pulmonary artery. The radiographs demonstrated the presence of a large, almost totally occlusive intraluminal filling defect. The patient did not have any contraindications to therapy with a thrombolytic agent, and recombinant tissue plasminogen activator was given intravenously (100 mg over 2 hours). The patient improved dramatically. His blood pressure improved, allowing the dobutamine to be stopped, and his oxygenation also improved. Heparin therapy was resumed and the partial thromboplastin time maintained at 1.5–2 times control.

References

1 Bell WR, Simon TL and DeMets DL. The clinical features of submassive and massive pulmonary emboli. *American Journal of Medicine* (1977) **62**: 355–360.
2 Moser KM. Venous thromboembolism. *American Review of Respiratory Diseases* (1990) **141**: 235–249.
3 Stein PD, Terrin ML, Hales CA, Palevsky HI, Saltzman HA, Thompson BT and Weg JG. Clinical, laboratory, roentgenographic, and electrocardiographic findings in patients with acute pulmonary embolism and no pre-existing cardiac or pulmonary disease. *Chest* (1991) **100**: 598–603.
4 Stein PD, Dalen JE, McIntyre KM, Sasahara AA, Wenger NK and Willis PW. The electrocardiogram in acute pulmonary embolism. *Progress in Cardiovascular Diseases* (1975) **17**: 247–257.
5 Goldhaber SZ. Recent advances in the diagnosis and lytic therapy of pulmonary embolism. *Chest* (1991) **99**: 173S–179S.
6 Dalen JE and Hirsh J. Third ACCP consensus conference on antithrombotic therapy. *Chest* (1992) **102**: 303S–549S.
7 Come PC, Kim D, Parker JA, Goldhaber SZ, Braunwald E, Markis JE and participating investigators. Early reversal of right ventricular dysfunction in patients with acute pulmonary embolism after treatment with intravenous tissue plasminogen activator. *Journal of the American College of Cardiology* (1987) **10**: 971–978.
8 Greenfield LJ and DeLucia A. Endovascular therapy of venous thromboembolic disease. *Surgical Clinics of North America* (1992) **72**: 969–989.
9 Masters RG, Koshal A, Higginson LA and Keon WJ. Ongoing role of pulmonary embolectomy. *Canadian Journal of Cardiology* (1988) **4**: 347–351.
10 Kasper W, Meinertz T, Henkel B, Eissner D, Hahn K, Hofmann T, Zeiher A and Just H. Echocardiographic findings in patients with proved pulmonary embolism. *American Heart Journal* (1986) **112**: 1284–1290.

1.4 Arrhythmias after Thrombolytic Therapy for Myocardial Infarction

R.W. Vandivier and R.E. Cunnion

History

A 50-year-old woman with known coronary artery disease came to the emergency department one hour after the onset of crushing substernal pain, associated with sweating, mild shortness of breath and extreme anxiety. Just three months earlier she had suffered a small myocardial infarction, which had been treated with streptokinase. She had not experienced angina pectoris after her myocardial infarction, and her health was otherwise excellent.

On initial examination she appeared distressed, lying on a trolley, receiving oxygen by nasal cannulae. Her blood pressure was 140/90 mmHg, her pulse rate 90/minute and her respiratory rate 28/minute. Her jugular veins were flat. No crackles, murmurs, gallops or rubs were heard. An electrocardiogram showed tall, peaked T waves and 3–4 mm of ST segment elevation in leads V1, V2 and V3, consistent with acute anterior myocardial injury. A chest radiograph was interpreted as normal.

The chest pain was not relieved by three 0.4 mg doses of sublingual nitroglycerin. An intravenous nitroglycerin infusion was started, and aliquots of morphine sulfate were given to a total of 8 mg, with partial relief of pain.[1,2]

The emergency department physician concluded, on clinical and electro-cardiographic grounds, that this patient was having an acute anterior infarction and there were no contraindications to therapy with a thrombolytic agent.[3] He ordered intravenous streptokinase 1.5 million units to be given over one hour. However, the pharmacist discovered that the streptokinase lot in stock had expired and replacement stock had not yet arrived.

Accordingly, the physician instead ordered intravenous recombinant tissue plasminogen activator (rtPA), 100 mg in a 'front-loaded' dosing regimen: 15 mg over 2 minutes, then 50 mg over 30 minutes, and then 35 mg over 60 minutes.[3,4] The patient was transported from the emergency department to the coronary care unit.

Forty-five minutes after starting the rtPA infusion, her chest pain was subsiding, and the coronary care unit nurse obtained another electrocardiogram. As the tracing was being recorded (Figure 1.4.1), the patient suddenly became unresponsive, with a rhythm interpreted as ventricular tachycardia. Immediate defibrillation with 200 Joules restored a normal sinus rhythm. A 100 mg bolus of lidocaine [lignocaine] was given, followed by an infusion of 3 mg min^{-1}. The nitroglycerin infusion was continued, and the rtPA infusion was stopped.

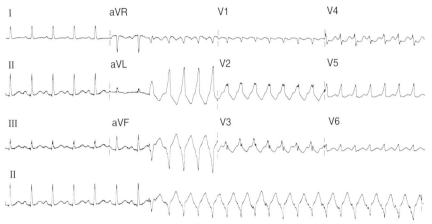

Figure 1.4.1. As this 12-lead electrocardiogram was being recorded the patient developed a wide-complex tachycardia, identified as ventricular tachycardia. Along the bottom is a rhythm strip from lead 2.

Traps

- Effective thrombolytic agents for acute myocardial infarction include streptokinase, rtPA, urokinase and anisoylated plasminogen–streptokinase activator complex (APSAC). The relative merits of the various agents continue to be a matter of some controversy.[3] It is clear, however, that the emergency department physician should not have considered streptokinase for this particular patient. Patients who have received streptokinase within the past six months or so should not receive it again. Administration of streptokinase induces neutralizing antibodies that can reduce its effectiveness (and the effectiveness of APSAC as well).[3]

- When thrombolytic therapy is successful, reperfusion of the occluded coronary artery is frequently accompanied by arrhythmias, as well as by relief of chest pain and ST segments returning toward normal.[5] Perhaps the most common reperfusion arrhythmia is accelerated idioventricular rhythm (AIVR), which differs from ventricular tachycardia only in having a slower rate ($\leqslant 100$/minute) and which generally is well-tolerated hemodynamically.[6] In this patient, the development of ventricular tachycardia, while needing defibrillation and antiarrhythmic therapy, was certainly no reason to terminate the rtPA infusion prematurely.

- The emergency department physician erred in not administering *aspirin*. The antiplatelet effects of aspirin are a crucial adjunct in the routine therapy of acute myocardial infarction.[1,3] In the ISIS-2 trial, aspirin in a dose of 162.5 mg reduced overall mortality from myocardial infarction by 23%.[7]

- It is important to give anticoagulation therapy with heparin in conjunction with rtPA.[3,4] Although optimal timing and dosage of heparin have not been firmly established, it is reasonable to administer a 5000 U intravenous bolus concomitant with the rtPA, followed by an infusion of $1000\,U\,h^{-1}$. Data concerning the usefulness of heparin as an adjunct to streptokinase and to APSAC are equivocal.[3]

Tricks

Only a minority of patients with acute myocardial infarction are candidates for thrombolytic therapy. Many patients present late; thrombolytic therapy is most effective when given within a few hours after the onset of pain, before the myocardium is extensively and irreversibly damaged. Some patients have electrocardiographic features (such as ST segment depression) that are not typical of myocardial infarction; thrombolytic therapy has been proven effective only in patients with ST segment elevations or with new bundle branch blocks. Many patients have contraindications to thrombolytic therapy, such as hypertension, central nervous system pathology or a bleeding disorder; such patients may be candidates for primary percutaneous transluminal coronary angioplasty.[1,3]

For patients who *are* candidates for thrombolytic therapy, a large literature addresses issues of relative safety and effectiveness among the available agents.[3] In two large trials, GISSI-2 and ISIS-3, that compared streptokinase and rtPA directly, the benefits were similar.[3] In a third large trial, GUSTO, the 'front-loaded' dosing regimen of rtPA was combined with heparin therapy. In this trial, rtPA produced a greater reduction in mortality than streptokinase, although the reduction was partially offset by a higher incidence of hemorrhagic stroke with rtPA.[4]

Acknowledging that the GUSTO results suggest slightly better efficacy for rtPA, the much lower cost of streptokinase may be a determining factor for many hospitals. Ultimately, the choice of thrombolytic agent is less important than the speed with which administration is started. Giving thrombolytic agents earlier allows more myocardium to be salvaged.[1,3]

The frequent occurrence of reperfusion arrhythmias has prompted some clinicians to use prophylactic lidocaine infusions as a routine adjunct to thrombolytic therapy. In the past, the use of prophylactic lidocaine for *all* patients with suspected myocardial infarction was standard practice in many coronary care units, with the goal of reducing the incidence of ventricular fibrillation and the hope of reducing mortality. However, as data accumulated it became clear that the prophylactic use of lidocaine was unwise and that its use was best confined to patients with specific indications.[1,2,8] Whether patients receiving thrombolytic therapy benefit from routine lidocaine prophylaxis remains unanswered.

As already mentioned, arrhythmias are a fairly specific (albeit insensitive) marker of successful reperfusion.[5] In managing a patient receiving thrombolytic therapy, as in managing any patient, the clinician must be careful to identify the arrhythmia correctly (e.g. the crucial distinction between ventricular tachycardia and supraventricular tachycardia with aberrancy),[9] to gauge the seriousness of the arrhythmia (e.g. the generally benign AIVR versus the more ominous ventricular tachycardia)[6] and to assess the need for emergent intervention (e.g. in this case, the need to defibrillate an unresponsive patient without delaying even to set up for synchronized cardioversion).

Beta adrenergic blocking agents are widely used in the management of patients with acute myocardial infarction.[1,2] Acute intravenous beta blockade is of value in patients, with no signs of congestive heart failure, who have continuing ischemia or such manifestations of increased adrenergic activity as tachycardia or hypertension. There are data suggesting that, among patients receiving rtPA, such early intravenous beta blockade may benefit even those who do *not* manifest continuing ischemia or increased adrenergic activity.[10] Long-term oral beta blockers are started routinely within the first few days after myocardial infarction, as secondary prevention in all patients who do not have contraindications.[1,2]

Follow-up

After defibrillation, the patient remained in normal sinus rhythm. Her rtPA was restarted and the full 100 mg dose completed; she was also given aspirin and anticoagulated with heparin. Her chest pain had resolved entirely by the completion of the rtPA infusion but, since she continued to have a mild tachycardia and to be hypertensive, an intravenous beta blocker was given (3 doses of metoprolol, 5 mg each, 5 minutes apart), and she was then started on oral metoprolol. Her ECG later showed small Q waves in leads V1, V2 and V3, with a peak creatine phosphokinase level of $1244\,\text{IU}\,\text{mL}^{-1}$ [$21\,\mu\text{mol}\,\text{L}^{-1}$].

After 24 hours, she had had no recurrent arrhythmias or chest pain and she had no signs of congestive heart failure. The infusions of nitroglycerin, lidocaine and heparin were stopped.

After eight days of progressive ambulation in the hospital, she was scheduled for a submaximal treadmill exercise test. If this test were negative for inducible ischemia, the expectation was that she would go home without requiring cardiac catheterization.[10] However, she developed chest discomfort and the ECG showed ischemic changes at peak exercise. Accordingly, she underwent coronary arteriography, which revealed an 80% stenosis of the mid-left anterior descending coronary artery distal to the first diagonal branch. Percutaneous transluminal coronary angioplasty was successfully performed, and she was then discharged on a regimen of aspirin, beta blockers and risk factor modification.

References

1 The American College of Cardiology/American Heart Association Task Force. Guidelines for the early management of patients with acute myocardial infarction. *Circulation* (1990) **82**: 664–707.
2 Jain P and Vlay SC. Pharmacological management of acute myocardial infarction. *Clinical Cardiology* (1992) **15**: 795–803.
3 Anderson HV and Willerson JT. Thrombolysis in acute myocardial infarction. *New England Journal of Medicine* (1993) **329**: 703–709.
4 The GUSTO Investigators. An international randomized trial comparing four

thrombolytic strategies for acute myocardial infarction. *New England Journal of Medicine* (1993) **329**: 673–682.

5 Shah PK, Cercek B, Lew AS and Ganz W. Angiographic validation of bedside markers of reperfusion. *Journal of the American College of Cardiology* (1993) **21**: 55–61.

6 Marriott HJL. Accelerated idioventricular rhythm and parasystole. In: *Practical Electrocardiography*, 7th edn. Baltimore, Williams and Wilkins, pp 244–255, 1983.

7 ISIS (Second International Study of Infarct Survival) Collaborative Group. Randomized trial of intravenous streptokinase, oral aspirin, both or neither among 17 187 cases of suspected acute myocardial infarction: ISIS-2. *Lancet* (1988) **2**: 349–360.

8 MacMahon S, Collins R, Peto R, Koster RW and Yusuf S. Effects of prophylactic lidocaine in suspected acute myocardial infarction: an overview of results from the randomized, controlled trials. *Journal of the American Medical Association* (1988) **260**: 1910–1916.

9 Wellens HJJ. The wide QRS tachycardia. *Annals of Internal Medicine* (1986) **104**: 879.

10 Williams DO, Braunwald E, Knatterud G, Babb J, Bresnahan J, Greenberg MA, Raizner A, Wasserman A, Robertson J, Ross R and TIMI investigators. One-year results of the thrombolysis in myocardial infarction investigation (TIMI) phase II trial. *Circulation* (1992) **85**: 533–542.

1.5 Hypotension, Acute Pulmonary Edema, and a Pansystolic Murmur after Acute Myocardial Infarction

R.W. Vandivier and R.E. Cunnion

History

A 60-year-old woman, with no prior history of cardiac disease, was admitted with an acute myocardial infarction to the coronary care unit, where she was treated with oxygen, nitroglycerin, streptokinase, aspirin and metoprolol.[1] She did not develop any recurrent chest pain nor any signs of congestive heart failure. However, she did have a transient episode of type II second degree atrioventricular block, which did not need pacing and which resolved when the metoprolol was stopped. Her electrocardiogram (Figure 1.5.1) developed the changes of a transmural anterior infarction; her creatine phosphokinase peaked at 1898 IU mL^{-1} [32 µmol L^{-1}].

On the fourth hospital day, as she was preparing for transfer to an ambulatory telemetry unit, her blood pressure abruptly decreased to 75/45 mmHg. A 12-lead electrocardiogram revealed sinus tachycardia, without new ischemic changes. Physical examination was notable for jugular venous distension, pulmonary rales, a summation gallop and a loud holosystolic (pansystolic) murmur. The intern ordered a 500 mL bolus of 0.9% saline, asked that the resident be paged urgently, and requested that a pericardiocentesis tray be brought to the bedside.

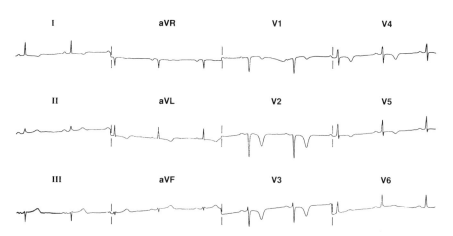

Figure 1.5.1. An abnormal 12-lead electrocardiogram showing evolution of an anterior myocardial infarction. Of note are the Q waves in leads V1 and V2, and the inverted T waves in leads V1 through V5.

TO DO / TO BUY

- ↳ Digital Piano
- ↳ Snowboarding Lesson
  Llandudno
- ↳ Helen McGreavy dance lessons
- ↳ Laura Bell Yoga
- ↳ Swedish massage course
  (Llandrillo)
- ↳ Valet car.
- ↳ ✳ RENEW HOME INSURANCE ✳

Traps

- In approaching this patient, the intern was sensible in seeking the counsel of more experienced physicians, who could guide him through an orderly diagnostic and therapeutic sequence while discouraging a premature attempt at pericardiocentesis.

  Hypotension after infarction usually has one of six causes: (1) extensive left ventricular damage leading to cardiogenic shock; (2) right ventricular infarction; (3) left ventricular free wall rupture with pericardial tamponade; (4) papillary muscle rupture with severe mitral regurgitation; (5) rupture of the interventricular septum; and (6) arrhythmias. In developing a differential diagnosis, potential non-cardiac causes, such as sepsis, hemorrhage or pulmonary embolism, should also be considered.[1–3]

- Massive infarction is the most common cause of cardiogenic shock, which usually develops when the acute infarction (or the combination of acute and previous infarctions) involves 40% or more of the left ventricular myocardium.[1,2] Acute mechanical complications (ventricular free wall rupture, ventricular septal rupture and papillary muscle rupture) account for only about one-third of infarct-related deaths.[3]

- In this setting, therapeutic and diagnostic measures must be undertaken simultaneously and rapidly.[2] Immediate therapeutic measures, aimed at restoring hemodynamic stability, typically include both pharmacologic support (i.e. inotropes and vasodilators) and mechanical support (i.e. intra-aortic balloon counterpulsation).[1,2,4,5] The most valuable immediate diagnostic measure, beyond the physical examination and the electro-cardiogram, is an echocardiogram, which can be performed as equipment is being set up for right-sided heart catheterization.

Tricks

Echocardiography can yield an enormous amount of diagnostic information in a matter of minutes. It allows non-invasive assessment of chamber sizes and wall thicknesses, regional and global contractility, valvular structure and function, and the presence or absence of intracardiac shunts and of pericardial fluid.[6] As such, acute mechanical complications can readily be identified or excluded, and appropriate decisions can be made concerning further diagnostic and therapeutic directions.

In the setting of acute infarction, a hypotensive patient, particularly one who does not respond immediately to a fluid challenge, can be managed much more confidently with the aid of invasive monitoring. Data from *right-sided heart catheterization* can be useful not only therapeutically (using the pulmonary artery occlusion pressure and the cardiac index to guide titration of fluids, diuretics, vasodilators and inotropic agents) but also diagnostically.[1,2]

Since most patients with cardiogenic shock have pump failure without acute mechanical complications, right-sided heart catheterization usually will show a high pulmonary artery occlusion pressure and a low cardiac index. Some patients, though, will manifest particular hemodynamic profiles.

- High right atrial and right ventricular diastolic pressures with a low pulmonary artery occlusion pressure suggest right ventricular infarction.[2]
- Elevation and equalization of pressures (right atrial, right ventricular end-diastolic, pulmonary artery diastolic and pulmonary artery occlusion) suggest pericardial tamponade, as found in ventricular free wall rupture.[2]
- A high pulmonary artery occlusion pressure with prominent *v* waves, albeit non-specific, suggests acute mitral regurgitation.[7]
- If blood samples are taken from the right atrium, right ventricle and pulmonary artery, left-to-right shunts can be detected by documenting abnormal increments in oxygen content.[8]
- Very high pulmonary artery pressures with a low pulmonary artery occlusion pressure suggests pulmonary embolism or another process associated with pulmonary hypertension.
- An unexpectedly high cardiac output in a patient with low blood pressure (and hence a low systemic vascular resistance) suggests the presence of sepsis or some other form of distributive shock.

The intern managing this patient, in calling for a pericardiocentesis tray, was displaying concern for possible *ventricular free wall rupture* with consequent hemopericardium and tamponade.[2,3] Given the clinical picture of sudden hypotension with jugular venous distension, this was a reasonable consideration, even though the systolic murmur would be unexplained. Other common presenting signs of tamponade include pulsus paradoxus and distant heart sounds.

Ventricular free wall rupture is most common among elderly women suffering a first transmural infarction, appears to be more common among patients who have received thrombolytic therapy, and usually occurs within the first week.[2,3] While ventricular rupture is usually a catastrophic event, with very rapid development of electromechanical dissociation, in some patients the rupture is sealed by pericardium and organizing thrombus, and the presentation may be less dramatic.

Echocardiography will confirm the presence of fluid in the pericardial sac; diastolic collapse of the right atrium and the right ventricular free wall are sensitive and specific echocardiographic markers for tamponade.[6] When these findings of ventricular free wall rupture are present, it is not necessary or desirable to take additional time to perform right-sided heart catheterization or coronary arteriography. Ventricular free wall rupture has a fatal outcome in 90% of patients, and salvage is possible only with prompt recognition, pericardiocentesis and urgent thoracotomy.[2,3]

Given this woman's acute hypotension and her pansystolic murmur, *acute mitral regurgitation* was another important diagnostic consideration.[2,3,9] Systolic murmurs due to *papillary muscle dysfunction* are very common within the first few days after myocardial infarction, but fortunately these murmurs usually do not signify hemodynamically significant mitral regurgitation. *Papillary muscle rupture* (or very severe papillary muscle dysfunction), by comparison, is relatively rare and far more serious, causing sudden, massive mitral regurgitation and marked hemodynamic decompensation.

Papillary muscle rupture, classically occurring within the first four days after myocardial infarction, usually is marked by chest pain, rapid development of pulmonary edema and shock.[9] On physical examination, a loud pansystolic murmur is audible at the apex. Echocardiographic demonstration of a flail mitral leaflet is diagnostic, and Doppler ultrasound can be used to assess the severity of regurgitation.[6,9] When right-sided heart catheterization is performed, the pulmonary artery occlusion pressure tracing will show large *v* waves, reflecting regurgitation of blood into a non-compliant left atrium. Importantly, while such *v* waves are sensitive for acute mitral regurgitation, they are not specific and may occur even in its absence.[7,9]

Patients in whom severe acute mitral regurgitation develops should be supported with intra-aortic balloon counterpulsation and a positive inotropic agent, such as dobutamine.[2,4,5,9] To the extent that blood pressure permits, an afterload-reducing agent such as nitroprusside can be very useful in increasing forward flow and minimizing regurgitant flow. If systemic perfusion fails to improve, the patient is at risk of developing multiple organ system failure, and surgery to repair or replace the valve must not be delayed. However, if the patient can be successfully stabilized on pharmacologic therapy alone, it may be desirable to delay surgery for 4–6 weeks to allow some healing to occur.[2,3,9]

Rupture of the ventricular septum after myocardial infarction usually presents as severe heart failure and low cardiac output, occurring acutely within the first week, more commonly with anterior than with inferior or inferoposterior infarctions.[2,3,10] Virtually every patient has an audible pansystolic murmur and more than half will have a parasternal thrill. Conduction disturbances are common. The degree of hemodynamic decompensation varies with the extent of the underlying infarction and with the amount of left-to-right shunting, which in turn depends on the size of the defect.

The diagnosis of septal rupture can be established on the basis of physical findings together with echocardiography and/or right-sided heart catheterization.[2,10] The widespread availability of color flow Doppler echocardiography permits sensitive and specific visualization of left-to-right shunting of blood across the septal defect.[6,10] Right-sided heart catheterization may sometimes create confusion, because septal rupture may be associated with large *v* waves in the pulmonary artery occlusion pressure tracing that are indistinguishable from those of acute mitral regurgitation.[7,10] However, when blood samples are obtained for oximetry, the elevation of oxygen saturation in right ventricular blood eliminates any uncertainty.[7,10]

The initial treatment of septal rupture is pharmacologic stabilization with inotropic agents and, if possible, vasodilators.[2,4,10] If the patient does not improve, intra-aortic balloon counterpulsation should be started. In patients with cardiogenic shock after septal rupture, the prognosis without urgent surgery is uniformly poor.[2,3,10] Some patients with septal rupture develop congestive heart failure but not cardiogenic shock. In such cases, surgery can sometimes be delayed for a time. The goal in such patients is to obtain optimal hemodynamic stability with pharmacologic therapy to minimize the operative risks. Survival is ultimately determined primarily by the size of the infarct rather than by the size of the defect.

Follow-up

As soon as he spoke with the intern, the resident notified the cardiology staff. The patient's blood pressure had improved only slightly, to 80/50 mmHg, with the fluid bolus. On re-examination a parasternal thrill was appreciated. A 50% oxygen mask was applied, an infusion of dobutamine was started at 10 μg kg^{-1} min^{-1}, and a radial artery catheter was inserted.

Two-dimensional echocardiography, performed at the bedside, revealed a large area of anteroseptal akinesis, a visible defect in the interventricular septum and moderate enlargement of the right ventricle. Color flow Doppler echocardiography demonstrated the presence of a large, high-velocity systolic flow jet originating from the left ventricular side of the defect and crossing the septum.[6]

Dobutamine was titrated to 25 μg kg^{-1} min^{-1}. Blood pressure still was only 85/55 mmHg, and an infusion of amrinone was started. Right-sided heart catheterization was performed; samples of blood were obtained for measurement of oxygen saturations (Table 1.5.1). Given the clear-cut elevation of saturations from approximately 60% in the right atrium to approximately 70% in the right ventricle, the data were felt to corroborate the echocardiographic diagnosis of ventricular septal rupture.[8,10]

Because of the patient's hemodynamic instability, she was taken to the cardiac catheterization laboratory, where coronary arteriography revealed complete proximal occlusion of the left anterior descending coronary artery. The left circumflex and right coronary arteries were patent, and the distal left anterior descending artery opacified faintly via collaterals.

The arteriography sheath was replaced with an intra-aortic balloon pump. In this clinical setting, the purpose of the balloon pump was to enhance coronary perfusion pressure and to reduce afterload, thereby increasing myocardial oxygen

Table 1.5.1. Oxygen saturation measurements from right-sided heart catheterization

Inferior vena cava	64%
Superior vena cava	59%
Right atrium	60%
Right ventricular inflow	69%
Right ventricular apex	71%
Right ventricular outflow	72%
Pulmonary artery	72%
Radial artery	91%

supply and reducing myocardial oxygen demand, concomitantly reducing blood flow across the septal defect.[5] With dobutamine at $25\,\mu g\,kg^{-1}\,min^{-1}$, amrinone at $10\,\mu g\,kg^{-1}\,min^{-1}$ and intra-aortic counterpulsation at $1:1$, the patient's blood pressure increased to $95/65\,mmHg$.[4]

The patient was taken to the operating room shortly thereafter and underwent closure of the septal defect with internal mammary artery grafting to the distal left anterior descending coronary artery. She was weaned from cardiopulmonary bypass without difficulty, recovered uneventfully and went home on the twelfth hospital day.

References

1 The American College of Cardiology/American Heart Association Task Force. Guidelines for the early management of patients with acute myocardial infarction. *Circulation* (1990) **82**: 664–707.

2 Domanski MJ. Management of cardiogenic shock complicating acute myocardial infarction. *Primary Cardiology* (1995) **21**: 11–17.

3 Weintraub RM. Post-MI mechanical complications: when to summon the cardiac surgeon. *Journal of Critical Illness* (1991) **6**: 435–440.

4 Om A and Hess ML. Inotropic therapy of the failing myocardium. *Clinical Cardiology* (1992) **16**: 5–14.

5 Scheidt S, Collins M, Goldstein J and Fisher J. Mechanical circulatory assistance with the intraaortic balloon pump and other counterpulsation devices. *Progress in Cardiovascular Diseases* (1982) **25**: 55–76.

6 Missri J. Evaluation and management of ischemic heart disease. In: *Clinical Doppler Echocardiography.* New York, McGraw-Hill, pp 207–222, 1990.

7 Pichard AD, Kay R, Smith H, Rentrop P, Holt J and Gorlin R. Large *v* waves in the pulmonary wedge pressure tracing in the absence of mitral regurgitation. *American Journal of Cardiology* (1982) **50**: 1044–1050.

8 Grossman W. Cardiac catheterization. In: Braunwald E (ed.) *Heart Disease*, 4th edn. Philadelphia, W.B. Saunders, pp 191–193, 1992.

9 Clements SD, Story WE, Hurst JW, Craver JM and Jones EL. Ruptured papillary muscle, a complication of myocardial infarction: clinical presentation, diagnosis, and treatment. *Clinical Cardiology* (1985) **8**: 93–103.

10 Lemery R, Smith HC, Giuliani ER and Gersh BJ. Prognosis in rupture of the interventricular septum after acute myocardial infarction and role of early surgical intervention. *American Journal of Cardiology* (1992) **70**: 147–151.

1.6 Hypotension Complicating Anterior Chest Trauma

R.W. Vandivier and R.E. Cunnion

History

A 22-year-old lumberjack working in a remote area of the American Pacific Northwest fell 40 feet from a tree when his ropes failed. As he fell his chest struck a large limb before impact with the ground. He remained conscious and was quickly taken in the back of a truck to the camp infirmary, where a physician immediately applied a hard cervical collar. He continued to be fully alert, complaining of pain over his anterior chest, lower back and right hip. Even though he appeared stable, the physician considered the mode of injury and the remote geographic location to need immediate helicopter transport to a regional trauma center.

During transport the patient developed tachycardia and shortness of breath; his oxygen saturation decreased to 90% while on $2\,L\,min^{-1}$ of oxygen by nasal cannula. The paramedics could find no evidence of a tension pneumothorax; he had audible breath sounds bilaterally and his blood pressure remained stable. They replaced the nasal cannula with 50% oxygen by face mask and his oxygen saturation increased to 94%. An infusion of Ringer's lactate at $200\,mL\,h^{-1}$ was also started through one of the two large bore intravenous catheters already in place.

Ninety minutes after the accident occurred, the patient arrived at the trauma center. During the flight he had become agitated, his tachypnea had worsened to 50 breaths/minute and his oxygen saturation had decreased to 89%, even though his oxygen face mask had been increased to 100%. His blood pressure was 90/60 mmHg, his pulse rate was 120/minute and he continued to have audible breath sounds bilaterally. The trauma resident decided to perform tracheal intubation and mechanical ventilation for respiratory failure, and a bolus of 1000 mL of Ringer's lactate was given for the hypotension. The initial post-intubation chest radiograph was of poor quality but showed no pneumothorax. There was an alveolar infiltrative pattern at both lung bases.

The patient's oxygenation improved immediately on mechanical ventilation and his blood pressure increased to 110/60 mmHg following the crystalloid bolus. Repeated physical examination was remarkable for tenderness, but no crepitus, over the entire anterior chest. Heart sounds were normal, without murmurs, rubs or gallops. Bowel sounds were absent and the right hip and lower back were tender to palpation. A 12-lead electrocardiogram (Figure 1.6.1) showed T wave inversions in the inferior leads.

To help distinguish between cardiac and non-cardiac causes for the hypotension and pulmonary edema, the trauma resident ordered a pulmonary artery catheter, two-dimensional echocardiography, serial blood specimens for creatine phosphokinase with MB isoenzymes, and a cardiology consultation.[1,2]

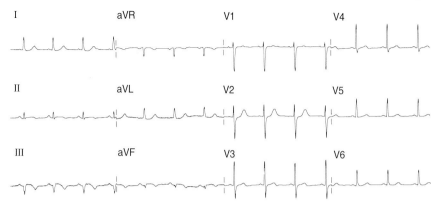

Figure 1.6.1. A 12-lead electrocardiogram obtained on arrival, notable for T wave inversions in leads III and aVF. These abnormalities, while non-specific, are consistent with right ventricular or inferior left ventricular contusion.

Hemodynamic measurements from the pulmonary artery catheter, obtained after the fluid bolus (Table 1.6.1), were consistent with hypovolemia, with a low right artrial pressure. There was no evidence of equalization of diastolic pressures to suggest pericardial tamponade and no elevation in the pulmonary artery occlusion pressure to suggest left ventricular dysfunction.[3]

A repeat chest radiograph (Figure 1.6.2) showed diffuse alveolar infiltrates. The film also showed fractures of the clavicle and second rib on the left, normal cardiac and great vessel contours, and no pneumothoraces. The echocardiogram showed a dilated, moderately hypokinetic right ventricle, with no evidence of pericardial effusion, valvular disruption, myocardial dissection, mural thrombus, or intramural hematoma.[4] Diagnoses of myocardial contusion, pulmonary contusion and hypovolemia were made, and computed tomogram of the abdomen and pelvis was performed to investigate for a source of the probable blood loss. It showed an accumulation of retroperitoneal blood of approximately 700–1000 mL, but no other abnormal collections, organ damage or pelvic fractures. The patient

Table 1.6.1. Hemodynamic measurements after a 1000 mL bolus of Ringer's lactate

Arterial pressure	110/60 mmHg
Heart rate	100/minute
Right atrial pressure	3 mmHg
Right ventricular pressure	38/2 mmHg
Right ventricular end-diastolic pressure	5 mmHg
Pulmonary artery pressure	39/12 mmHg
Pulmonary artery occlusion pressure	9 mmHg
Cardiac output	$3.4 \, \text{L min}^{-1}$
Cardiac index	$2.0 \, \text{L min}^{-1} \, \text{m}^{-2}$
Systemic vascular resistance	$1686 \, \text{dyn-sec cm}^{-5}$
Systemic vascular resistance index	$2867 \, \text{dyn-sec cm}^{-5} \, \text{m}^{-2}$

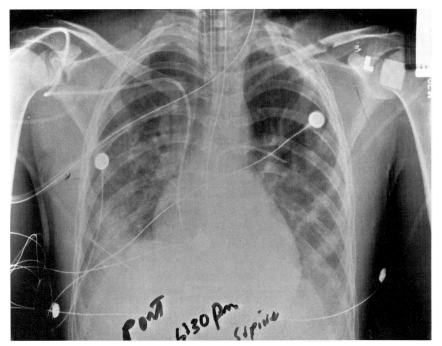

Figure 1.6.2. Chest radiograph obtained following endotracheal intubation and placement of a pulmonary artery catheter. Diffuse alveolar infiltrates are present, consistent with pulmonary contusions and/or adult respiratory distress syndrome. The cardiac silhouette is not enlarged. Fractures are seen in the left clavicle and left second rib, but there is no pneumothorax.

was transferred to the surgical intensive care unit for respiratory and cardiovascular monitoring and serial blood counts.

Traps

• Hypotension after multiple trauma carries a broad list of differential diagnoses.[3] Not infrequently, more than one cause of hypotension may be present, making an orderly, complete approach to the trauma victim crucial. While hemorrhage from abdominal organs, pelvis and long bones, great vessels or soft tissues is the most common cause of hypotension after multiple trauma, other potential causes need to be ruled out. Relatively small amounts of hemorrhage into the pericardium from disrupted epicardial vessels may produce pericardial tamponade. Other mechanisms of hypotension may not entail blood loss at all, e.g. tension pneumothorax or loss of autonomic vascular tone after spinal cord injury. In this patient, hypovolemia was appropriately recognized from the clinical and hemo-dynamic data, and a source of blood loss was sought even though the echocardiogram was indicative of a significant contusion of the right ventricle.[5,6]

- No single test has been accepted as a gold standard for the diagnosis of myocardial contusion, since none has demonstrated the required sensitivity and specificity.[1,3–5,7] In one prospective trial, 68 patients were evaluated to assess the relative merits of three tests commonly used to diagnose myocardial contusion.[8] The data showed that 44% of those with evidence of myocardial dysfunction by two-dimensional echocardiography had no evidence of injury by electrocardiography or creatine phosphokinase isoenzymes, and 67% of those with evidence of myocardial injury by creatine phosphokinase isoenzymes had no dysfunction apparent on echocardiography.[8] The trauma resident in this case prudently decided to use more than one mode of testing to evaluate the presence and extent of myocardial injury in a hemodynamically unstable patient whose history was consistent with significant thoracic trauma.

Tricks

In the USA, blunt cardiac trauma is most frequently seen in motor vehicle accidents, where it is estimated to be the primary cause of up to 5% of deaths.[4] However, any form of forceful injury to the thorax can cause cardiac injury.[6] The overall incidence of cardiac injury reported among victims of significant blunt trauma varies widely, from 16 to 76%. Much of this variation is likely to be due to differing clinical diagnostic criteria and the imperfect testing methods that are used.[3,9]

Important clinical clues that should alert the physician to the possibility of an underlying cardiac injury include both the mechanism of injury and the presence of any physical signs that correlate with the force of impact. Any blow to the thorax or rapid deceleration can cause cardiac injury, particularly if it occurs during a motor vehicle accident. Thoracic injuries such as fractures of the first, second or multiple ribs, fractures of the sternum or scapula, or widening of the mediastinal or cardiac contours are indicators of an injury forceful enough to inflict myocardial damage.[4] If any of these signs are found, a more thorough search for cardiac injury should be made, although it must be remembered that significant injury to the myocardium can occur even in the absence of such signs.[4]

Blunt cardiac trauma most commonly affects the right ventricle and atrium, because of their anterior position behind the sternum; however, all four chambers can be involved.[3,4] The heart may become compressed between the sternum and vertebrae, or a violent deceleration may cause an internal compression of the heart against either bony structure alone.[9] The spectrum of potential injury is quite broad with contusion being the most common. The full thickness or only a portion of the myocardial wall may be injured, but in all cases small vessel disruption, myocardial necrosis and red blood cell leakage into muscle fibers are present.[6] Most fatal outcomes, however, are not caused by the myocardial contusion itself but rather by acute or delayed rupture.[3] Other, less common injuries to the heart include coronary artery laceration, pericardial trauma, valvular disruption, ventricular aneurysm and myocardial dissection.[9]

The diagnosis of myocardial contusion, even though it is the most common traumatic heart injury, can be the most difficult to make.[3,4] Electrocardiography, creatine phosphokinase isoenzyme analysis, two-dimensional echocardiography and radionuclide angiography are the diagnostic tests used most often, but all are problematic with respect to both sensitivity and specificity.

Electrocardiography and cardiac monitoring are abnormal in a majority of patients who have sustained significant blunt thoracic trauma, showing a wide variety of manifestations including non-specific ST and T wave abnormalities (such as the inferior T wave inversions in this case), ectopic beats, supraventricular and ventricular arrhythmias, and conduction disturbances.[3-5] The correlation of these findings with the underlying cardiac injury can be misleading, since other coexisting conditions such as electrolyte imbalances, altered autonomic tone and head injury are frequently present and can cause confounding electrocardiographic abnormalities.

Creatine phosphokinase isoenzyme analysis is widely used to detect evidence of myocardial necrosis, either by finding total levels of MB (the isoenzyme found predominantly in the myocardium) above $100\,\text{IU}\,\text{mL}^{-1}$ [$2\,\mu\text{mol}\,\text{L}^{-1}$] or by finding MB, as a fraction of total creatine phosphokinase, above 5%.[3] Multiple trauma victims frequently have elevated total creatine phosphokinase levels from skeletal muscle injury.[10] These elevated levels may camouflage myocardial injury by diluting the myocardial MB fraction to less than 5%. Alternatively, since up to 4% of the creatine phosphokinase in skeletal muscle may be MB, a false diagnosis of myocardial injury could be reached if reliance were placed solely on absolute levels of MB.[5,10]

Echocardiography has become an important, useful alternative to electrocardiography or creatine phosphokinase isoenzyme analysis for the diagnosis of cardiac injury, since it offers a non-invasive method of imaging the heart to determine the extent of structural and physiologic impairment of cardiac chambers, valves and the pericardium.[5] However, technical limitations can arise in patients with pneumothoraces and multiple rib fractures that may reduce its usefulness in some patients;[3] transesophageal echocardiography can be helpful in such situations. Another test occasionally used is *radionuclide cineangiography*, which has relatively good sensitivity and specificity for myocardial contusion, but its use is limited because of the difficulty of performing it on the most severely injured patients.[3]

In the case of this patient, hypotension resulted from the combination of retroperitoneal hemmorhage and right ventricular contusion. If a patient presented with severe right ventricular contusion, but without significant hemorrhage, one would expect central venous pressure to be elevated. In a normovolemic patient, the hemodynamic profile of right ventricular contusion resembles that of acute right ventricular infarction, i.e. elevated right atrial and right ventricular end-diastolic pressures, normal pulmonary artery occlusion pressure and decreased cardiac output.

The physician must assimilate all of the information from these imperfect tests and integrate this with the clinical setting and mechanism of injury to make the diagnosis of cardiac damage. While the most severe cardiac traumas or those associated with multiple injuries will require intensive care unit monitoring, more limited forms of injury, such as suspected myocardial contusion without arrhythmia, may be best cared for on a telemetry unit.[1]

Follow-up

Following his transfer to the intensive care unit, the patient's retroperitoneal bleeding quickly stopped without further intervention. Transfusion of packed red blood cells and crystalloid stabilized his heart rate and blood pressure, and support with inotropic and vasopressor agents was not needed. Occasional ventricular ectopic beats and one brief run of an accelerated idioventricular rhythm were seen during the first 24 hours, but these did not affect blood pressure and were not treated with antiarrhythmic agents. Total creatine phosphokinase peaked within the first 24 hours to $4000\,IU\,mL^{-1}$ [$67\,\mu mol\,L^{-1}$] with an MB fraction of 4%, or $160\,IU\,mL^{-1}$ [$3\,\mu mol\,L^{-1}$].

The pulmonary artery catheter, placed initially for diagnostic purposes, was used to monitor hydration closely, allowing right atrial pressure and cardiac output to be optimized while avoiding elevation of the pulmonary artery occlusion pressure to levels that might compromise oxygenation further (Table 1.6.2). By the third hospital day his oxygen requirement had decreased, his radiographic infiltrates had improved and his trachea was extubated.

A follow-up echocardiogram was done seven days after the accident to look for delayed complications of blunt cardiac injury. The right ventricular dilation and hypokinesis seen on the first examination had largely resolved, except for some mild residual hypokinesis, and there was no indication that ventricular aneurysm, mural thrombus or valvular insufficiency had developed. Three days later he was discharged home and made a full recovery.

Table 1.6.2. Hemodynamic measurements 24 hours after admission

Arterial pressure	$122/72\,mmHg$
Heart rate	85/minute
Right atrial pressure	$12\,mmHg$
Right ventricular pressure	$41/4\,mmHg$
Right ventricular end-diastolic pressure	$10\,mmHg$
Pulmonary artery pressure	$40/15\,mmHg$
Pulmonary artery occlusion pressure	$10\,mmHg$
Cardiac output	$3.9\,L\,min^{-1}$
Cardiac index	$2.3\,L\,min^{-1}\,m^{-2}$
Systemic vascular resistance	$1573\,dyn\text{-}sec\,cm^{-5}$
Systemic vascular resistance index	$2667\,dyn\text{-}sec\,cm^{-5}\,m^{-2}$

References

1 Norton MJ, Stanford GG and Weigelt JA. Early detection of myocardial contusion and its complications in patients with blunt trauma. *American Journal of Surgery* (1990) **160**: 577–582.

2 Krasna MJ and Flancbaum L. Blunt cardiac trauma: clinical manifestations and management. *Seminars in Thoracic and Cardiovascular Surgery* (1992) **4**: 195–202.

3 Moore EE, Feliciano DV, Reines HD, *et al.* Chest trauma. In: Fuhrman BP, Shoemaker WL (eds) *Critical Care: State of the Art*. Society of Critical Care Medicine, Fullerton, pp 57–68, 1989.

4 Anonymous. Traumatic injury of the heart [editorial]. *Lancet* (1990) **336**: 1287–1289.

5 Paone RF, Peacock JB and Smith DLT. Diagnosis of myocardial contusion. *Southern Medical Journal* (1993) **86**: 867–870.

6 Nirgiotis JG, Colon R and Sweeney MS. Blunt trauma to the heart: the pathophysiology of injury. *Journal of Emergency Medicine* **8**: 617–623.

7 Liuzza GE. Diagnosis of myocardial contusion. *Southern Medical Journal* (1994) **87**: 419–420.

8 Helling TS, Duke P, Beggs CW and Crouse LJ. A prospective evaluation of 68 patients suffering blunt chest trauma for evidence of cardiac injury. *Journal of Trauma* (1989) **29**: 961–966.

9 Blintz M, Gall WE and Harbin D. Blunt myocardial disruption: report of an unusual case and literature review. *Journal of Trauma* (1992) **33**: 933–934.

10 Biffl WL, Moore FA, Moore EE, Savaia A, Read RA and Burch JM. Cardiac enzymes are irrelevant in the patient with suspected myocardial contusion. *American Journal of Surgery* (1994) **169**: 523–528.

2 Hemodynamic Monitoring

2.1 Decreasing Urine Output after Pelvic and Abdominal Trauma

Michael R. Pinsky

History

A 19-year-old male college student with no previous medical problems was out with his room mates one Saturday night drinking beer. He attempted to climb a flag pole on a dare from his friends. He got two-thirds of the way up the flag pole (approximately 35 feet [11 meters]) when the flag pole began to sway and then broke near its base. The young man fell onto the concrete surface hitting his left side. According to witnesses he was knocked unconscious by the impact.

His friends immediately called for help and placed the patient in a supine position and covered him with a coat. The paramedics arrived within 10 minutes of the call and found a young male, pale and unconscious. There was clotted blood in his mouth and nose. The pupils were equal and reactive, and there was left frontal facial ecchymosis. There were no signs of cyanosis or respiratory distress. His systolic blood pressure was palpable at 80 mmHg, his pulse 120/minute and respiration 20/minute and unlabored. His neck was stabilized, electrocardiograph monitoring begun and an intravenous catheter inserted from an antecubital vein. An infusion of Ringer's lactate was started at 250 mL h^{-1} and he was transported to the emergency department.

Examination in the emergency department revealed a blood pressure of 90/40 mmHg and a pulse of 110/minute. The pupils were equal and reactive with full concordant scanning of both eyes to all fields. No obvious abnormalities of the airway, head or neck were seen. The abdomen was silent with minimal guarding and rebound. Initial survey radiographs and a head CT scan revealed an undisplaced pelvic fracture-dislocation of the right pubic ramus and left sacro-iliac joint. The left mid-lung had alveolar and reticular lung opacities with a left-sided pleural effusion and fractures of left ribs 7 through 10. No intracranial or cervical pathology was identified.

Initial hematocrit was 45% and an arterial blood gas taken on a 35% face mask revealed pH 7.50 [H$^+$ 36 nmol L^{-1}], $P_a\text{CO}_2$ 28 mmHg [3.7 kPa] and $P_a\text{O}_2$ 135 mmHg [18 kPa], and he had a blood alcohol level of 25 mg dL^{-1} [5.4 mmol L^{-1}]. Physical examination after the radiographic examinations showed that he was that intermittently awake after painful stimuli. When awake he was confused but complaining of diffuse abdominal, pelvic and right leg pain. Breath sounds on the left side were diminished and his abdomen silent and slightly distended with mild guarding and rebound. No additional abnormalities in laboratory or physical examination were found. A paracentesis was performed and revealed gross blood in the abdomen. Insertion of a urinary catheter revealed no gross hematuria and an initial volume of 1200 mL straw-colored fluid. Based on these findings the patient was rapidly fluid-resuscitated with crystalloid solution, typed and cross matched for blood. After this he went to the operating room for an exploratory laparotomy for presumed splenic rupture.

Surgical findings at laparotomy included a ruptured spleen and a 3 cm anterior tear in the left hemidiaphragm. A splenectomy was performed and the diaphragmatic tear repaired with insertion of a left thoracostomy tube and abdominal drains into the lesser sac and perisplenic bed. During surgery the patient required 4 units of packed red blood cells and a total of 3000 mL of crystalloid to maintain hemodynamic stability (mean arterial pressure >70 mmHg, pulse <90/minute). Estimated blood loss was 2000 mL.

The patient was then transferred directly to the intensive care unit with an indwelling central venous catheter and radial arterial catheter, with his trachea intubated on mechanical ventilatory support. A nasogastric tube and a left-sided tube thoracostomy with -15 cmH$_2$O suction (with no air leak) were also present. His pelvic fracture had been stabilized with sand bags. The orthopedic surgeons had asked for complete pelvic immobilization without hip flexion or torso rotation for the next 48 hours. The patient was stable on awakening from general anesthesia, with mean arterial pressure 75 mmHg, pulse 85/minute, sinus rhythm, urine output over 75 mL h^{-1} and a hematocrit of 38%. Over the next 12 hours as the patient gradually awoke, he was weaned from mechanical ventilation and his trachea extubated. Fluid management was started during the immediate postoperative period with dextroses 0.9% NaCl with 30 mEq L^{-1} KCl at 125 mL h^{-1}. Repeat laboratory studies at 12 hours after the operation revealed a hematocrit of 35%, hemoglobin 11.6 g dL^{-1}, with a normal prothrombin time, partial thromboplastin time and platelet count. Serum electrolytes, BUN and creatinine were within normal limits and unchanged from initial values taken immediately preoperatively. The patient's mean arterial pressure was 80 mmHg and his pulse 95/minute.

Over the next 12 hours the patient's urine output progressively decreased from 75 to 35 mL h^{-1}, while both his mean arterial pressure and pulse, though variable from hour to hour, if anything increased slightly. Transcutaneous pulse oximetry showed a progressive decrease in arterial oxygen saturation from an initial postoperative value of 99% to between 89 and 92% at 24 hours after operation on 35% oxygen by face mask. The patient complained of generalized abdominal and left chest pain and became increasingly more agitated and tachypneic, necessitating intermittent doses of midazolam (1 mg IV) and fentanyl by continuous infusion (50 μg h^{-1}). At this time, 24 hours after surgery, a repeat chest radiograph revealed a diffuse left mid-lung field infiltrate, left tube thoracostomy and elevated left hemidiaphragm with blunted lateral aspect, but without evidence of pneumothorax.

An urgent abdominal ultrasound was ordered to rule out ureteral obstruction because of the decreasing urinary output associated with complaints of abdominal pain. The patient was also given an additional dose of fentanyl (100 μg IV) for pain. Immediately after the fentanyl, the patient became acutely hypotensive, tachycardic, with increased agitation requiring upper extremity restraint.

Traps

- The physicians relied on mean arterial pressure to assess intravascular volume status in a previously healthy patient. This variable is an insensitive indicator of volume status.[1] Normal homeostatic baroreceptor mechanisms function to maintain a near constant mean arterial pressure despite widely varying cardiac outputs and intravascular volume states. This is especially true in otherwise healthy young adults. Hemorrhage or heart failure do not initially manifest their presence as hypotension, but rather as signs of increased sympathetic tone (resting tachycardia) and decreased urine output. In this patient's situation pain, postsurgical stress and anxiety may all lead to increased sympathetic tone complicating the heart rate–blood pressure responses to volume loss.
- The physicians taking care of this patient were focused on the pelvic fracture as a source of postrenal obstruction and did not adequately appreciate the marked fluid requirements of an injured patient. Although a potential problem, pelvic fractures usually involve the bladder wall or urethra and rarely manifest themselves as progressive obstruction. More likely, they either continue to bleed from the pelvic fracture, or leak from the capillaries. This capillary leak is caused by the generalized endothelial injury following trauma. Both induce a decrease in intravascular blood volume.

   Agitation and decreasing urine output were the only signs of hypovolemia. The high resting sympathetic tone was reduced by the sympatholytic effects of the bolus of fentanyl. This abrupt sympathetic withdrawal allowed the hypovolemia to manifest itself as hypotension. In this patient, the intravascular fluid resuscitation, although initially adequate, was inadequate for the continuing fluid requirements associated with fluid shifts from intravascular to interstitial spaces. Agitation, decreasing urine output and other signs of increased sympathetic tone associated with progressive hypovolemia were all ignored in this patient until the sympatholytic effect of the bolus of fentanyl unmasked it.

Tricks

Although it is not wise to use mean arterial pressure and heart rate as the primary markers of an adequate cardiac output, their change in response to a volume challenge is useful in defining intravascular volume status.[2] The body's homeostatic mechanisms defend blood pressure (vital organ perfusion) by increasing vasomotor tone, strongly masking either blood loss or decreased ventricular pump function.[1] Whenever possible, the physician should use multiple signs to assess both the level of sympathetic tone and cardiovascular reserve.

   The usual response to progressively decreasing urine output is either to give a bolus fluid challenge or to increase fluid resuscitation rates. The physicians taking care of this patient were understandably concerned about increasing the patient's volume status because of the increasing left lung infiltrate and progressive hypoxemia. If these changes reflected pulmonary capillary leak then further fluid resuscitation would only make the pulmonary edema and hypoxemia worse. Even so, a transient fluid challenge test could have been performed. The traditional transient fluid challenge involves either sitting the patient up to decrease venous return or lifting the legs to increase venous return. A positive response to sitting up, meaning decreased circulating blood volume, could be manifest by a variety of cardiovascular changes including a decrease in arterial pressure and signs of central hypoperfusion (dizziness, syncope). These changes are usually associated with an increased sympathetic tone-induced increase in heart rate. The leg-raising test would induce the opposite changes if a low rate of venous return were inducing a reflex increase in sympathetic tone. The advantage of a transient fluid challenge test lies in its reversality and rapidity, whereas the negative aspects of this challenge lie in its minimal and transient nature and the need to monitor vital signs which may not change due to the baseline level of sympathetic tone.

The assessment of 'postural changes' in heart rate and blood pressure were briefly considered by the physicians taking care of this patient, but were discarded as a diagnostic option in this case because of the desire not to flex the hip joint in a patient with a pelvic fracture. However, the physicians could have easily given a postural challenge in this patient without flexing the hip or stressing the pelvis simply by tilting the bed upward (reverse Trendelenburg maneuver) to reduce venous return. This bed tilt maneuver is an equally useful gravitational stress test and can be applied in any patient, even in a patient in a full body cast. If such a tilt test had been done in this patient, a tachycardia and hypotension would likely have developed, given the profound effects that fentanyl produced.

The head-down (Trendelenburg position) maneuver incorrectly used by many critical care practitioners is not recommended as a method to increase venous return. Placing the head in the dependent position increases intracranial pressure, induces baroreceptor withdrawal of sympathetic tone and actually decreases cerebral blood flow.[3] The increase in mean arterial pressure seen with this maneuver is an artefact of the increased column of arterial blood produced by leg elevation which is matched by an equal amount of increased venous pressure. Thus, the routine use of the head-down Trendelenberg maneuver in hypotensive patients should be avoided. If transient increases in venous return are required, raising the legs will induce similar increases in venous return without the negative effects of the head-down maneuver of baroreceptor-induced vasomotor tone and intracranial pressure. If the leg-raising maneuver cannot be done, as in this patient, a fluid challenge may be justified. Although the physicians may have had justifiable fears of worsening gas exchange if a fluid challenge had been given, because of the probable left-sided lung contusion, a tilt test would carry no such risk and would have been diagnostic.

In an otherwise healthy patient, there is little additional benefit gained from more invasive hemodynamic monitoring, such as pulmonary arterial catheterization. End-organ functional measures, such as urine output, level of consciousness, and capillary filling if previously available are usually sufficient to guide cardiovascular therapy in the previously healthy patient.

As an additional point, a decreasing urine output in a patient whose bladder is catheterized could reflect either bilateral ureteric obstruction or extrinsic bladder compression from an expanding anterior pelvic hematoma. But both these conditions are very rare. Simple studies, like measuring the urine specific gravity and microscopic examination of the urinary sediment for evidence of red blood cells may aid considerably in establishing the correct diagnosis. In catheterized patients with otherwise normal renal function, it is reasonable to assume that decreasing urine output is not the result of postrenal causes.

Follow-up

The patient was rapidly resuscitated with two boluses of 500 mL 0.9% saline IV which resulted in a decrease in his heart rate to 85/minute and an increase in his mean arterial pressure to 75 mmHg. Ultrasound studies of the pelvis showed no uretheral distension, normal sized kidneys and no evidence of a peripelvic hematoma. Urine specific gravity was measured and found to be 1.030 when the urine output had improved. No preresuscitation urine sample (when the urine output was low) was available for comparison. Repeat hematocrit was 33%. The patient's fluid replacement rate was increased to $175\,\mathrm{mL\,h}^{-1}$, which included 3000 mL per day of hyperalimentation solution.

Follow-up examinations over the next few days revealed a gradually increasing hematocrit. The left-sided chest tube was removed on the morning of the third hospital day and the patient transferred out of the intensive care unit that afternoon. Following a prolonged rehabilitation interval, he returned to normal activities.

References

1 Shippy CR, Appel PL and Shoemaker WC. Reliability of clinical monitoring to assess blood volume in critically ill patients. *Critical Care Medicine* (1984) **12**: 107–115.
2 Shoemaker WC, Matsuda T and State D. Relative hemodynamic effectiveness of whole blood and plasma expanders in burn patients. *Surgical Gynecology and Obstetrics* (1973) **144**: 909–915.
3 Sibbald WJ, Paterson NAM, Holliday RI, *et al*. The Trendelenberg position: hemodynamic effects in hypotensive and normotensive patients. *Critical Care Medicine* (1979) **7**: 218–224.

2.2 Hypotension, Hypoxemia and Venous Return in an Immunocompromised Host
Michael R. Pinksy

History

A 56-year-old truck driver with a greater than 60 pack-year smoking history saw his physician for new-onset blood-tinged sputum following a prolonged chest cold. A chest radiograph showed a right mid-lung density and right perihilar fullness. Chest computed tomographic (CT) examination revealed a single 1.5 cm right mid-lung field mass and right hilar and paratracheal adenopathy. Sputum cytology and fiber-optic bronchoscopy were negative for endobronchial pathology, infectious causes, or malignant cells. A medistinoscopy was performed and the diagnosis of small cell carcinoma of the lung made. To see if he had metastatic disease, a head CT scan, bone scan, liver–spleen scan and serum chemistry were performed. They were all negative. The patient was transferred to an oncology center where he was placed in a combined local radiation therapy–chemotherapy protocol, which included upper mantle irradiation and cisplatin.

Three weeks into his second cycle of chemotherapy, the patient presented to the emergency department complaining of fever, chills, myalgias and increasing dyspnea of two days' duration. On examination, he was acutely ill, pale, in mild respiratory distress, but without jaundice or cyanosis. His temperature was 39°C, pulse 120/minute, blood pressure 85/60 mmHg and respiration 30/minute. Relevant physical examination findings included sweating, decreased right-sided breath sounds anteriorly with dullness to percussion over the right scapula and back associated with tubular breath sounds and the suggestion of a right-sided pleural rub. The patient was unable to produce sputum either spontaneously or after induction with hypertonic saline.

Pertinent laboratory findings included a white blood cell count of $4 \times 10^4 \, \text{L}^{-1}$ ($400 \, \text{dL}^{-1}$), platelets of $6.5 \times 10^4 \, \text{L}^{-1}$ ($65\,000 \, \text{dL}^{-1}$), and a hematocrit of 33%. Arterial blood gas analysis while the patient was breathing 6 L per minute oxygen by nasal prongs was pH 7.33 [H^+ 46 nmol L^{-1}], $P_a\text{O}_2$ 65 mmHg [8.7 kPa] and $P_a\text{CO}_2$ 35 mmHg [4.7 kPa]. A chest radiograph confirmed the presence of a right middle and right lower lobe alveolar filling process, without lung volume loss, and with air bronchograms to the mid-lung fields. A right pleural effusion was questioned by the radiologist reading the films.

The patient was admitted to the medical intensive care unit with the diagnosis of probable pneumonia in an immunocompromised host. Samples of blood, sputum and urine were sent for microbiological examination. A central venous catheter was inserted to sample venous blood, serve as a site for drug infusion and to monitor central venous pressure (CVP). The patient was placed on broad spectrum antibiotics, resuscitated with 5% dextrose and 0.45% saline at $200 \, \text{mL h}^{-1}$ and placed on a 0.4 $F_I\text{O}_2$ face mask. Blood pressure increased initially following admission to 105/55 mmHg and CVP increased from the time of insertion of the central venous catheter until two hours later (2–6 cmH$_2$O). However, over the next two hours (six hours after admission) the patient became progressively more hypotensive (systolic arterial pressure 75 mmHg), confused, combative and dyspneic. CVP readings were difficult to interpret because of the vigorous respiratory efforts but were believed not to be elevated. Repeat arterial blood gas analysis revealed a pH 7.25 [H$^+$ 56 nmol L^{-1}], P$_a$O$_2$ 45 mmHg [6 kPa] and a P$_a$CO$_2$ of 35 mmHg [4.7 kPa]. Because of the patient's confused and agitated state and worsening hypoxemia, despite enriched F$_I$O$_2$, the decision was made not to attempt non-invasive ventilatory support with continuous positive airway pressure by face mask, but to sedate him and intubate his trachea, and give him positive-pressure ventilation with positive end-expiratory pressure (PEEP) and an enriched F$_I$O$_2$. Furthermore, fluid resuscitation was stopped once the decision to intubate was made because of concern that vigorous fluid resuscitation may worsen hypoxemia. The plan was to start fluid resuscitation after starting mechanical ventilatory support.

Immediately upon intubation of the trachea and starting positive-pressure ventilation with a tidal volume of 800 mL and 10 cmH$_2$O PEEP, the patient became profoundly hypotensive (systolic arterial pressure of 40 mmHg). He rapidly progressed to ventricular fibrillation over the next few minutes. Vigorous cardiopulmonary resuscitative (CPR) efforts, including intracardiac epinephrine [adrenaline] and transthoracic pacing, were unable to restore spontaneous circulatory state after more than 60 minutes, despite arterial blood gas analyses during resuscitation revealing no hypoxemia or metabolic acidosis. The patient was pronounced dead after one hour of unsuccessful CPR. Permission for an autopsy was refused by the wife who witnessed most of the events described above.

Traps

- The first problem was not appreciating the profound reduction in circulating blood volume with a CVP of 10 cmH$_2$O and its interactions with both gas exchange efficiency and ventilation. The switch from spontaneous to positive-pressure ventilation invariably reduces the pressure gradient for systemic venous return decreasing left ventricular filling even further.[1] Cardiovascular instability after starting positive-pressure ventilation can be profound in hypovolemic patients and needs to be considered before tracheal intubation. This will enable effective counter-measures, such as bolus fluid resuscitation and alternative forms of ventilatory support to be used. CVP is an inaccurate measure of intravascular volume status. Perhaps its best use is to exclude volume hypovolemia if it is greater than 20 cmH$_2$O.[1]

- Two processes probably contributed to the worsening of arterial oxygenation in this patient. First, the pneumonitis by itself increased intrapulmonary shunt blood flow by minimizing the effectivity of the local hypoxic pulmonary vasoconstrictive response.[2] Normally, collapsed or flooded lung, as seen in patients with bronchial obstructions (lung cancer), do not cause profound hypoxemia because of concomitant pulmonary vasoconstriction. However, if inflammation is also present, as with acute pneumonitis, then inflammatory vasodilating mediators increase blood flow to flooded alveoli increasing the intrapulmonary shunt. Second, hypovolemia-induced decreased cardiac output and increased muscular activity (increased respiratory effort) result in increased oxygen extraction across the systemic bed decreasing mixed venous oxygen saturation. Thus, for the same amount of intrapulmonary shunt, hypovolemia and increased respiratory efforts will worsen further arterial oxygenation.

- Profound cardiovascular insufficiency after starting mechanical ventilation support may occur in patients with reduced effective circulating blood volume.[3] The causes of this instability are multiple, but include sedation-induced loss of sympathetic tone, positive-pressure ventilation-induced increased intrathoracic pressure and lung volume. All of these processes will further reduce, either directly or indirectly, the pressure gradient for systemic venous return. Sedation reduces sympathetic tone allowing blood to pool in the periphery. Increased intrathoracic pressure, or more appropriately the loss of the spontaneous ventilation-induced decrease in intrathoracic pressure increases CVP, which is the back pressure to venous return. Finally, increasing lung volume may increase pulmonary vascular resistance impeding right ventricular ejection or simply compress the heart, limiting diastolic filling. As in this patient, the combined results of starting mechanical ventilation can be tragic.

Tricks

Understanding that a low cardiac output may play a role worsening gas exchange, measures of cardiac output or organ perfusion should be sought. In this case, the patient did not have an indwelling urinary bladder catheter inserted, thus the physicians did not know that the patient was effectively anuric for the six hours of his last hospital admission. Second, the increased confusion and agitation, although potentially caused by sepsis, could also have been caused by cerebral ischemia. *Never ignore a treatable diagnosis even if the possibility of a non-treatable diagnosis is more likely.*

In this patient the initial management should have included more aggressive fluid resuscitation to restore arterial pressure toward normal. If in attempting this, the patient becomes more hypoxemic, then a pulmonary artery catheter should have been inserted to measure the back pressure to pulmonary blood flow, pulmonary artery occlusion pressure. These measurements will aid in diagnosing the cause of pulmonary edema (high or low pressure edema), as well as allowing the physician to measure both cardiac output and mixed venous oxygen saturation. These measurements, along with measures of arterial oxygenation would allow for the calculation of shunt, systemic oxygen transport and systemic oxygen uptake. Although we will never know what the exact cause of cardiovascular collapse was in this patient, the likely diagnosis and sequence of events was:

1. Chemotherapy-induced immunosuppression.
2. Community-acquired pneumonia (most likely Gram-positive organism).
3. Sepsis syndrome progressing to septic shock as the effective intravascular volume decreased.
4. Increased oxygen demand by the respiratory muscles exacerbating arterial hypoxemia.
5. Sedation, positive-pressure ventilation and PEEP inducing a further reduction in venous return, decreasing cardiac perfusion pressure.
6. Cardiac arrest.

It is unclear if aggressive fluid resuscitation would have helped this patient, but it is clear that starting mechanical ventilatory support, without the addition of fluid resuscitation, hastened the patient's death.

References

1 Guyton AC. Effect on cardiac output of respiration, opening the chest, and tamponade. In: Guyton AC, Jones CE, Coleman THE (eds) *Cardiac Output and Its Regulation*, 2nd edn. Philadelphia, W. B. Saunders, pp 427–482, 1973.
2 Marshall BE and Marshall C. Continuity of response to hypoxic pulmonary vasoconstriction. *Journal of Applied Physiology* (1980) **49**: 189–196.
3 Pinsky MR. Cardiopulmonary Interactions. In: Dantzker M (ed.) *Cardiopulmonary Critical Care*, 2nd edn. Philadelphia, W. B. Saunders, pp 87–120, 1991.

2.3 Sepsis, Hypotension and Elevated Arterial Blood Lactate

Michael R. Pinsky

History

A 44-year-old housewife with a history of recurrent postprandial epigastric epigastric discomfort and bloating for over five years presented to her local doctor with severe unrelenting abdominal pain of 4 hours' duration. The patient had not sought medical help sooner because of her responsibilities to her four young children, aged 2 to 10. This time, however, the pain was different and more severe. It started as usual with diffuse epigastric dull aching pain, nausea and tenderness making her change from wearing jeans to a loose-fitting house coat. However, after about an hour the pain increased suddenly and was generalized to most of her abdomen and lower back region, making her light-headed and forcing her to lie down. She denied any vomiting, diarrhea, constipation or change in the color of her stools, which were usually dark brown in color. No other relevant medical, social or travel history was elicited.

On examination, she was a moderately overweight female in acute distress lying quietly on the examination table. Her temperature was $39°C$, pulse 105/minute, blood pressure 175/110 mmHg and respiration 22/minute. Her abdomen was rigid without bowel sounds and with marked guarding and rebound. An erect abdominal radiograph taken at the physician's office revealed ileus and questionable evidence of free air under the right hemidiaphragm. The tentative diagnosis of hollow viscous perforation was made and the patient transferred by ambulance from the doctor's office to the hospital where surgical consultation was obtained.

Supplemental laboratory findings obtained on admission to the hospital included a white blood cell count of $1.05 \times 10^4 \, L^{-1}$ ($10\,500 \, dL^{-1}$) with 20% band forms, hematocrit 42% and $22.5 \times 10^4 \, L^{-1}$ ($225\,000 \, dL^{-1}$) platelets. Serum transaminase levels were slightly elevated whereas serum alkaline phosphatase and direct bilirubin levels were markedly elevated. Following collection of blood for microbiological studies and type and crossing for potential transfusion needs, the patient was given ampicillin (1 g IV) and gentamycin (250 mg IV) and then taken to the operating room where an exploratory laboratory was performed for a presumed ruptured gall bladder. At the operation there was diffuse bile staining of the abdominal contents, a thickened gall bladder wall with multiple small dark brown stones in the head of the gall bladder. No obvious site of the bile leak was identified. Cultures of abdominal fluid and bile were taken and a cholecystectomy was performed with T-tube drainage. The abdomen was flushed with 0.9% saline, drains placed and the abdomen closed with retention sutures.

The patient did remarkably well for the next two days with her temperature decreasing, return of occasional bowel sounds and reduced, but not abolished, abdominal pain. She was rapidly weaned from mechanical ventilatory support in the postanesthetic recovery room and except for a transient interval during induction of general anesthesia, required no vasopressor support to maintain a mean arterial blood pressure above 70 mmHg. On the first two postoperative days serum transaminase levels remained slightly elevated. Admission blood culture results grew *Haemophilus influenzae* in one of four bottles. Nasogastric aspiration remained high postoperatively, averaging over 50 mL h^{-1}. The gentamycin had been stopped after the initial dosage, but the ampicillin had been continued (500 mg IV 4 hourly). Hyperalimentation and electrolyte replacement were started on the first day after operation and the patient's hemodynamic status, urine output and electrolyte balance were considered reasonable.

In the early morning hours of the third postoperative day, she suddenly developed a violent shaking chill followed by an acute confusional febrile state (temperature 38.5°C). Her blood pressure which had been 135/90 mmHg, and pulse of 82/minute were now 80/45 mmHg and 115/minute, respectively. The patient was transferred to the surgical intensive care unit where in rapid succession she was rehydrated (1000 mL Ringer's lactate and 250 mL hydroxy-ethylstarch), specimens were taken for microbiological culture, and she was started on broad spectrum antibiotics. Immediate blood examinations revealed a white blood cell count of 1.5×10^4 L^{-1} (15 000 dL^{-1}), hematocrit of 33%, platelets 15×10^4 L^{-1} (150 000 dL^{-1}), arterial lactate of 3.5 mmol L^{-1}, and arterial blood gas on an F_IO_2 of 0.4 of: pH 7.38 [42 nmol L^{-1}], P_aO_2 128 mmHg [17.1 kPa] and P_aCO_2 38 mmHg [5.1 kPa]. Her urine output was questionable so an indwelling urinary catheter was inserted which revealed 50 mL of reddish brown liquid, specific gravity 1.030, positive for bilirubin and protein, with white blood cells and debris seen on microscopic examination. Neither her blood pressure nor her urine output increased in response to this fluid challenge. Pulse oximetry estimates of arterial oxygen saturation decreased from 99 to 93%. Thus, the decision was made to insert both a balloon-flotation pulmonary artery catheter to assess left ventricular filling pressures and cardiac output, and a radial artery catheter to monitor her hemodynamic status.

Initial data from these catheterizations revealed a cardiac index of 3.5 L min^{-1} m^{-2}, mixed venous oxygen saturation of 85%, pulmonary artery occlusion pressure of about 10–15 mmHg (difficult to interpret because of the marked respiratory artefact), pulse of 105/minute, blood pressure of 92/50 mmHg and mean arterial pressure of 58 mmHg. Arterial blood gas analysis revealed a pH of 7.41 [H$^+$41 nmol L^{-1}], P_aO_2 of 135 mmHg [18 kPa] on a 0.4 F_IO_2, and a P_aCO_2 of 38 mmHg [5.1 kPa]. Concomitant with these data the patient's urine output increased to 85 mL h^{-1} and she became more lucid. Arterial lactate levels remained elevated at 3.1 mmol L^{-1}. Because of the continuing hyperlactacemia and hypotension, despite apparently adequate fluid resuscitation, dopamine was started and the dose increased in an attempt to maintain a mean arterial pressure of 80 mmHg. However, mean arterial pressure could only be increased to a mean value of 70 mmHg at 20 μg kg^{-1} min^{-1} dopamine and urine output decreased to less than 20 mL h^{-1} despite a maintaining of cardiac index at about 3.2 L min^{-1} m^{-2}. Because of a persistently elevated arterial lactate level

$(3.2 \, \text{mmol} \, \text{L}^{-1}$ on remeasurement) in the setting of clear evidence of systemic hypotension and end-organ hypoperfusion the decision was made to start an epinephrine [adrenaline] infusion for presumed severe septic shock and cardiovascular collapse.

Traps

The first error was an over-reliance on mean arterial pressure and serum lactate levels to assess organ perfusion in a patient with previously normal end-organ function. In support of the actions of the physicians, hypotension during sepsis is a common occurrence. It is thought to be caused by the release of potent vasodilating substances by the endothelium and activated formed cellular elements.[1] Persistent hyperlactacemia predicts a poor prognosis.[2] However, a mean arterial pressure of 55 mmHg may be adequate in many patients. This lady showed evidence of adequate end-organ flow as manifest by normal cerebration and urine output. In the setting of high to high-normal cardiac index and adequate organ function, a mean arterial pressure of 55 mmHg may be acceptable so long as diastolic arterial pressure is not so low as to compromise coronary blood flow. Furthermore, the hyperlactacemia was not associated with metabolic acidosis suggesting that these changes reflected non-specific metabolic effects of sepsis rather than ischemic circulatory shock. Serum lactate levels are sensitive, but not specific, markers of tissue ischemia. The common occurrence of increased serum lactate levels in critically ill, but resuscitated patients, suggests that processes other than tissue ischemia are responsible for hyperlactacemia in a majority of these patients.[3] Although insensitive as a marker of regional blood flow, the presence of a high mixed venous oxygen saturation (85%) and cardiac index $(3.5 \, \text{L} \, \text{min}^{-1} \, \text{m}^{-2})$ argues against significant global tissue ischemia. Finally, the use of either dopamine or epinephrine in this setting will induce a decrease, not an increase, in renal and splanchnic blood flow promoting, not preventing, end-organ dysfunction. Although essential in maintaining organ perfusion pressure when mean arterial pressure and organ perfusion pressures are very low (<55 mmHg), the benefit of these potent vasopressor agents in otherwise stable patients has not been documented. In this patient, the decision to use epinephrine resulted in a worsening of renal blood flow.

Tricks

Whenever possible, rely on primary measures of the adequacy of peripheral blood flow. Such measures include level of consciousness, gut function (bowel sounds), urine output and normal physical activity. Surrogate measures of regional function may include EEG for the brain, gastric tonometry for the gut, 2 hourly creatinine clearance studies for the kidney, and ketone body ratios (acetoacetic acid/β hydroxybutyric acid) for hepatic function. In this patient, the treatment focused on maintenance of cardiac index at its present level or at most attempting therapeutic trials to increase it further; noting how such interventions altered urine output, mentation, serum lactate levels and other measures of ischemia, such as gastric tonometry and ketone body ratios, could have facilitated resuscitative efforts. There is no magic cardiac index, but there is a minimal organ perfusion pressure below which autoregulation of blood flow occurs:[4] that pressure level varies among subjects but probably occurs in most subjects at or above a mean arterial pressure of 55 mmHg.

Follow-up

When epinephrine was started, urine output decreased to less than $5 \, mL \, h^{-1}$. The vasopressor therapy was stopped and mean arterial blood pressure maintained by fluid resuscitation alone. The epinephrine was rapidly weaned off in one hour and the dopamine reduced to $5 \, \mu g \, kg^{-1} \, min^{-1}$. Fluids were given intravenously to keep the pulmonary artery occlusion pressure at approximately 15 mmHg. With this approach, the patient's urine output progressively increased to $>125 \, mL \, h^{-1}$ and her serum lactate level decreased to $2.3 \, mmol \, L^{-1}$. Blood cultures from the initial septic episode were positive for *Escherichia coli* sensitive to the aminoglycoside being used. She never developed clinically significant abnormalities with gas exchange. The serum creatinine increased on the following day from 0.9 $[68 \, \mu mol \, L^{-1}]$ to $1.5 \, mg \, dL^{-1}$ $[114 \, \mu mol \, L^{-1}]$ returning to normal the following day. By two days following the acute hypotensive episode she had recovered enough for her invasive monitoring to be stopped. She was transferred to a regular ward bed the next morning, and discharged home four days later.

References

1 Kilbourn RO, Gross SS and Jubran A. *N*-Methyl-L-arginine inhibits tumor necrosis factor-induced hypotension: implications for the involvement of nitric oxide. *Proceedings of the National Academy of Science, USA* (1990) **87**: 3629–3632.
2 Perez DI, MacGregor M, Dossetor JB, *et al.* Lactic acidosis: a clinically significant aspect of shock. *Canadian Medical Association Journal* (1964) **90**: 673–675.
3 Hotchkiss RS and Karl IE. Reevaluation of the role of cellular hypoxia and bioenergic failure in sepsis. *Journal of the American Medical Association* (1992) **267**: 1503–1510.
4 Pinsky MR. The meaning of cardiac output. *Intensive Care Medicine* (1990) **16**: 415–417.

3 Increased Intrathoracic Pressure

3.1 The Many Disguises of PEEP
Adelaida M. Miro

History

A 26-year-old man with a long-standing history of steroid-dependent bronchial asthma was seen in the emergency department with an acute exacerbation secondary to an upper respiratory tract infection. The acute bronchospasm was treated with aerosolized bronchodilators, intravenous theophylline and cortico-steroids with only partial improvement. Because he had previously needed tracheal intubation and mechanical ventilation for an acute asthma attack, he was admitted to the intensive care unit for further observation and management.

Upon arrival in the ICU, he was restless and markedly dyspneic. Vital signs showed a temperature of 39°C, heart rate of 130/minute, arterial blood pressure of 156/100 mmHg and a respiratory frequency of 35 breaths/minute. On physical examination there was poor bilateral air entry on inspiration and expiratory wheezing. Pulse oximetry showed the oxygen saturation to be 98% while breathing 2 L of oxygen by nasal cannula. An arterial blood gas revealed a pH of 7.33 [H^+ 47 nmol L^{-1}], P_aCO_2 of 48 mmHg [6 kPa], and P_aO_2 of 122 mmHg [16.3 kPa]. A decision was made to intubate this patient's trachea because he had not responded to maximal medical management and was developing respiratory failure.

The patient was premedicated with intravenous fentanyl 150 µg and midazolam 4 mg before tracheal intubation. Once he appeared sedated, tracheal intubation was attempted. During laryngoscopy, the patient rapidly awoke from the sedation and became agitated. Despite the agitation, the physician was able to successfully pass the tracheal tube. He was verbally reassured by the physician in attempts to calm his anxiety and his upper extremities were restrained to avoid self-extubation. The patient was then placed on assist-control ventilation at a tidal volume of 10 mL kg^{-1} per breath and a rate of 12 breaths/minute without any positive end-expiratory pressure (PEEP).

Examination a few minutes after tracheal intubation revealed a restless and agitated patient with a heart rate of 135 beats/minute, blood pressure of 85/60 mmHg and respiratory frequency of 30 breaths/minute.

Trap

Hypotension after tracheal intubation and positive-pressure ventilation is extremely common.[1] It has many causes, but there are certain risk factors that should be identified and avoided. Knowing that hypotension can develop and why represents a central aspect of the cardiopulmonary management of patients with severe airflow obstruction.

Tricks

The transition from spontaneous breathing to positive-pressure ventilation is one of the most common causes of hypotension in these circumstances. During spontaneous respiration, intrathoracic pressure decreases to subatmospheric values and systemic venous return (ventricular preload) increases. Conversely, during positive-pressure ventilation, intrathoracic pressure becomes more positive which, by reducing the pressure gradient for venous return, in turn decreases cardiac output. If a patient is normo- or hypervolemic, this decrease in venous return is usually not associated with any significant hypotension. However, when patients are even mildly hypovolemic or dehydrated from their acute illness, the transition to positive-pressure ventilation can lead to a severe cardiovascular embarrassment.

This patient was hypovolemic because of his febrile, upper respiratory tract infection and acute asthma. In general, patients who are suspected of being intravascularly depleted (fever, dry mucous membranes, orthostatic changes in blood pressure) should receive supplemental intravenous crystalloid or colloid fluid resuscitation before tracheal intubation whenever possible. Alternatively, fluid can be given after starting mechanical ventilation to facilitate restoration of normal arterial blood pressure.

A second mechanism which further increases intrathoracic pressure, decreases venous return and ultimately results in hypotension, is the development of hyperinflation or 'auto-PEEP'.[2-5] The term 'auto-PEEP' or 'intrinsic PEEP' was coined to describe the phenomenon of a positive alveolar pressure at the end of exhalation. This increases the functional residual capacity (FRC) despite positive end-expiratory pressure (PEEP) not being set on the ventilator (external PEEP).

Auto-PEEP develops because of insufficient expiratory time to expel the tidal breath. In patients with emphysema, auto-PEEP occurs because of a loss of elastic recoil of the pulmonary parenchyma, while in patients with acute asthma or chronic bronchitis, auto-PEEP develops secondary to increases in airway resistance. Irrespective of the mechanism, the increase in end-expiratory alveolar pressures decreases venous return, identical to that caused by applying external PEEP to a ventilator circuit. This increase in lung volume increases intrathoracic pressure, which reduces the pressure gradient for venous return back to the right atrium. If lung volume increases enough, pulmonary vascular resistance also increases. These two mechanisms decrease venous return to the right ventricle, just when it needs the extra volume to overcome the increase in pulmonary vascular resistance. Eventually cardiac output and systemic arterial blood pressure decrease.

The amount of auto-PEEP can be measured by several techniques. The simplest and most widely used, in mechanically ventilated patients, is the end-expiratory occlusion method described by Pepe and Marini.[2] With this technique, the expiratory port of the ventilator is manually occluded for a fraction of a second, immediately before delivery of the next ventilator breath. After occlusion, any increases in airway pressure above the end-expiratory level is measured by the airway pressure manometer and represents the amount of auto-PEEP that is present. Normally, there should be no measurable auto-PEEP. The timing of the occlusion is important, since occluding the expiratory port too early can cause a falsely elevated estimate of auto-PEEP.

It is also important to recognize that even patients without any evidence of obstructive airway disease and normal pulmonary function can develop auto-PEEP.[6] This is a common occurrence in the critically ill – a subject that has received a disproportionately small amount of attention. One common scenario is with agitated or combative patients whose tracheas are intubated and who are breathing at rapid respiratory rates while on a fully supported ventilatory mode such as assist-control. In these patients, with every inspiratory effort, the ventilator delivers a full tidal volume breath, usually in the order of $10–12\,mL\,kg^{-1}$ per breath. Since expiratory time is reduced because of the tachypnea, the lungs become hyperinflated and, ultimately, the cascade of increasing end-expiratory alveolar pressure and intrathoracic pressures leads to a decrease in cardiac output and hypotension. An identical mechanism of hyperinflation and hypotension can result if minute ventilation is intentionally increased, such as when attempting to lower P_aCO_2 to compensate for a metabolic acidosis or to reduce intracranial hypertension.[7,8]

In summary, there are several mechanisms that can lead to cardiovascular compromise when patients are placed on mechanical ventilation. Intravascular volume should be restored before tracheal intubation whenever possible. Auto-PEEP can be minimized by treatment of the underlying disease (bronchodilators, steroids, etc.) and providing sedation and anxiolytics to agitated patients to minimize respiratory effort and global carbon dioxide production. Finally, 'therapeutic' hyperventilation should be undertaken with extreme care, since this may also lead to an unfavorable reduction in cardiac output and arterial blood pressure.

Follow-up

The physician caring for this patient identified the hyperinflation as the cause of cardiovascular insufficiency and took measures to reduce auto-PEEP. The patient was sedated and the ventilatory mode switched from assist-control to synchronous intermittent mandatory ventilation (SIMV). With this, the minute ventilation and respiratory rate decreased, but the P_aCO_2 remained constant at 45 mmHg [6 kPa]. Within the next 24 hours, the bronchospasm lessened, and the trachea was extubated 36 hours after tracheal intubation. He was discharged home five days following admission after being switched to oral bronchodilator agents and metered dose inhalers for β_2-adrenergic agonists and beclomethasone.

References

1 Miro AM and Pinsky MR. Heart–lung interactions. In: Tobin MJ (ed.) *Principles and Practice of Mechanical Ventilation*. St Louis, McGraw-Hill, pp 647–671, 1994.

2 Pepe PE and Marini JJ. Occult positive end-expiratory pressure in mechanically ventilated patients with airflow obstruction. *American Review of Respiratory Diseases* (1982) **126**: 166–170.

3 Smith JC and Marini JJ. Impact of PEEP on lung mechanics and work of breathing in severe airflow obstruction. *Journal of Applied Physiology* (1988) **65**: 1488–1499.

4 Benson MS and Pierson DJ. Auto-PEEP during mechanical ventilation of adults. *Respiratory Care* (1988) **33**: 557–568.

5 Pinsky MR. Through the past darkly: the ventilatory management of patients with COPD [editorial]. *Critical Care Medicine* (1994) **22**: 1714–1717.

6 Marini JJ. Should PEEP be used in airflow obstruction [editorial]. *American Review of Respiratory Diseases* (1989) **140**: 1–3.

7 Rogers PL, Schlichtig R, Miro A and Pinsky M. Auto PEEP during CPR: an 'occult' cause of electromechanical dissociation? *Chest* (1991) **99**: 492–493.

8 Scott LR, Benson MS and Bishop MJ. Relationship of endotracheal tube size to auto-PEEP at high minute ventilation. *Respiratory Care* (1986) **31**: 1080–1082.

3.2 Hypotension in a Mechanically Ventilated Asthmatic

Steven M. Scharf

History

A 31-year-old, white, female with a long history of asthma was admitted to the hospital through the emergency department because of a severe exacerbation of asthma, probably triggered by a viral infection. Her home asthma regimen consisted of inhaled steroids and bronchodilators. Despite therapy with inhaled beta agonists and intravenous methylprednisolone, she failed to improve.

On admission, she was afebrile and appeared in moderate to severe distress using her accessory muscles, blood pressure 130/80 mmHg, pulse 110/minute, 20 mmHg pulsus paradoxus, respiratory rate of 35/minute. Auscultation of the lungs revealed bilateral wheezing, but the breath sounds were mildly decreased. Peak expiratory flow rate was $80 \, L \, min^{-1}$. Chest radiography showed hyperinflation, but no other acute changes. Arterial blood gases (ABGs) on $4 \, L \, min^{-1}$ oxygen by nasal cannula administered oxygen showed P_aO_2 of 75 mmHg [10 kPa], P_aCO_2 of 46 mmHg [6.1 kPa], and a pH of 7.37 [$H^+44 \, nmol \, L^{-1}$].

Several hours later, she appeared dusky and lethargic. ABGs showed P_aO_2 68 mmHg [9.1 kPa], P_aCO_2 53 mmHg [7.1 kPa], pH 7.31 [$H^+49 \, nmol \, L^{-1}$]. Her trachea was intubated and she was placed on positive-pressure ventilation and transferred to the intensive care unit.

In the intensive care unit she was heavily sedated and paralyzed. Ventilator settings were F_IO_2 0.6, tidal volume $12 \, mL \, kg^{-1}$, rate 16/minute, peak inflation pressure $58 \, cmH_2O$. ABGs showed: P_aO_2 90 mmHg [12 kPa], P_aCO_2 45 mmHg [6 kPa], pH 7.38 [$H^+ \, 42 \, nmol \, L^{-1}$], blood pressure 120/70 mmHg, pulse 110/minute. Treatment with inhaled beta agonists and intravenous steroids was continued. Two hours later ABGs showed P_aO_2 75 mmHg [10 kPa], P_aCO_2 55 mmHg [7.3 kPa], pH 7.31 [$H^+ \, 49 \, nmol \, L^{-1}$]. To compensate for the hypercapnia the ventilator rate was turned up to 20/minute. Repeat ABGs showed P_aO_2 70 mmHg [9.3 kPa], P_aCO_2 50 mmHg [6.7 kPa], pH 7.33 [$H^+ \, 43 \, nmol \, L^{-1}$]. The blood pressure was now 85/60 mmHg and pulse 120/minute. Because of continuing hypercapnia the ventilator rate was increased further to 24/minute. ABGs showed P_aO_2 70 mmHg [9.3 kPa], P_aCO_2 48 mmHg [6.4 kPa], pH 7.35 [$H^+ \, 45 \, nmol \, L^{-1}$]. The systolic blood pressure was 70 mmHg, pulse 135/minute, the trachea was mid-line. Because of bilateral hyperresonance and shock, tension pneumothorax, possibly bilateral, was suspected. Preparations were made to drain the presumed pneumothorax and a chest radiograph was ordered.

Traps

This patient was not experiencing a tension pneumothorax, one dreaded complication in asthmatic patients on a ventilator. Rather, she was experiencing dynamic hyperinflation of the lungs. In patients with severe airways obstruction, exhalation time (T_e) is prolonged. It may be so prolonged that all the tidal volume (V_t) may not be exhaled in the allotted T_e, which is set by the ventilatory rate and the inspiratory : expiratory ratio. As respiratory rate is increased, T_e decreases. This leads to less of the set inspiratory tidal volume being exhaled and, as a consequence, lung volume at end-expiration (functional residual capacity – FRC) increases. FRC will increase until the additional recoil of the respiratory system coupled with the decrease in airways resistance associated with increased lung volume allows all of the V_t to be exhaled in the allotted T_e. Since asthmatic patients usually have elevated baseline FRC because of their disease process,[1] the additional dynamic increase in lung volume can push FRC up close to total lung capacity!

The consequences of severely increasing lung volume in this manner are similar to severely increasing lung volume by any other means, for example applying high levels of positive end-expiratory pressure. These include increased risk of barotrauma[2] and cardiovascular collapse.[3] The hemodynamics of dynamic hyperventilation can resemble those of tension pneumothorax, pneumomediastinum or cardiac failure, with increased central venous and pulmonary wedge pressures, decreased cardiac output, decreased blood pressure and possibly increased systemic vascular resistance. The mistake here was to continue to shorten T_e (increase respiratory rate) in order to maintain a normal arterial P_{CO_2}, thus increasing dynamic hyperinflation and resulting in severe hemodynamic compromise.

Tricks

The trick in this patient is not to aim for a normal P_{aCO_2}. The ventilator was disconnected for approximately 30 seconds until dynamic hyperinflation was eliminated. Ventilation was then restarted at V_t 8 mL kg^{-1}, rate 14/minute (total ventilation 112 mL kg^{-1} min^{-1}), F_{IO_2} 0.7. Peak inflation pressure was 38 cmH$_2$O. Blood pressure increased almost immediately to 135/80 mmHg and pulse decreased to 100/minute. On the new mode of ventilation, ABGs were P_{aO_2} 95 mmHg [12.7 kPa], P_{aCO_2} 60 mmHg [8 kPa], pH 7.29 [H$^+$ 51 nmol L^{-1}].

In this case, it was decided to allow the patient to remain hypercapnic (thus the name 'permissive hypercapnia') and maintain oxygenation. The hemodynamic consequences of dynamic hyperinflation can be so severe that one must sometimes pay the price of hypoventilation for hemodynamic stability. Dynamic hyperinflation is probably relatively common in asthmatic patients requiring mechanical ventilation.[2,4,5] A ventilatory strategy which attempts to minimize this by increasing T_e (decreasing ventilatory rate at constant inspiratory : expiratory time ratio) and decreasing V_t, has been shown in at least one controlled trial to decrease the morbidity and possibly mortality associated with mechanical ventilation.[6] In this trial, dynamic hyperinflation was regulated such that lung volume was limited to $\leqslant 20\,\mathrm{mL\,kg^{-1}}$ above FRC by a combination of decreased rate and V_t.

Further gain may be had by decreasing inspiratory time, by increasing inspiratory flow rate, at the same ventilatory rate, hence preserving overall ventilation. This maneuver will increase peak inspiratory pressure. However, this should not result in increased risk of barotrauma since the pressure increase is totally caused by flow-resistive pressure drops across the large airways. The increased pressure should therefore be dissipated along the airway, resulting in no increase in end-expiratory alveolar pressure (measured as inspiratory plateau pressure). However, rapid inflation of the lung could be associated with abnormalities of distribution of ventilation, thus worsening gas exchange.[7] High inspiratory flows are still favored by some,[8] and the matter remains controversial.

Low tidal volume has been recommended such that total ventilation remains $\leqslant 115\,\mathrm{mL\,kg^{-1}\,min^{-1}}$[,2,4,6] which results in an average $P_a\mathrm{CO_2}$ of $77\pm23\,\mathrm{mmHg}$ $[10.3\pm3.1\,\mathrm{kPa}]$ and pH of 7.17 ± 0.13 $[\mathrm{H^+}\;67\pm1\,\mathrm{nmol\,L^{-1}}]$ in adults.[2] A V_t of $8\,\mathrm{mL\,kg^{-1}}$ produces the lowest level of dynamic hyperinflation compared with higher V_t lower rate combinations.[4] Thus, starting with a V_t of this level and respiratory rate of 10–14 seems a reasonable initial ventilator strategy. $F_{I}\mathrm{O_2}$ should be set at a level adequate to achieve an arterial oxyen saturation of at least 90–92%. In some patients with severe airways plugging and occasional shunting, a saturation of 85–90% may need to be accepted even with an $F_{I}\mathrm{O_2}$ of 1. It should be remembered that owing to the Bohr shift of the oxyhemoglobin dissociation curve, oxygen saturation will be less at any given $P_a\mathrm{O_2}$ during hypercapnic acidosis than when pH is normal. Thus, a $P_a\mathrm{O_2}$ which was adequate to achieve arterial oxygen saturation of 90–92% with normal pH will not be adequate during acidosis. Since pure ventilation/perfusion deficits can be overcome with oxygen, an $F_{I}\mathrm{O_2}$ of 0.4–0.6 is usually adequate for oxygenation during permissive hypercapnia. Because of further increasing lung volume and hence the risk of barotrauma, PEEP is dangerous during mechanical ventilation in asthmatics and should be avoided.

While some patients may tolerate permissive hypercapnia and acidosis without discomfort, most patients will feel very dyspneic, at least during the first stages of hypoventilation. Patients allowed to trigger the ventilator (assist-control mode) or to breathe spontaneously between machine-delivered breaths (intermittent mandatory ventilation) may have high respiratory rates. The respiratory rate may increase such that dynamic hyperinflation again becomes a problem. Thus, heavy sedation sometimes with neuromuscular blockade paralysis is usually necessary at first.

There is no universally agreed upon set of guidelines for targeting the level of ventilation during permissive hypercapnia. Interestingly enough, the actual $P_a\mathrm{CO_2}$ is probably not the most useful target, but rather the changes in respiratory volume seem to be the most important indicators of mortality and morbidity with this mode of ventilation. Some have recommended maintaining peak inflation pressure at less than $50\,cmH_2O$.[9] However, as pointed out above, because of flow-resistive pressure losses down the airway (including the tracheal tube), this value does not represent the alveolar pressure – the pressure which represents the risk of barotrauma. A better measure might be airway plateau pressure during an inspiratory hold maneuver, which does measure alveolar pressure (no flow condition) at end-inspiration. However, without knowledge of lung compliance this number cannot be translated into a change in lung volume. Studies have not yet been done which relate end-inspiratory plateau pressure to risk for barotrauma.

In one study, a dynamic increase in lung volume of $\geqslant 20\,mL\,kg^{-1}$ was associated with increased morbidity and possibly mortality.[2] Thus, it is reasonable to measure the increase in lung volume caused by dynamic hyperinflation. One way to do this is to turn the ventilator off at end-expiration (paralyzed patient) and measure exhaled volume. Unfortunately, most ventilators measure exhaled volume with a flow measuring device, and many flow measuring devices underestimate flows when flow is low. Thus, the exhaled volume will be underestimated. A water-seal or dry spirometer could be attached to the exhalation port to measure actual volume expired, but this is often impractical. The volume of dynamic hyperinflation could also be calculated by calculating respiratory system compliance (C) from measurements of end-inspiratory plateau pressure and intrinsic PEEP (=$PEEP_i$, the airway pressure at zero flow conditions at end-expiration).

$$C = V_t/(P_{plat} - PEEP_i) = VHI/P_{plat}$$

where VHI = volume of dynamic hyperinflation. Rearranging:

$$VHI = (V_t)(P_{plat})/(P_{plat} - PEEP_i)$$

This formula assumes, of course, that compliance is linear over the range of alveolar pressure = 0 to the end-tidal volume. Since lung compliance is not linear, the assumption may not hold over the relevant range. However, this may be a convenient way for estimating the volume of hyperinflation to determine how far one is above or below the level of $20\,mL\,kg^{-1}$.

Finally, hypoventilation may be undertaken empirically, with changes in ventilator setting dependent on clinical and physiological recovery. This is probably the most commonly used method. One should bear in mind that in this case hypoventilation may be either excessive or not enough.

In general, during hypercapnic ventilation, cardiac output increases, systemic vascular resistance decreases and blood pressure is relatively well maintained,[10] primarily due to sympathoadrenal stimulation. Hypercapnic acidosis is a well-known potent pulmonary vasoconstrictor.[10] Hypercapnia *per se* can decrease cardiac contractility, although this effect is usually overcome *in situ* by sympathoadrenal stimulation. These considerations suggest that caution should be exercised using permissive hypercapnia when there is inhibition of the sympathoadrenal axis, as with the concomitant administration of beta adrenergic blockers, or coexisting severe cardiomyopathy. Hypercapnia is a potent cerebral vasodilator. Permissive hypercapnia should be considered contraindicated when there is a coexisting condition causing increased intracranial pressure and/or cerebral ischemia. Intracranial pressure monitoring should be considered if permissive hypercapnia is unavoidable under these circumstances. Concomitant metabolic acidosis may make the acidosis resulting from permissive hypercapnia unacceptable. Finally, the biochemical effects of hypercapnic acidosis such as hyperkalemia, increased free serum calcium, altered drug (especially aminoglycosides[11]) pharmacokinetics should be borne in mind.

It is now recognized that the mechanical sequelae of mechanical ventilation are potentially as serious as the condition for which mechanical ventilation was undertaken in the first place. It is now accepted that the pursuit of normal ABGs under all circumstances is not desirable under certain conditions in which there is very severe airways obstruction. Permissive hypercapnia with maintenance of oxygenation is a ventilatory strategy under these conditions and represents an important new addition to the treatment of ventilatory failure.

Follow-up

Over the next 24 hours the patient's condition improved and weaning from the ventilator was accomplished uneventfully two days later.

References

1 Woolcock A and Read J. Lung volumes in exacerbations of asthma. *American Journal of Medicine* (1966) **41**: 259–273.
2 Williams T, Tuxen D, Scheinkestel C and Bowes G. Risk factors for morbidity in mechanically ventilated patients with acute severe asthma. *American Review of Respiratory Diseases* (1992) **146**: 607–615.
3 Scharf SM. Cardiovascular effects of positive pressure ventilation. *Journal of Critical Care* (1992) **7**: 168–279.
4 Tuxen D and Lane S. The effects of ventilatory pattern on hyperinflation, airway pressures, and circulation in mechanical ventilation of patients with severe airflow obstruction. *American Review of Respiratory Diseases* (1987) **136**: 872–879.
5 Higgens B, Greening A and Crompton C. Assisted ventilation in severe acute asthma. *Thorax* (1986) **41**: 464–467.
6 Tuxen D. Permissive hypercapnia. *American Journal of Respiratory and Critical Care Medicine* (1994) **150**: 870–874.
7 Luksza AR, Smith P, Coakley J, Gordon IJ and Atherton ST. Acute severe asthma treated by mechanical ventilation: 10 years' experience from a district hospital. *Thorax* (1986) **41**: 459–463.
8 Hall J and Wood L. Management of the critically ill asthmatic patient. *Medical Clinics of North America* (1990) **74**: 779–796.
9 Mansel J, Stogner S, Petrini M and Norman J. Mechanical ventilation in patients with acute severe asthma. *American Journal of Medicine* (1990) **89**: 42–48.
10 Cullen D and Eger E. Cardiovascular effects of carbon dioxide in man. *Anesthesiology* (1974) **41**: 345–349.
11 Bryan L. Mechanisms of action of aminoglycosides antibiotics. In: Root R, Sande M (eds) *New Dimensions in Antimicrobial Therapy.* Contemporary Issues in Infectious Disease Series. New York, Churchill Livingston, pp 17–36, 1984.

3.3 Two Problems with Positive End-expiratory Pressure (PEEP) and the Heart during Acute Respiratory Distress Syndrome (ARDS)

Hamid R. Sadaghdar

History

A 68-year-old retired painter with a history of benign prostatic hypertrophy was admitted to the hospital with a two-day history of fever, chills and increasing dysuria. On examination, the patient was tachypneic with a respiratory rate of 30/minute, blood pressure 100/60 mmHg, temperature of 39°C, and he was mentally disoriented. His chest radiograph was normal. Arterial blood gas in room air showed a pH of 7.38 [H^+ 41 nmol L^{-1}], a P_aCO_2 of 34 mmHg [4.5 kPa], a P_aO_2 of 65 mmHg [8.7 kPa], and HCO_3 of 20 mmol L^{-1}. Gram stain of the urine showed many white cells and Gram-negative rods. Blood cultures were taken. Broad spectrum antibiotic therapy was started, and he was admitted to the intensive care unit with the presumed diagnosis of septic syndrome secondary to urinary tract infection.

During the next 24 hours the patient's condition deteriorated. His respiratory rate increased to 45/minute, blood pressure decreased to 85/50 mmHg and his S_pO_2 was 85%. His was trachea was intubated for respiratory support and he was given 2 L of 0.9% saline IV. A chest radiograph showed diffuse bilateral interstitial infiltrates compatible with ARDS. After the initial fluid resuscitation he remained hypotensive. A norepinephrine [noradrenaline] infusion was added and titrated to maintain a systolic blood pressure of $\geqslant 100$ mmHg. Arterial blood gas analysis, with an F_IO_2 of 1.0 showed a pH of 7.30 [H^+ 50 nmol L^{-1}], a P_aCO_2 of 28 mmHg [3.7 kPa], a P_aO_2 of 60 mmHg [8 kPa], with HCO_3^- of 15 mmol L^{-1}.

A pulmonary artery catheter was inserted for hemodynamic evaluation. The first measurement showed a pulmonary artery occlusion pressure (PAOP) of 10 mmHg, a cardiac output of 9.5 L min^{-1}, and a heart rate of 120/minute with sinus rhythm. The cardiac index (CI) and systemic vascular resistance were, respectively, 5.2 L $min^{-1}m^2$ and 480 dyn-sec cm^{-5}. PEEP was added and gradually increased to improve the oxygenation. Arterial blood gas analysis, with an F_IO_2 of 0.8 and a PEEP of 15 cmH$_2$O, showed a P_aO_2 of 65 mmHg. To improve further the oxygenation and decrease the risk of oxygen toxicity, PEEP was increased to 20 cmH$_2$O. Arterial oxygenation improved but the patient's blood pressure decreased to 80/50 mmHg. Hemodynamic evaluation showed a PAOP of 16 mmHg, a CI of 3.2 L $min^{-1}m^{-2}$, and a heart rate of 120/minute with sinus rhythm. At this point, the patient's cardiac filling pressure was considered adequate and norepinephrine infusion rate was increased to support the blood pressure. After this intervention, the blood pressure increased to 85/60 mmHg,

PAOP and cardiac index remained the same and heart rate increased to 132/minute with sinus rhythm. Urine output, which was $50 \, mL \, h^{-1}$ before the increase of PEEP, decreased to $10 \, mL \, h^{-1}$ for the next 2 hours.

Trap 1

There was overreliance on PAOP to estimate left ventricular filling pressure during mechanical ventilation with moderate to high levels of PEEP.

Trick 1

It is important to follow indices of peripheral organ perfusion such as urine output and mental state. After this initial evaluation, or if the evaluation of peripheral organ perfusion cannot be performed accurately because of the presence of concomitant diseases, left ventricular filling pressure (LVFP) can be estimated by measuring PAOP after a brief disconnection (3 seconds) from the ventilator (off-PEEP or nadir PAOP).

Pulmonary artery occlusion pressure is often used as an estimate of left atrial pressure and therefore of LVFP. In the normal heart, mean left atrial pressure is similar to left ventricular end-diastolic pressure, and normally provides a good estimate of both pulmonary venous pressure and LVFP.[1,2] The accuracy of this correlation has been questioned during mechanical ventilation with moderate to high levels of PEEP (~$15 \, cmH_2O$). In this condition, LVFP measured by PAOP can be overestimated because of transmission of PEEP to the pulmonary microvasculature and to the intrapleural space. On the other hand, in patients with diffuse non-homogeneous lung disease, such as ARDS, hyperinflation of the alveoli can occur during the application of moderate to high levels of PEEP. This hyperinflation can cause the collapse of alveolar capillaries leading to formation of alveolar dead space (West zones 1 and 2). In these conditions the PAOP reflects alveolar rather than mean left atrial pressure.[3] Although the best way of measuring PAOP when using moderate to high levels of PEEP remains controversial, measurement of PAOP after disconnection from the ventilator (nadir or off-PEEP PAOP) may be an alternative for better estimation of LVFP. This technique consists of PAOP measurement immediately (within 2 seconds) after abrupt disconnection of the patient from the ventilator. The immediate decrease of PAOP (nadir PAOP) will be independent of the hemodynamic changes associated with this abrupt withdrawal of PEEP, such as changes in left ventricular preload and afterload.

In a dog model of ARDS,[4] ventilated with PEEP up to $15 \, cmH_2O$, nadir PAOP reflected left atrial transmural pressure (P_{latm}) better than on-PEEP PAOP at low LVFP ($\leqslant 9 \, mmHg$). At higher levels of LVFP ($\geqslant 9 \, mmHg$), on-PEEP PAOP correlated better than nadir PAOP with P_{latm}. In man, this technique has been used in patients after cardiac surgery with no significant lung function abnormalities.[5] In this study, nadir PAOP correlated well with P_{latm} after disconnection from the ventilator with PEEP up to $15 \, cmH_2O$. Although nadir

PAOP has not been validated in humans with ARDS, this technique may be an alternative in this patient population for better estimation of LVFP during the application of moderate to high levels of PEEP. In this patient, nadir PAOP was 10 mmHg, not 16 mmHg recorded on PEEP. The increase of PAOP from nadir to on-PEEP values was most probably the result of transmission of high intrathoracic pressure to the pulmonary artery catheter rather than the improvement of LVFP. Overlooking this interaction between PEEP and PAOP may result in over-estimation of LVFP during the application of moderate to high levels of PEEP, and may inhibit a more aggressive fluid resuscitation needed by these patients.

Trap 2

Overlooking the effect of high intrathoracic pressure on cardiac output.

Trick 2

Intravascular volume expansion is important to compensate for PEEP-induced hypotension secondary to the decrease of cardiac output. In patients with normal heart function, reduction of cardiac output during the application of moderate to high levels of PEEP is mainly because of an increase in intrathoracic pressure which reduces venous return.[6] The effect of PEEP on hemodynamics is attributed to transmission of airway pressure to intrapleural space. Both lung and chest-wall compliance influence the transmission of airway pressure to the intrapleural space but in opposite directions.[7] A decrease in lung compliance, as in ARDS, reduces this transmission. Reduction of chest-wall compliance, such as abdominal distension, ascites, abdominal splinting or increased chest-wall muscle tone, enhance transmission of airway pressure to the pleural space. In patients with acute lung injury, the reduction of cardiac output with increasing PEEP is not compensated for by an increase in heart rate.[8] The reason that heart rate fails to increase despite a decrease in cardiac output with PEEP remains unclear. Thus, the reduction of stroke volume as a consequence of a decrease in preload is the most common cause of the decrease of cardiac output during the application of PEEP. Decreased venous return to the right heart, increased right ventricular afterload and decreased ventricular contractility have been proposed to explain the observed decrease in left ventricular preload. during the use of PEEP. Among these factors, decrease in venous return to the right heart secondary to the increase in intrapleural pressure plays the major role in the reduction of left ventricular preload.[8,9] Expansion of intravascular volume, by intravenous fluid administration, will increase venous return and stroke volume, and consequently restore the cardiac output. The increase in right ventricular afterload is insignificant in most patients with acute lung injury treated with moderate levels of PEEP. At higher levels of PEEP ($\geqslant 25$ cmH$_2$O), right ventricular afterload may be increased enough to contribute to the reduction of left ventricular preload through the mechanism of ventricular interdependence.[10] Although in patients with normal myocardial function there is no evidence that myocardial contractility is adversely affected,[8,10,11] previous or concomitant cardiac abnormalities may jeopardize the normal response to PEEP.

Follow-up

Once the nadir PAOP was measured, intravascular bolus fluid challenges were given. After an initial 1200 mL of fluid resuscitation, heart rate decreased to 90/minute, urine output increased to 50 mL h^{-1}, and the norepinephrine infusion was first reduced and then stopped. The patient's gas exchange slowly improved. Although his recovery was subsequently delayed by the development of a nosocomial pneumonia, he was gradually weaned off PEEP and the trachea extubated on the fourteenth hospital day. He was discharged home one week later. One month later, he had fully recovered, except for a little breathlessness.

References

1 O'Quin R and Marini JJ. Pulmonary artery occlusion pressure: clinical physiology, measurement, and interpretation. *American Review of Respiratory Diseases* (1983) **128**: 319–326.

2 Lappas D, Lell WA, Gabel JC, Civetta JM and Lowenstein E. Indirect measurement of left atrial pressure in surgical patients. Pulmonary-capillary wedge and pulmonary-artery diastolic pressures compared with left-atrial pressure. *Anesthesiology* (1973) **38**: 394–397.

3 Guyton RA, Chiavarelli M, Padgett CA, Cheung EH, Staton GW and Hatcher CR Jr. The influence of positive end-expiratory pressure on intrapericardial pressure and cardiac function after coronary artery bypass surgery. *Journal of Cardiothoracic Anesthesiology* (1987) **1**: 98–107.

4 Carter RS, Snyder JV and Pinsky MR. LV filling pressure during PEEP measured by nadir wedge pressure after airway disconnection. *American Journal of Physiology* (1985) **249**: H770–776.

5 Pinsky MR, Vincent JL and de Smet JM. Estimating left ventricular filling pressure during positive end-expiratory pressure in humans. *American Review of Respiratory Diseases* (1991) **143**: 25–31.

6 Fewell JE, Abendschein DR, Carlson CJ, Rapaport E and Murray JF. Mechanism of decreased right and left end-diastolic volume during continuous positive pressure ventilation in dog. *Circulation Research* (1980) **47**: 467–472.

7 O'Quin RJ, Marini JJ, Culver BH and Butler J. Transmission of airway pressure to pleural space during edema and chest wall restriction. *Journal of Applied Physiology* (1985) **59**: 1171–1177.

8 Dhainault JF, Devaux JY, Monsallier JF, Brunet F, Villemant D and Huyghebaert MF. Mechanisms of decreased left ventricular preload during continuous positive-pressure ventilation in ARDS. *Chest* (1986) **90**: 74–80.

9 Viquerat CE, Righetti A and Suter PM. Biventricular volumes and function in patients with adult respiratory distress syndrome ventilated with PEEP. *Chest* (1983) **83**: 509–514.

10 Jardin F, Farcot JC, Boisante L, Curien N, Margairaz A and Bourdarias JP. Influence of positive end-expiratory pressure on left ventricular performance. *New England Journal of Medicine* (1981) **304**: 387–392.

11 Van Trigt P, Spray TL, Pasque MK, *et al.* The effect of PEEP on left ventricular diastolic dimensions and systolic performance following myocardial revascularisation. *Annals of Thoracic Surgery* (1982) **33**: 583–592.

3.4 Management of Unilateral Pulmonary Disease
G. Daniel Martich and Morris I. Bierman[†]

History

A 54-year-old man was found by emergency medical service (EMS) personnel lying in an alley on his right side with vomitus coming out of his mouth. His 'friends' told the EMS that the patient had been drinking through the night and that they found him this morning arousable, but confused and with difficulty breathing. The EMS transported him to the hospital where his trachea was intubated, stabilized in the emergency department, and brought to the intensive care unit (ICU) for further management of his presumed aspiration of gastric contents.

He was noted to be a disheveled, unshaven, malodorous man in moderate respiratory distress. At this time his vital signs were: blood pressure 100/48 mmHg, pulse rate 124/minute, respiratory rate 28/minute (SIMV 16), temperature 38.5°C. He was edentulous, otherwise examination of his head revealed no evidence of trauma or abnormal findings. On auscultation of the chest, crackles and markedly decreased breath sounds were heard on the right, with vesicular breath sounds and good air movement on the left. His fingertips were tar-stained. He was confused and combative, and moved all four extremities spontaneously.

Laboratory investigations revealed a white blood cell count of $14 \times 10^9\,L^{-1}$ with a left shift. Arterial blood gas (ABG) analyses are summarized in Table 3.4.1.

A portable chest radiograph showed a correctly positioned tracheal tube. The right lung had diffuse alveolar infiltrates, while the left lung revealed moderate hyperinflation and was clear of infiltrates.[1]

Table 3.4.1. Arterial blood gas analyses

	F_IO_2	PEEP (cmH$_2$O)	Position	pH	H$^+$ (nmol L^{-1})	P_aCO_2 (mmHg/kPa)	P_aO_2 (mmHg/kPa)	HCO$_3^-$ (mEq L^{-1})
#1	0.2	Mask	Supine	7.33	47	48/6.4	38/5.1	28
#2	1.0	Mask	Supine	7.32	48	50/6.7	40/5.3	28
#3	1.0	5	Supine	7.35	45	45/6.0	42/5.6	26
#4	1.0	10	Supine	7.32	48	50/6.7	36/4.8	26
#5	1.0	5	Supine	7.35	45	42/5.6	50/0.7	24
#6	1.0	10R/5L	Lateral	7.42	38	40/5.3	195/26	24

R, Right; L, left.

[†] Deceased

Trap

Increasing amounts of PEEP were added with no improvement in oxygenation (Table 3.4.1, ABG #4). The patient became more agitated and tachypneic on $10\,cmH_2O$ of PEEP and cardiac output decreased.

Trick

While trying to splint open the injured lung, the physiologic consequences of overdistending relatively normal lung units must be prevented. As early as the mid-1970s, several investigators observed that patients with unilateral lung disease may require special ventilatory needs when increasing levels of PEEP worsen oxygenation.[2]

The concept of overdistending normal alveoli is not limited to unilateral pulmonary disease. Patients with ARDS have been shown to have a relatively heterogeneous distribution of affected lung units despite the radiographic appearance of a diffuse alveolar pattern.[3] By increasing PEEP in our patient, we paradoxically increased shunting through the diseased lung through overdistension of normal alveoli. Furthermore, the ratio of ventilation to perfusion (V/Q) may increase in the overdistended lung units, causing an increase in the ratio of deadspace to tidal volume (V_d/V_t).

The good compliance of the healthy lung may prevent any meaningful V/Q improvement through the application of increased PEEP. The decrease in cardiac output is a common consequence of decreasing venous return caused by increasing intrathoracic pressure.

The morbidity and mortality after aspiration of gastric contents depends principally on two factors: the volume and the pH of the aspirated fluid.[1] Large volumes of stomach contents aspirated into the lungs generally cause greater pulmonary pathology and lead to a more prolonged recovery. Aspiration of fluid with a pH of <2.5 [H^+ 56 nmol L^{-1}] causes a pattern of pulmonary edema from diffuse capillary leak, damage to type I pneumocytes and an intense inflammatory response with infiltration of neutrophils into the alveoli (e.g. the acute respiratory distress syndrome, ARDS).

Unilateral aspiration and bacterial pneumonias requiring mechanical ventilatory support are not common. They pose difficult management problems. Patients suffering from unilateral intraparenchymal hemorrhage or single lung transplant recipients whose allograft has suffered injury (i.e. reperfusion, ischemia, infection, or rejection) may similarly present with severe respiratory distress and unilateral radiographic findings.

Despite intubation and mechanical ventilation, this patient remained hypoxemic with a predominantly unilateral pulmonary injury. The level of PEEP was reduced to $5\,cmH_2O$. This was associated with an immediate return of the cardiac output to baseline, but he remained agitated and hypoxemic. Sedation and therapeutic neuromuscular blockade were added to decrease the patient's anxiety, eliminate chest wall muscle tone as a source of poor compliance, and reduce global oxygen demand. Next, the patient was turned from the supine position to the left lateral decubitus position where his diseased lung was uppermost and the 'normal' lung dependent.

Positioning the diseased lung uppermost and the unaffected lung dependent to it may increase blood flow to the 'normal' lung and improve ventilation/perfusion matching. A recent study compared the use of lateral position alone against the effects of almitrine bismesylate in patients with unilateral bacterial pneumonia and severe hypoxemia.[4] Almitrine bismesylate, a respiratory stimulant, which acts on peripheral chemoreceptors, induces pulmonary vasoconstriction in normal and diseased lungs. The presumption of the study was that in patients with unilateral pulmonary disease, hypoxic vasoconstriction is absent; therefore by causing vasoconstriction in the diseased lung, shunting of blood through non-ventilated alveoli would decrease. The study concluded that significant increases in oxygenation were noted in the lateral position group and that no beneficial effects were observed in the almitrine group. This logic forms the basis for the expression 'Down with the good lung'.

Although oxygenation improved slightly with positioning, the patient remained hypoxemic (Table 3.4.1, ABG #5). The housestaff considered differential lung ventilation (DLV) with or without selective PEEP application as the only additional ventilatory modality that may be useful. A double lumen tracheal tube (DL-TT) was placed. Extracorporeal membrane oxygenation (ECMO) for refractory hypoxemia and carbon dioxide removal is used in a small number of teaching institutions with variable success, but is not yet indicated in this patient. The attending physician chose a 39 French (adult sizes from 35 to 41 Fr in odd numbers) left bronchial tube.

Left-sided DL-TTs are indicated for almost all clinical situations in the critically ill patient, except when left bronchial mainstem narrowing or obstruction, or thoracic aortic aneurysms preclude placement. The short length of the right mainstem bronchus before the origin of the right upper-lobe orifice makes a right DL-TT more difficult to position and maintain in position. A fiberoptic intubating bronchoscope is used during placement of the DL-TT to assure proper position of the bronchial balloon. The relationships between ventilation–perfusion and atelectasis formation in various positions during conventional and differential lung ventilation have been recently reported.[5] Fifteen patients undergoing elective surgery for non-pulmonary pathology were evaluated under five conditions: (1) supine, awake; (2) supine during anesthesia with conventional mechanical ventilation (CV), no PEEP; (3) lateral position during CV, no PEEP; (4) lateral position during CV with $10\,cmH_2O$ PEEP; (5) lateral position during differential ventilation with selective PEEP applied to the dependent lung.

The authors recorded systemic and pulmonary hemodynamics, venous admixture and arterial blood gases. Additionally, serial computerized tomographs of the chest were obtained in six patients and the percentage of atelectatic area was noted under each condition. Compared to CV, differential ventilation with selective PEEP applied to the dependent lung improved oxygenation, decreased CT evidence of atelectasis and decreased both the alveolar–arterial oxygen gradient and venous admixture.

Follow-up

The patient's oxygenation continued to improve after starting DLV with selective application of PEEP to the diseased right lung (Table 3.4.1, ABG #6). After 36 hours of DLV, the physiologic differences between the two lungs had diminished, which allowed return to conventional single lumen ventilation. This was accomplished initially by simply deflating the bronchial balloon cuff and using a 'Y' adapter to connect the two lumens to a single ventilator. Because weaning was expected to occur over several days, the patient's trachea was reintubated with a conventional tracheal tube to reduce the work of breathing (DL-TTs are longer than conventional tracheal tubes). This also improves the ability to suction the airways (small catheters must be used with the DL-TT as each lumen is small) and may improve patient comfort. The patient was weaned from mechanical ventilation over the next several days. He was discharged from the intensive care unit to an alcohol rehabilitation unit for further care on the fifteenth hospital day.

References

1 Modell JH and Boysen PG. Pulmonary aspiration of stomach contents. In: Shoemaker WC, Ayres S, Grenvik A, Holbrook PR, Thompson WL (eds) *Textbook of Critical Care*, 2nd edn. Philadelphia, W. B. Saunders, pp 565–567, 1989.
2 Kanarek DJ and Shannon DC. Adverse effect of positive end-expiratory pressure on pulmonary perfusion and arterial oxygenation. *American Review of Respiratory Diseases* (1975) **112**: 457–459.
3 Maunder RJ, Shuman WP, McHugh JW, Marglin SI and Butler J. Preservation of normal lung regions in the adult respiratory distress syndrome. *Journal of the American Medical Association* (1986) **255**: 2463–2465.
4 Dreyfuss D, Kjedaini K, Lanore J-J, Mier L, Froidevaux R and Coste F. A comparative study of the effects of almitrine bismesylate and lateral position during unilateral bacterial pneumonia with severe hypoxemia. *American Review of Respiratory Diseases* (1992) **146**: 295–299.
5 Klingstedt C, Hedenstierna G, Baehrendtz S, Lundqvist H, Strandberg A, Tokics L and Brismar B. Ventilation–perfusion relationships and atelectasis formation in the supine and lateral positions during conventional mechanical and differential ventilation. *Acta Anaesthesiolica Scandinavia* (1990) **34**: 421–429.
6 Chandler JM, Bierman MI and Stein KL. Independent lung ventilation. In: Shoemaker WC, Ayres S, Grenvik A, Holbrook PR, Thompson WL (eds) *Textbook of Critical Care*, 3rd edn. Philadelphia, W. B. Saunders, ch 100, 1995.

3.5 The Effects of PEEP on Carbon Dioxide Clearance

Stephen A. Bowles

History

A 67-year-old male patient underwent a radical neck dissection for a tumor of the posterior pharynx. He had a long and significant history of chronic obstructive pulmonary disease, requiring steroid therapy over the past three years, a history of coronary artery disease with an inferolateral myocardial infarction eight years before and a three-vessel coronary artery bypass surgery five years ago. He drank 4 or 5 beers daily although he claimed not to have drunk over the past two months and had smoked on average a pack and a half of cigarettes each day for the past fifty years. At home he used an albuterol metered dose inhaler, and took prednisone 10 mg every other day.

After an uncomplicated surgical procedure he was admitted to the intensive care unit (ICU) for continued mechanical ventilation. At that time his examination revealed an elderly appearing male with surgical wounds on his neck with a drain in place. There was an old scar over his sternum and a scaphoid abdomen. On auscultation the second heart sound was loud and his breath sounds were quiet. Laboratory tests showed a white blood cell count of $14.2 \times 10^9 \, L^{-1}$ ($14.2 \times 10^3 \, dl.^{-1}$) and a hematocrit of 25%. The chest radiograph showed hyperinflated lungs but was otherwise normal. He was begun on clindamycin 600 mg IV eight hourly, albuterol inhaler treatment four hourly, and hydrocortisone 50 mg IV six hourly. On the second postoperative day his trachea was extubated and the hydrocortisone dose was decreased to 25 mg six hourly. Nasogastric tube feedings were started.

The following day he was noted to be dyspneic with a respiratory rate of 30/minute. Examination showed labored breathing with crackles in the right base and wheezes in all lung fields. Arterial blood gases on an aerosol face mask delivering an F_IO_2 of 0.6 were: pH 7.21 [H^+ 61 nmol L^{-1}], P_aCO_2 74 mmHg [9.9 kPa] and P_aO_2 48 mmHg [6.4 kPa] (Table 3.5.1). His trachea was re-intubated with a 7 Fr orotracheal tube. After tracheal intubation, material resembling tube feedings were suctioned from his lungs. A chest radiograph showed a right-sided infiltrate in both the lower and apical lung fields with the tip of the tracheal tube located 3 cm above the carina. A presumptive diagnosis of acute aspiration pneumonia was made.

The initial ventilator settings were: SIMV, a rate of 12/minute, a tidal volume of 650 mL, a PEEP of 5 cmH$_2$O, and an F_IO_2 of 1.0. The patient was very agitated, hypertensive to 220/120 mmHg, with a respiratory rate of 35–45/minute. The peak airway pressures ranged from 60 to 65 cmH$_2$O. Because of concerns over the possibility of alcohol withdrawal, a continuous intravenous infusion of midazolam was started. One hour later, despite being unresponsive, he

Table 3.5.1. Respiratory care flow sheet

Time	Mode	F_IO_2	RR	PEEP (cmH$_2$O)	Paw	pH	H$^+$ (nmol L^{-1})	P_aCO_2 (mmHg)	P_aCO_2 (kPa)	P_aO_2 (mmHg)	P_aO_2 (kPa)	HCO$_3^-$
14.12	AFM	0.6	32	—	—	7.21	62	74	9.9	48	6.4	28.6
15.11	SIMV	1.0	42	5	62	7.30	50	58	7.7	81	10.8	27.9
17.00	SIMV	0.6	12/12	5	34	7.36	46	50	6.7	94	12.5	—
19.00	SIMV	0.6	12/12	5	36	7.34	42	56	7.5	68	9.1	29.6
20.35	SIMV	0.6	12/12	10	39	7.38	46	51	6.8	74	9.9	29.1
24.00	SIMV	0.6	12/12	15	44	7.34	50	58	7.7	64	8.5	30.7
00.42	SIMV	0.6	16/16	15	50	7.30	58	62	8.3	63	8.4	29.8
01.12	SIMV	1.0	16/16	20	57	7.24	79	68	9.1	61	8.1	28.2
01.26	SIMV	1.0	20/20	20	65	7.10	—	84	11.2	52	6.9	24.9

SIMV, Synchronous intermittent mandatory ventilation; **AFM**, Aerosol face mask; **Paw**, Peak airway pressure.

continued to breathe rapidly and out of phase with the ventilator with peak airway pressures at times exceeding $70 \, cmH_2O$. Neuromuscular paralysis with a vecuronium infusion was begun and his paralysis was titrated to one twitch out of four with a train of four monitor. Starting therapeutic paralysis reduced his peak airway pressures to $34 \, cmH_2O$ and over a two hour period the F_IO_2 was decreased to 0.6 and the S_pO_2 was consistently 96%. A repeat arterial blood gas gave a pH of 7.36 [H^+ 44 nmol L^{-1}], a P_aCO_2 of 50 mmHg [6.7 kPa], and a P_aO_2 of 94 mmHg [12.5 kPa].

That evening his S_pO_2 dropped to a low value of 90%. Examination revealed wheezing in all fields, and crackles primarily in the right base. A chest radiograph showed a minimal increase in the right-sided densities and a new patchy infiltrate throughout the left lung. An arterial blood gas taken on an F_IO_2 of 0.6, a respiratory rate of 12/minute and a PEEP of $5 \, cmH_2O$, showed a pH of 7.34 [H^+ 46 nmol L^{-1}], a P_aCO_2 of 56 mmHg [7.5 kPa] and a P_aO_2 of 68 mmHg [9.1 kPa]. The level of PEEP was increased to $10 \, cmH_2O$ in an attempt to increase oxygenation, and an arterial blood gas 90 minutes later revealed that the P_aCO_2 had decreased while the P_aO_2 had increased. The pulse oximeter revealed a 96% oxygen saturation. Three hours later the arterial oxygen saturation acutely decreased to 93%. No blood gases were obtained, but because of the decreased saturation the PEEP was increased to $15 \, cmH_2O$. An arterial blood gas obtained 30 minutes later showed a pH of 7.34 [H^+ 46 nmol L^{-1}], the P_aO_2 had decreased to 64 mmHg [8.5 kPa] and the P_aCO_2 had increased from 51 to 58 mmHg [6.8 to 7.7 kPa]. Because of the increasing P_aCO_2 and the decreasing pH, the respiratory rate was increased to 16/minute. Despite this intervention, the blood gas obtained 30 minutes later revealed a further decrease in the pH to 7.30 [H^+ 50 nmol L^{-1}], the P_aCO_2 was now 62 mmHg [8.3 kPa], and the P_aO_2 was virtually unchanged at 63 mmHg [8.4 kPa]. At the same time it was noted that the peak airway pressure had increased back up to $50 \, cmH_2O$. Despite this increase in peak airway pressure and the maintenance of the S_pO_2 greater than 90%, the PEEP was further increased to $20 \, cmH_2O$ and the F_IO_2 was increased to 1.0. A blood gas taken on these ventilator settings revealed a pH of 7.24 [H^+ 57 nmol L^{-1}], a P_aCO_2 of 68 mmHg [9.1 kPa] and a P_aO_2 of 61 mmHg [8.1 kPa]. The respiratory rate was then increased to 20/minute. Ten minutes later the patient's blood pressure had decreased from 132/80 to 94/54 mmHg and the arterial oxygen saturation had decreased into the eighties. An ECG, and a chest radiograph to evaluate for the presence of a pneumothorax were ordered. A dopamine infusion was started, and an additional dose of hydrocortisone was given. An arterial blood gas taken during this unstable period revealed a pH of 7.10 [H^+ 80 nmol L^{-1}], a P_aCO_2 of 84 mmHg [11.2 kPa] and a P_aO_2 of 52 mmHg [6.9 kPa]. Before the chest radiograph or ECG could be obtained, the patient's blood pressure dropped further and ventricular tachycardia was noted. Cardiopulmonary resuscitation was begun.

Trap

PEEP applied by the ventilator and auto-PEEP generated by increasing the respiratory rate can interfere with carbon dioxide elimination.

Tricks

To understand why the patient continued to worsen despite what at first glance may have appeared to be appropriate changes in the ventilator settings, an understanding of the effects of PEEP on pulmonary physiology and gas exchange is needed. The effects of PEEP on oxygenation and the physiology behind these effects are frequently considered by clinicians. PEEP also has effects on carbon dioxide removal which are often neglected. These effects should be understood and considered.

An overall index of the efficiency of carbon dioxide removal, the efficiency of ventilation, is the physiologic dead space ($V_D/V_T CO_2$) as calculated by the Enghoff modification of the Bohr equation.[1] Physiologic dead space is calculated as:

$$(P_a CO_2 - P_E CO_2)/P_a CO_2$$

where $P_a CO_2$ is the arterial partial pressure of carbon dioxide and $P_E CO_2$ is the partial pressure of carbon dioxide in the expired air. Physiologic dead space, also known as functional dead space, is a theoretical volume; it is not a volume that conforms to any anatomic structure, but represents the portion of a tidal volume in which no gas exchange occurs, if in the remaining portion of the tidal volume gas exchange is theoretically 100% complete. Anatomical dead space, in comparison, is the combined volume of all airways in which gas exchange is minimal and consists of the upper airway down to, but not including, the respiratory bronchioles. In mechanically ventilated patients the anatomical dead space also includes any portions of the ventilator circuit, such as the tracheal tube, through which both inspired and expired air pass. Anatomical dead space is only a portion of the physiologic dead space. Physiologic dead space is the more important volume when considering gas exchange.

The physiologic dead space is determined by several factors:

- The anatomic dead space. The entire volume of the airways that has little or no blood flow to it for gas exchange.[2]
- The venous admixture. The shunt fraction affects carbon dioxide removal as there is no carbon dioxide removal from blood 'shunted around' the lung.[3]
- The distribution of ventilation : perfusion ratios. Under normal conditions ventilation and perfusion are closely matched but when this matching is disturbed and there is an increase in the portion of the lung which is either of high or low V/Q, then carbon dioxide elimination will be reduced.[4]
- The Haldane effect. When oxygen binds to hemoglobin, the solubility of carbon dioxide within the blood is reduced. Because of this, when the blood is poorly oxygenated then the solubility of carbon dioxide in the blood remains high and carbon dioxide elimination is diminished.[5]

All of these factors are affected by acute lung injury and chronic airflow obstruction and are variably affected by the application of PEEP during positive-pressure breathing. Because of the multiple factors involved, the effect of PEEP on carbon dioxide elimination is not consistent and it varies from patient to patient. In patients with acute lung injury V_D/V_TCO_2 is increased. The application of low levels of PEEP (5–10 cmH$_2$O) frequently reduces V_D/V_TCO_2 through a reduction of shunt blood flow.[6] At higher levels of PEEP the effects appear to be more variable and unpredictable. Anatomical dead space as measured by the Fowler technique or the inert gas method, has been shown to increase with the application of higher levels of PEEP, presumably as a result of the distension of the conducting airways. PEEP can also cause a redistribution of the ventilation : perfusion ratios. At higher levels of PEEP, generally 15 cmH$_2$O and above, a greater proportion of the ventilation may go to high V/Q regions. Carbon dioxide elimination is impaired when an increased proportion of the ventilation is distributed to regions with high V/Q ratio.[6–9] The cause of this redistribution of ventilation : perfusion ratios may be a reduction of cardiac output. Increasing intrathoracic pressure decreases venous return causing a reduction of cardiac output and pulmonary perfusion. The decrease in pulmonary blood flow results in a decrease in the perfusion of well-ventilated regions in the upper lung fields. Alternatively, the increase in physiologic dead space may be caused by direct compression of alveolar capillaries in contact with well-ventilated but hyperexpanded alveoli, causing a decrease in flow to these lung units thus increasing the area of lung that is ventilated but not perfused, the so-called West Zone 1 of the lung.[10] The hyperinflation of alveoli with direct compression of adjacent capillaries can also cause a redistribution of flow from well-ventilated alveoli to poorly ventilated alveoli resulting in impaired oxygenation, with impaired oxygenation leading to a reduction in carbon dioxide removal due to the Haldane effect.[6]

In this patient an improvement in carbon dioxide elimination and oxygenation was seen when the PEEP was increased from 5 to 10 cmH$_2$O, presumably because of a reduction in the shunt. When the PEEP was subsequently increased to 15 cmH$_2$O the P_aCO_2 increased. In paralyzed patients the increase in V_D/V_TCO_2 is more apparent because a compensatory increase in minute ventilation does not occur. In this patient the ventilation rate was then increased in an attempt to increase alveolar ventilation and carbon dioxide removal but the next blood gas revealed a further increase in the P_aCO_2. This may appear paradoxical; however, increasing the ventilator rate in a patient with known obstructive lung disease and audible wheezes will shorten the expiratory time which may lead to inadequate time for complete expiration. The end result is hyperinflation and auto-PEEP. The increase in the peak airway pressure that occurred in this patient when the ventilator rate was increased supports this theory and should have served as a clue that auto-PEEP was present. This auto-PEEP may have lead to a further increase in V_D/V_TCO_2. At this time a reduction of the patient's respiratory rate and the addition of measures to treat any reversible component of his obstructive pulmonary disease would have been appropriate. The next two ventilator changes, increasing the PEEP and then increasing the ventilator rate, only resulted in further increases in the V_D/V_TCO_2 and a deterioration of the patient's condition.

This patient may appear to present an impossible dilemma in ventilator management. To treat this patient optimally, the adverse effects of PEEP need to be recognized and the aims of treatment re-evaluated. First, the patient's oxygen saturations were 90% or higher at all times. Increasing the oxygen saturation to higher levels leads to a minimal improvement in the oxygen content of the blood. Transfusing the patient with blood to increase his hematocrit from 25% would have had a greater impact on his oxygen delivery. Attempts to increase the saturation by increasing the PEEP resulted in significant increases in $V_D/V_T co_2$.

Second, there is little evidence to indicate that a respiratory acidosis of the degree seen in this patient is harmful. Attempts to correct it were unnecessary and led to auto-PEEP. The auto-PEEP had the same effect as the exogenously applied PEEP. If the adverse effects of PEEP on carbon dioxide elimination had been recognized, management of this patient's ventilations may have been altered and the adverse events that followed could have been prevented. In patients with severe obstructive lung disease complicated by acute lung injury, such as this patient, a balance between permissive hypercapnia, auto-PEEP and adequate gas exchange needs to be made. In this patient the decision to increase minute ventilation led to the patient's cardiac arrest.

Follow-up

At first, cardiopulmonary resuscitation (CPR) restored sinus rhythm with palpable peripheral pulses. After that there was increasing difficulty ventilating the patient with a self-inflating bag because of the high pressures needed. An arterial blood gas at this time showed a worsening hypercarbic acidosis, a metabolic acidosis and adequate oxygenation. The patient became pulseless despite a supraventricular rhythm and then asystolic. CPR was resumed. After 45 minutes of CPR it was stopped and the patient pronounced dead. An autopsy revealed cerebral atrophy, no evidence of residual tumor in the neck, no evidence of a pneumothorax, patchy consolidation of all lung fields, no evidence of pulmonary embolism and cardiomegaly with evidence of an old myocardial infarction but no evidence of a recent myocardial infarction.

References

1 Enghoff H. Volumen inefficax. Bermekungen zur Frage des schädlichen Raumes. *Uppsala Lak Forhandlung* (1938) **44**: 191–218.
2 Severinghaus JW and Stuppel M. Alveolar dead space as an index of distribution of blood flow in pulmonary capillaries. *Journal of Applied Physiology* (1957) **10**: 335–348.
3 Kuawabara S and Duncalf D. Effect of anatomic shunt on physiologic dead space to tidal volume ratio – a new equation. *Anesthesiology* (1969) **31**: 575–577.
4 West JB. Causes of carbon dioxide retention in lung disease. *New England Journal of Medicine* (1971) **284**: 1232–1236.
5 Hlasta MP and Robertson HT. Inert gas elimination characteristics of the normal and

abnormal lung. *Journal of Applied Physiology: Respiratory Environment in Exercise Physiology* (1978) **44**: 258–266.

6 Coffey Rl, Albert RK and Robertson HT. Mechanisms of physiologic dead space response to acute oleic acid lung injury. *Journal of Applied Physiology: Respiratory Environment in Exercise Physiology* (1983) **55**: 1550–1557.

7 Dueck R, Wagner PD and West JB. Effects of positive end-expiratory pressure on gas exchange in dogs with normal and edematous lungs. *Anesthesiology* (1977) **47**: 359–366.

8 Hedenstierna G, White FC, Mazzone and Wagner P. Redistribution of pulmonary blood flow in the dog with PEEP ventilation. *Journal of Applied Physiology: Respiratory Environment in Exercise Physiology* (1979) **46**: 278–287.

9 Dantzker DR, Brook CJ, Dehart P, Lynch JP and Weg JG. Ventilation–perfusion distribution in the adult respiratory distress syndrome. *American Review of Respiratory Diseases* (1979) **120**: 1039–1052.

10 Nieman BS, Paskanik AM and Bredenberg CE. Effect of positive end-expiratory pressure on alveolar capillary perfusion. *Journal of Thoracic and Cardiovascular Surgery* (1988) **95**: 712–716.

3.6 Dynamic Hyperinflation and Shock
Philippe Rico and Derek C. Angus

History

A 60-year-old obese female was brought to the emergency room by ambulance with severe abdominal pain, hypotension (80 mmHg systolic), tachycardia (130/minute), tachypnea (respiratory rate 40/minute) and hypoxia (S_pO_2 87%). The neighbor who called the ambulance knew her to be a heavy smoker (at least 2 packs/day), and a heavy drinker (whisky). No other medical history was available. Her trachea was intubated, and her blood pressure (BP) was increased to 90/50 mmHg with intravenous fluids.

She was transferred to the intensive care unit (ICU) 45 minutes later with a strong peripheral pulse at 120/minute. Assist-control ventilation was used with a tidal volume of 700 mL, a rate of 10/minute, an inspiratory flow rate of 50 L min^{-1}, a positive end-expiratory pressure (PEEP) of 5 cmH$_2$O, and an F_1O_2 of 0.5. She was breathing at 14 breaths/minute with peak pressures of 30 cmH$_2$O. Her pulse oximeter read 92% with the following arterial blood gas and lactate values: pH 7.32 [H$^+$ 48 nmol L^{-1}], P_aCO_2 48 mmHg [6.4 kPa], P_aO_2 72 mmHg [9.6 kPa], HCO$_3$ 24 mmol L^{-1}, and lactate 3.5 mmol L^{-1}. Her abdomen was diffusely tender and firm. A serum amylase was reported as 840 IU L^{-1}. Central venous and arterial catheters were inserted for vascular access and monitoring. The initial central venous pressure (CVP) was 8 mmHg and BP was now 100/60 mmHg after a total of 2 L of intravenous crystalloid solution. A portable chest radiograph showed good central line and tracheal tube position, mild bilateral hyperinflation, and no focal infiltrates.

The patient was then transported to the CT scanning suite where she received a total of 400 μg of fentanyl intravenously in 50 and 100 μg boluses for pain and agitation. During transfer back to the ICU, the respiratory therapist found the patient increasingly difficult to hand-ventilate and so increased the F_1O_2 to 0.75 to maintain the S_pO_2 above 92%.

On arrival in the ICU, she was hypotensive. The systolic BP had decreased to 80 mmHg with a heart rate of 130/minute and a prominent pulsus paradoxus (>20 mmHg). Her temperature was 38.3°C and her CVP was 16 mmHg. She had remained oliguric with a urine output below 25 mL h^{-1} since admission. Though unrousable, she appeared to be in respiratory distress, making shallow inspiratory efforts at about 30 breaths/minute. The ventilator, however, recorded only 6 breaths/minute over the set rate of 14. Peak airway pressures were now 50 cmH$_2$O on the same settings for PEEP, tidal volume and flow as before. The S_pO_2 had decreased to 90% (F_1O_2 0.75). Diminished bilateral breath sounds were present on auscultation with minimal end-expiratory wheezes. The abdominal CT scan demonstrated severe acute pancreatitis and no evidence of bowel perforation.

The patient was given calcium chloride 1 g intravenously with no effect on blood pressure. A dopamine infusion was started at $5\,\mu g\,kg^{-1}\,min^{-1}$, but no additional intravenous fluids were given because of the elevated CVP, the associated hypoxia, and 1 mm ST segment depression seen on leads V4 to V6. The systolic blood pressure increased to 90 mmHg and the dopamine was increased to maintain a systolic BP above 100 mmHg. After one aerosolized beta-agonist bronchodilator treatment (albuterol 2.5 mg), the peak airway pressures decreased slightly to $45\,cmH_2O$. A small amount of thick, purulent secretion was suctioned from the tracheal tube. A repeat chest radiograph showed no change.

Twenty minutes later, the dopamine was at $20\,\mu g\,kg^{-1}\,min^{-1}$. The systolic blood pressure was 105 mmHg and the heart rate was 135/minute. A pulmonary artery catheter was placed: the CVP was 16 mmHg, the pulmonary arterial occlusion pressure (PAOP) was 18 mmHg, the pulmonary arterial pressure was 35/21 mmHg, and the cardiac index was $3.8\,L\,min^{-1}\,m^{-2}$. The patient's extremities showed severe **livedo reticularis** and she was now anuric.

Trap

This patient was suffering from cardiovascular insufficiency secondary to iatrogenic dynamic hyperinflation (auto-PEEP) induced by an inappropriately high minute ventilation in the face of expiratory air flow limitation (chronic obstructive airways disease).[1] This probably occurred during transport while she was being hand-ventilated with large tidal breaths. The gradual overdistension led to decreased oxygenation (increased ventilation–perfusion mismatch). This was not recognized by the respiratory therapist who further aggravated the situation by inappropriately increasing the tidal volume and the respiratory frequency – a reasonable ventilatory strategy if the patient's problem had been atelectasis. The overdistension increased intrathoracic pressure, decreasing venous return, cardiac output and blood pressure. Because intrathoracic pressure was high, left ventricular filling pressures appeared artefactually elevated. Failure to understand this phenomenon led to a misinterpretation of the significance of the elevated vascular filling pressures and to the inappropriate treatment of a preload dependent hemodynamic state with vasopressors thereby compounding end-organ ischemia (anuria). While this trap may therefore have been less likely if a portable ventilator had been used during transport, this situation could have occurred during any episode of hand-ventilation (such as during bronchoscopy or while moving the patient from bed to chair).

Trick

Attention should have been focused in this patient on the unexplained increase in peak airway pressures. Although hypotension could have been associated with the acute pancreatic process alone, high peak airway pressures would only be a feature if either acute lung injury or massive pleural effusions developed. Neither of these processes were present at this early point in the patient's course. A more acute, potentially life-threatening process, such as a tension pneumothorax, has to be ruled out. Understanding why the peak airway pressure increased from 30 to 50 cmH_2O on the same ventilatory mode with the same tidal volume, flow and PEEP is key to the management of this patient's precarious hemodynamic status.

Two simple bedside tests will aid in the interpretation of raised peak airway pressures in ventilated patients when the cause is not immediately apparent: the inspiratory pause and the end-expiratory airway occlusion maneuver.

An increase in peak inspiratory airway pressure is caused by either an increase in inspiratory airway resistance or a decrease in lung compliance. These causes can be differentiated by assessing the dynamic (peak) and static (plateau) airway pressures during inspiration. The peak airway pressure represents the total pressure required to overcome: (1) the frictional resistance to airflow throughout the airways (ventilator circuit, tracheal tube and tracheobronchial tree); (2) the frictional resistance to lungs and chest wall motion; and (3) the elasticity of the lungs and chest wall. The static airway pressure represents only the pressure required to overcome the elasticity of the lungs and chest wall because it is measured during a no-flow state where frictional resistances are eliminated. These pressures can be measured easily at the bedside by transiently adding a 0.5 second end-inspiratory pause to the ventilator-delivered breath, and reading the peak pressure reached during inspiration followed by the plateau pressure maintained during the inspiratory pause (Figure 3.6.1).

The difference between the peak and plateau airway pressures (cmH_2O) divided by the inspiratory flow ($L s^{-1}$) equates the total inspiratory airway resistance (across the tracheobronchial tree, ventilator tubing, tracheal tube, lung

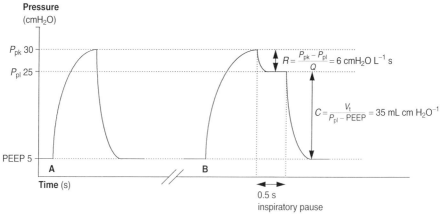

Figure 3.6.1. Pressure tracings from ventilator-delivered breaths over time. (A) Baseline state: tidal volume (V_t) = 700 mL; inspiratory flow (Q) = 0.83 L s^{-1}; PEEP = 5 cmH$_2$O. (B) Baseline state with end-inspiratory pause. By adding a short end-inspiratory pause to the machine-breath, the plateau pressure (P_{pl}) can be measured and the resistance (R) and compliance (C) of the respiratory system calculated. (P_{pk} = peak airway pressure; PEEP = positive end-expiratory airway pressure.)

and chest wall). The ratio of the tidal volume (mL) to the difference between the static airway pressure and the total positive end-expiratory pressure (total PEEP) represents the compliance of the lung–chest wall unit (thoracic compliance).[2] In this patient (Figure 3.6.1), the initial peak airway pressure was 30 cmH$_2$O with a plateau pressure of 25 cmH$_2$O, giving a reasonable inspiratory resistance of 6 cmH$_2$O L^{-1}s (normal is less than 4 cmH$_2$O L^{-1}s), and a compliance of 35 mL^{-1} cmH$_2$O$_1$ (normal is between 60 and 100 mL cmH$_2$O^{-1}). When her peak airway pressure increased to 50 cmH$_2$O, her plateau pressure also increased to 45 cmH$_2$O leaving the inspiratory resistance unchanged but the compliance markedly decreased at 17.5 mL cmH$_2$O^{-1} (Figure 3.6.2A,B), suggesting that an acute decrease in thoracic compliance was the explanation for the sudden increase in airway pressures.

There are few conditions that can cause an acute decrease in lung compliance. They include 'flash' pulmonary edema, massive hemorrhage in the tracheobronchial tree, tension pneumothorax, bronchial intubation or obstruction of a main bronchus, and dynamic hyperinflation. In this patient with chronic obstructive airways disease (COAD) (FEV$_1$: 35% of predicted), a relatively high

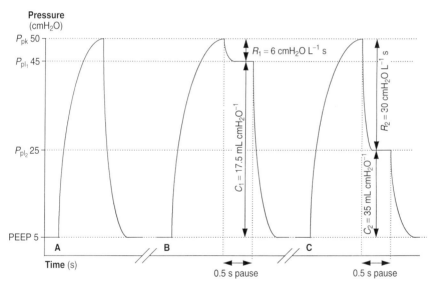

Figure 3.6.2. Pressure tracings from ventilator-delivered breaths over time. (A) Increased peak airway pressure state: tidal volume (V_t) = 700 mL; inspiratory flow (Q) = 0.83 L s^{-1}; **PEEP** = 5 cm H$_2$O. (B) and (C) Increased peak airway pressure state with end-inspiratory pause. By performing the end-inspiratory pause maneuver a decreased compliance state (B) can be differentiated from an increased resistance state (C). Compared with the baseline state described in Figure 3.6.1, in situation B here, resistance [$R_1 = (P_{pk} - P_{pl_1})/Q$] is unchanged but compliance [$C_1 = V_t/(P_{pl_1} - PEEP)$] appears to be lower. In situation C, however, compliance [$C_2 = V_t/(P_{pl_2} - PEEP)$] is unchanged but resistance [$R_2 = (P_{pk} - P_{pl_2})/Q$] has increased. An acute rise in airway resistance can result from bronchospasm, accumulation of secretions, kinking of the inspiratory limb of the breathing circuit, or from an inadvertent increase in the ventilator flow rate settings. (Abbreviations as in Figure 3.6.1.)

minute ventilation, and an unimpressive portable chest radiograph, dynamic hyperinflation is the most likely diagnosis and the easiest to treat.

Dynamic hyperinflation occurs when the expiratory time is insufficient to allow complete exhalation of the previous breath leading to a progressive increase in the functional residual capacity. This results in a residual flow-driving pressure at the end of expiration or auto-PEEP, also known as intrinsic PEEP or occult PEEP. This pressure is not detected by the ventilator manometer during normal cycling because the ventilator expiratory limb is open to the atmosphere. However, by manually occluding the expiratory limb of the breathing circuit at the very end of expiration (end-expiratory airway occlusion maneuver), pressure equilibration between the lung and the ventilator circuit occurs and the total PEEP in the breathing circuit can now be measured.[3] The difference between the measured total PEEP and any ventilator-set PEEP is the auto-PEEP (Figure 3.6.3). Note that if the maneuver is performed too early during expiration, total PEEP and auto-PEEP will be overestimated. For a reliable estimation of the auto-PEEP during the end-expiratory airway occlusion, it is often necessary to sedate or paralyze the tachypneic patient while delaying the next ventilator-delivered breath (by decreasing the respiratory rate). The end-expiratory airway occlusion maneuver in this patient demonstrated a total PEEP of 20 cmH$_2$O on a set PEEP of 5 cmH$_2$O (Figure 3.6.3, pattern 2).

Thus, the patient had developed 15 cmH$_2$O of auto-PEEP. Since it is the total PEEP that must be subtracted from the static pressure in the denominator of the compliance equation, her true thoracic compliance was not 17.5 but 28 mL/cmH$_2$O, which is only slightly decreased from her baseline state. Auto-PEEP was therefore the main factor responsible for the acute increase in peak airway pressure. Aggressive hand-ventilation without sufficient time for exhalation by an inexperienced respiratory therapist during transport had rapidly created a state of dynamic hyperinflation in this patient with severe COAD. This problem could still have occurred with a transport ventilator as dynamic hyperinflation can develop in an agitated patient who is breathing rapidly with ventilator settings that prevent adequate exhalation time (breath stalking).

Auto-PEEP is particularly likely in patients with COAD, because of the airway narrowing (inflammation and mucus production) and loss of elastic recoil (emphysematous changes) resulting in a prolonged expiratory phase. However, if minute ventilation is sufficiently large, auto-PEEP can occur even in the absence of COAD simply because of inadequate exhalation time.[4]

The patient's breathing pattern gives an additional clue to the presence of significant auto-PEEP. First, by watching the chest and listening to the breath sounds or simply by looking at her respiratory flow-time tracing on the ventilator, it would have been obvious that her exhalation time was insufficient as her expiratory flow continued uninterrupted until the next breathing effort. Thus, dynamic hyperinflation had to be occurring.

Furthermore, she could only trigger the ventilator 6 times over the set rate of 14 despite visibly trying to breathe at 30/minute. The triggering sensitivity set on the ventilator demand valve had not been changed (1.5 cmH$_2$O) but because of the presence of 15 cmH$_2$O of auto-PEEP, the effective triggering sensitivity of the

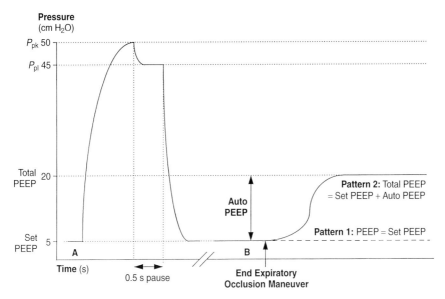

Figure 3.6.3. Pressure tracing from ventilator-delivered breaths over time. (A) Increased peak airway pressure state: tidal volume (V_t) = 700 mL; inspiratory flow (Q) = 0.83 L s^{-1}; **PEEP** = 5 cm H_2O. (B) End-expiratory airway occlusion maneuver. In a state of increased peak airway pressure, when compliance appears to be decreased (A), performing the end-expiratory airway occlusion maneuver allows detection of auto-PEEP (pattern 2) caused by dynamic hyperinflation. In this situation, the real positive end-expiratory airway pressure (total PEEP) is the sum of the ventilator set PEEP (5 cmH_2O) and the auto-PEEP (15 cmH_2O). As a consequence, the true static compliance is no longer 17.5 mL cmH_2O^{-1} but 28 mL cmH_2O^{-1} [$C- V_t/(P_{pl}$ – total PEEP)]. In the absence of auto-PEEP (pattern 1), the increased peak airway pressure state can be attributed to a decrease in compliance which can be seen acutely with pulmonary edema, tracheobronchial hemorrhage, bronchial intubation or tension pneumothorax.

demand valve was now 16.5 cmH_2O (set sensitivity plus auto-PEEP).[5] In other words, since the patient had hyperinflated her lungs to a volume equal to giving her 15 cmH_2O of PEEP, she needed to decrease her intrathoracic pressure by that amount before airway pressure would decrease. The ventilator trigger threshold would then be additive. Not surprisingly, this debilitated and sedated patient was unable to consistently generate a negative inspiratory pressure greater than 16.5 cmH_2O – which explains the discrepancy between her observed respiratory rate and that delivered by the ventilator.

As auto-PEEP develops, mean alveolar pressure increases. This, in turn, causes mean pleural and right atrial pressures to increase. As right atrial pressure increases, the pressure gradient for venous return decreases, ventricular preload is compromised, and cardiac output and BP decrease. This preload-dependent hemodynamic state may be difficult to recognize at first because the transmission of the increased alveolar pressure to vascular structures in the chest make the

CVP and the PAOP appear high despite intravascular volume depletion. [6] The addition of vasopressors in this setting is clearly not indicated and will further compromise end-organ perfusion and function. The worsening of the renal function on a high-dose dopamine infusion was therefore not unexpected.

Follow-up

After administration of sedatives and muscle relaxants, the patient was temporarily disconnected from the ventilator. The ensuing prolonged expiratory phase allowed her expiratory alveolar pressure to return to zero and her lung volume to re-equilibrate at her baseline functional residual capacity (FRC), dissipating the dynamic hyperinflation. Her CVP and PAOP decreased significantly, uncovering the previously undiagnosed hypovolemia. Despite this, her heart rate slowed and her systematic arterial pressure increased because her cardiac output increased with the increase in venous return. Clearly, the auto-PEEP she had developed was hemodynamically significant. Mechanical ventilation was restarted after approximately 30 seconds with the goal of maximizing the expiratory time. A lower tidal volume of 600 mL and a higher inspiratory flow of 90 L min^{-1} were chosen, and aerosolized bronchodilators were administered every four hours. One liter of crystalloids solution and 500 mL of colloid solution were rapidly infused intravenously and the dopamine was easily weaned to 2.5 µg kg^{-1} min^{-1} while the mean blood pressure stayed above 65 mmHg. Within the next hour urine output restarted while the peripheral **livedo reticularis** subsided.

The patient remained hemodynamically stable thereafter, simply needing large amounts of intravascular fluid over the first 48 hours. By the tenth hospital day her abdominal pain and pancreatic inflammation had subsided and she was successfully weaned from mechanical ventilation and her trachea extubated.

References

1 Pinsky MR. Through the past darkly: ventilatory management of patients with COPD. *Critical Care Medicine* (1994) **22**: 1714–1717.
2 Tobin MJ. Respiratory monitoring during mechanical ventilation. *Critical Care Clinics* (1990) **6**: 679–709.
3 Pepe PE and Marini JJ. Occult positive end-expiratory pressure in mechanically ventilated patients with airflow obstruction. *American Review of Respiratory Diseases* (1982) **126**: 166–170.
4 Scott LR, Benson MS and Bishop MJ. Relationship of endotracheal tube size to auto-PEEP at high minute ventilation. *Respiratory Care* (1986) **31**: 1080–1082.
5 Marini JJ. Should PEEP be used in airflow obstruction. *American Review of Respiratory Diseases* (1989) **140**: 1–3.
6 Rogers PL, Schlichtig R, Miro A and Pinsky M. Auto-PEEP during CPR; an occult cause of electromechanical dissociation. *Chest* (1991) **99**: 492–493.

4 Sepsis, Including MSOF

4.1 Acute Sepsis of Unknown Etiology; Strategies in Diagnosis and Management; Goals of Initial Therapy and What Questions to Ask First

Victor M. Chavez and George M. Matuschak

History

A 70-year-old white male was admitted to an outlying hospital with a 7-day history of fever, myalgias, bifrontal headache, nausea and intermittent epigastric pain. The patient was a retired railroad worker with no significant prior medical problems. On physical examination he was alert and normotensive, but in moderate respiratory distress with a respiratory rate of 26/minute; the pulse was 120/minute and the temperature 38.7°C. No skin lesions or lymphadenopathy were noted. Evaluation of the chest revealed clear lungs on auscultation, normal first and second heart sounds, and no murmurs or gallops. Diffuse epigastric tenderness was present. Bowel sounds were diminished but neither rebound tenderness nor flank pain were elicited. The stool did not contain occult blood. There were no focal neurologic abnormalities or signs of meningeal irritation.

Relevant laboratory findings included a modestly increased white blood cell (WBC) count $15.5 \times 10^9\,L^{-1}$ ($15\,500\,\mu L^{-1}$) with 34% immature neutrophils. Values for serum electrolytes, liver function tests, BUN, creatinine, creatine phosphokinase and amylase were all within normal limits. The ECG revealed sinus tachycardia and non-specific abnormalities of the ST segments and T waves. No infiltrates were detected on the chest radiograph; abdominal films were remarkable only for increases in intestinal gas without signs of ileus. Urinalysis showed 5 white blood cells, 1+ bacteria and a positive nitrite reaction. Based on these findings, a presumptive diagnosis of urosepsis was made. Two sets of blood cultures and a urine culture were obtained, after which an intravenous infusion of 0.9% saline was begun at $100\,mL\,h^{-1}$ and 2 g ampicillin sodium with 1 g sulbactam were given every 6 hours.

Over the next 48 hours, the patient's condition did not improve. Neither subjective symptoms nor pyrexia remitted. Although the physical examination was unchanged, the WBC increased to $18.4 \times 10^9\,L^{-1}$ ($18\,400\,\mu L^{-1}$) while the platelet count decreased to $98 \times 10^9\,L^{-1}$ ($98\,000\,\mu L^{-1}$). Blood cultures were repeated, and 1 g vancomycin IV every 12 hours along with $3\,mg\,kg^{-1}$ per day gentamicin IV every 8 hours were added to the antibiotic regimen. By the next day, arterial hypotension had supervened (systolic pressure 85 mmHg), along with increased dyspnea and acute oliguria. Bolus infusions of 0.9% saline (200 mL IV over 30 minutes) improved blood pressure only transiently. Although blood and urine cultures remained sterile, the patient was transferred to the intensive care unit (ICU) of a different institution for management of septic shock thought secondary to urosepsis.

Upon admission to the ICU, the patient was found to be stuporous, febrile to 39°C, and in moderately severe respiratory distress. The arterial blood pressure was 85/45 mmHg, the pulse 126 beats/minute, and the respiratory rate 36/minute. The skin and mucous membranes were warm and dry; no rashes, petechial or vesicular eruptions were noted. The sclerae were mildly icteric. Breath sounds were diminished over both lung fields and crackles were heard at both posterior lung bases. A grade II/VI systolic murmur was heard over the cardiac apex, along with an S_3 gallop. The abdomen was obese without tenderness or ascites; bowel sounds were diminished throughout. The rest of the physical examination was unremarkable. Blood and urine cultures were again obtained and dopamine was infused beginning at $5 \mu g \, kg^{-1} \, min^{-1}$, which was subsequently increased to $12 \mu g \, kg^{-1} \, min^{-1}$ to maintain the systolic blood pressure at > 90 mmHg. Arterial blood gases showed an acute uncompensated respiratory alkalosis and a P_aO_2 of 109 mmHg [14.1 kPa] with the patient on an F_IO_2 of 1.0 by face mask. Because of progressive arterial oxygen desaturation to $< 90\%$ by pulse oximetry, the patient's trachea was intubated and positive-pressure ventilation started in the assist-control mode at 12 breaths/minute at a tidal volume of $7 \, mL \, kg^{-1}$ with $5 \, cmH_2O$ positive end-expiratory pressure. A repeat blood gas analysis on an F_IO_2 of 0.4 showed a normal acid–base balance and an increase in the P_aO_2 to 122 mmHg [16.3 kPa] (P_aO_2/F_IO_2 ratio = 305).

Laboratory analyses revealed the following hematologic values: hemoglobin $12.2 \, g \, dL^{-1}$; WBC $6.2 \times 10^9 \, L^{-1}$ ($6 \, 200 \, mL^{-1}$) with 43% neutrophils, 56% band forms and 1% monocytes. Although the platelet count was $48 \times 10^9 \, L^{-1}$ ($48 \, 000 \, mL^{-1}$), the coagulation profile revealed normal prothrombin and partial thromboplastin times as well as fibrinogen and D-dimer results. A test for HIV was negative. All of the liver function tests were elevated: the alanine aminotransferase was $232 \, U \, L^{-1}$, the aspartate aminotransferase $225 \, U \, L^{-1}$, the alkaline phosphatase $208 \, U \, L^{-1}$ and the bilirubin $3.5 \, mg \, dL^{-1}$ [$59.5 \mu mol \, L^{-1}$]. Serum amylase and lipase values were normal. Azotemia was reflected by BUN and creatinine values of $50 \, mg \, dL^{-1}$ [$8.3 \mu mol \, L^{-1}$] and $4.7 \, mg \, dL^{-1}$ [$358.7 \mu mol \, L^{-1}$], respectively.

In addition to dopamine, aggressive fluid resuscitation was started and the patient received $5 \, L$ of 0.9% saline over the next 2 hours. However, oliguria persisted and hypotension recurred despite increasing the dopamine infusion to $18 \mu g \, kg^{-1} \, min^{-1}$. Cultures of blood, tracheal aspirate, cerebrospinal fluid and urine were obtained, after which the patient's antibiotic regimen was changed to include erythromycin, ceftriaxone and tobramycin. The ECG demonstrated sinus tachycardia but was otherwise unchanged from previously.

To assist in establishing an infectious focus of the presumed septic state, several radiological studies were performed. The chest radiograph showed modest cardiomegaly and mild pulmonary vascular congestion but no infiltrates; thoracentesis of a small right pleural effusion revealed a transudate with no evidence of infection. A computed tomographic scan of the abdomen revealed no abnormalities of the liver, gallbladder, kidneys or genitourinary tract. Likewise, ultrasonic examination showed no evidence of hepatobiliary or pancreatic abnormalities.

A radial artery and a balloon-directed pulmonary artery catheter were placed to assess the patient's volume status and cardiac function. The initial

Table 4.1.1. Cardiopulmonary data

Arterial pressure	95/45 mmHg
Heart rate	116/minute
Pulmonary artery pressure	28/12 mmHg
Mean pulmonary artery pressure	17 mmHg
Pulmonary artery occlusion pressure	16 mmHg
Right atrial pressure	10 mmHg
Cardiac index	4.39 L min^{-1} m^{-2}
Systemic vascular resistance index	1240 dyn-sec cm^{-5}
S_aO_2	94%
S_vO_2	61%

cardiopulmonary data (Table 4.1.1) were interpreted as indicating a hyperdynamic cardiovascular state and adequate fluid resuscitation. At this time, additional history was obtained from the patient's wife during discussion of prognostic issues. Two weeks before admission, she had found several ticks in the patient's clothes after a hunting trip. A presumptive diagnosis of tick-borne rickettsial disease (e.g. Rocky Mountain spotted fever or ehrlichiosis) was made and 100 mg doxycycline was given intravenously every 12 hours. Within 24 hours, the patient was afebrile and weaning of vasopressor support under way.

Trap

This otherwise healthy individual developed an acute febrile illness in which headache, myalgias, and gastrointestinal complaints were prominent initial symptoms. The rather non-specific presentation, first ascribed to genitourinary infection, was followed shortly thereafter by a fulminating clinical course that included life-threatening shock and progressive dysfunction of multiple organ systems. This case demonstrates two important traps that may complicate the management of patients with such severe illnesses, especially when they fail to respond to initial empiric therapy.

First, failure of the physicians to modify the list of differential diagnostic possibilities when circumstances so dictated. This resulted in a delay in diagnosis and starting specific treatment. Here the negative urine and blood cultures 24 and 48 hours after presentation did not induce reassessment of the possible causes of the unsuccessful therapy or consideration of alternate diagnoses. Reassessment is important, whether or not sepsis is considered to be the underlying problem, since conditions other than infection may give rise to similar clinical findings found in this patient including fever, as typified by the systemic inflammatory syndrome (SIRS).[1] Second, failure to obtain a detailed history, either on initial presentation or within the next 72 hours, may lead to oversimplification of the clinical problem. This contributed to the considerable delay in making the diagnosis of a tick-borne illness, which in the case of Rocky Mountain spotted fever is associated with increased long-term morbidity and mortality.[2,3]

Trick

A broad diversity of septic and non-septic critical illnesses are characterized by a presentation including fever and rapid progression to shock and multiple systems organ failure (Table 4.1.2). When sepsis is strongly suspected, vigorous volume resuscitation and broad spectrum antimicrobial therapy after obtaining appropriate cultures are key initial measures. However, as this case demonstrates, certain microbial infections associated with life-threatening shock and organ injury require specific treatment by antibiotics that are ordinarily not part of commonly used regimens. Among these are the two tick-borne diseases, Rocky Mountain spotted fever and ehrlichiosis, both of which are increasingly recognized to cause serious illness.[5–7] Because only approximately 50% of

Table 4.1.2. Common and uncommon causes of shock progressing to multiple organ failure[*]

Common causes
Sepsis (bacteremic, non-bacteremic, non-bacterial)
Trauma
Aspiration of gastric contents
Acute pancreatitis
Infective endocarditis
Heat stroke

Uncommon causes
Disseminated tuberculosis
Antiphospholipid antibody syndrome
Thrombotic thrombocytopenic purpura
Unusual microbial infections
  Rocky Mountain spotted fever
  Ehrlichiosis
  P. falciparum malaria
  Vibrio vulnificus sepsis
Intoxications/toxins
  Arsenic
  Ethylene glycol
  Organophosphates
  Mercury
  Methanol
  Amanita mushroom ingestion
  Scorpion, snake envenomation
Pheochromocytoma

[*] Modified from ref. (4).

infected individuals recall a tick bite,[5] these disorders should be considered in any patient presenting with fever and headache in conjunction with an undiagnosed illness and evidence of shock with multisystem involvement, irrespective of the presence of a rash. When present, the typically petechial rash of Rocky Mountain spotted fever beginning on the extremities and spreading centripetally is a helpful clue. However, this rash may be evanescent, and an additional 10% of individuals infected with *Rickettsia rickettsiae* may never develop one (e.g. Rocky Mountain 'spotless' fever).[5] Regardless, encephalopathy, hyponatremia, thrombocytopenia, increased values for liver function tests and elevated creatine phosphokinase levels are characteristic clinical features. Recently, increased serum levels of cytokines and intercellular adhesion molecule-1 have been reported in patients with Rocky Mountain spotted fever.[8] Most likely, these findings contribute to the observed derangements in cardiopulmonary function, formed blood elements, and biochemical indices of organ function in both Rocky Mountain spotted fever and ehrlichiosis.

Human ehrlichiosis, first reported in 1986, is caused by *Ehrlichia* spp. rickettsiae which have an incubation period of 1–21 days (mean 11–12 days).[6] Two forms of disease are recognized which share clinical features and responsiveness to specific antimicrobial therapy: human monocytic ehrlichiosis caused by *E. chaffeensis*[6,9] and human granulocytic ehrlichiosis caused by *E. phagocytophila/E. equi*.[10,11] An accompanying rash, if present, is usually petechial or maculopapular; pancytopenia and abnormalities of liver function are common.[5-7] Although first identified in the southeastern portion of the USA, human ehrlichiosis has now been reported in all sections of the USA and Europe.[12] Specific and effective treatment for both tick-borne diseases is tetracycline or doxycycline, 100 mg twice daily, or chloramphenicol, with therapy continued for 2–3 days after the patient becomes afebrile.

Follow-up

Over the next 48 hours after starting doxycycline, the patient's blood pressure, heart rate and cardiac index became normal without dopamine. Likewise, renal functional abnormalities rapidly resolved and his trachea was extubated uneventfully.

Initial IgG antibodies to *Ehrlichia* spp. were found to be elevated at a titer of 1:160 (normal <1:40, Specialty Laboratories Inc., Santa Monica, California). Seven days later the IgG antibody rose further to 1:640. Collectively, these results confirmed the diagnosis of ehrlichiosis.[6]

References

1 American College of Chest Physicians/Society of Critical Care Medicine Consensus Conference. Definitions for sepsis and organ failure and guidelines for the use of innovative therapies in sepsis. *Critical Care Medicine* (1992) **20**: 864–874.

2 Kirkland KB, Wilkinson WE and Sextin DJ. Therapeutic delay and mortality in cases of Rocky Mountain spotted fever. *Clinical Infectious Diseases* (1995) **20**: 1118–1121.

3 Archibald LK and Sexton DJ. Long-term sequelae of Rocky Mountain spotted fever. *Clinical Infectious Diseases* (1995) **20**: 1122–1125.

4 Matuschak GM. Multiple systems organ failure: clinical expression, pathogenesis, and therapy. In: JB Hall, GA Schmidt, LDH Wood (eds) *Principles of Critical Care*. St. Louis, McGraw-Hill, p 613–636, 1992.

5 Jantausch BA. Lyme disease, Rocky Mountain spotted fever, ehrlichiosis: emerging and established challenges for the clinician. *Annals of Allergy* (1994) **73**: 4–11.

6 Middleton DB. Tick-borne infections. What starts as a tiny bite may have a serious outcome. *Postgraduate Medicine* (1994) **95**: 131–139.

7 Dumler JS and Bakken JS. Ehrlichial diseases of humans: emerging tick-borne infections. *Clinical Infectious Diseases* (1995) **20**: 1102–1110.

8 Sessler CN, Schwartz M, Windsor AC and Fowler AA 3rd. Increased serum cytokines and intercellular adhesion molecule-1 in fulminant Rocky Mountain spotted fever. *Critical Care Medicine* (1995) **23**: 973–976.

9 Standaert SM, Dawson JE, Schaffner W, Childs JE, Biggie KL, Singleton J Jr, Gerhardt RR, Knight ML and Hutcheson RH. Ehrlichiosis in a golf-oriented retirement community. *New England Journal of Medicine* (1995) **333**: 420–425.

10 Bakken JS, Dumler JS, Chen SM, Eckman MR, Van Etta LL and Walker DH. Human granulocytic ehrlichiosis in the upper midwest United States. A new species emerging? *Journal of the American Medical Association* (1994) **72**: 212–218.

11 Goodman JL, Nelson C, Vitale B, Madigan JE, Dumler JS, Kurtti TJ and Munderloh UG. Direct cultivation of the causative agent of human granulocytic ehrlichiosis. *New England Journal of Medicine* (1996) **334**: 209–215.

12 Buonavoglia D, Sagaziio P, Gravino EA, de Caprariis D, Cerundolo R and Buonavoglia C. Serological evidence of *Ehrlichia canis* in dogs in southern Italy. *Microbiologica* (1995) **18**: 83–86.

4.2 Sepsis in Patients with Pre-existing Liver Dysfunction: Therapeutic and Prognostic Issues

George M. Matuschak

History

A 67-year-old sedentary male with biopsy-documented chronic hepatitis, treated chronically with prednisone 10 mg/day was transferred to the intensive care unit from another institution. This followed the acute onset of left calf pain one day before, which was accompanied by progressive edema of his left leg, dyspnea, hypoxemia and shock. The patient was intubated after arterial blood gases revealed a P_aO_2 of 50 mmHg [6.67 kPa] on an F_IO_2 of 0.9 by face mask. He was placed on mechanical ventilation (assist-control mode) of a V_T of 10 mL kg^{-1} and 5 cmH$_2$O positive end-expiratory pressure, with improvement in his arterial oxygenation (P_aO_2 127 mmHg [16.9 kPa]) on an F_IO_2 of 0.8. Before his transfer, a ventilation–perfusion scan was done. This was interpreted as indeterminate for pulmonary thromboembolism. The patient was transferred on mechanical ventilatory support and fluid resuscitation was continued.

On arrival, the patient was stuporose, icteric, jaundiced and afebrile. The heart rate was 130/minute, the blood pressure 85/0 mmHg by a Doppler exam, and the respiratory rate was 32/minute. There were scattered coarse breath sounds over both lung fields. The abdomen was obese, but no ascites was detected. The left calf was slightly warm and erythematous, and very tender to palpation without accompanying superficial venous thrombosis or crepitus. Mid-calf and mid-thigh circumferences were approximately 4 cm greater on the left than right lower extremity and the dorsum of the foot had 1 + pitting edema. No pathologic changes or subcutaneous emphysema were seen on anteroposterior films of the leg.

Despite intravascular fluid challenge with 2 liters of 0.9% saline, hypotension and oliguria persisted requiring dopamine 14 µg kg^{-1} min^{-1} and norepinephrine [noradrenaline] 0.1 µg kg^{-1} min^{-1} for stabilization. A subsequent ultrasound examination was negative for abscesses or fluid collections. A computed tomographic scan through the level of the upper thighs demonstrated minimal soft tissue edema of the left thigh and anteromedial aspect of the right thigh (Figure 4.2.1).

Pertinent laboratory data included: total serum bilirubin 12.2 mg dL^{-1} [208.6 µmol L^{-1}] and alanine aminotransferase 176 U L^{-1} [2.91 µkat L^{-1}], both of which were unchanged from previous outpatient values, and an anion gap of 17 mEq L^{-1} with an arterial lactate of 13 mmol L^{-1}. Repeat arterial blood gases on an F_IO_2 of 1.0 were: pH 7.18 [H$^+$66 nmol L^{-1}], P_aCO_2 28 mmHg [3.73 kPa] and P_aO_2, 81 mmHg [10.8 kPa]. The chest radiograph showed a normal cardiac silhouette, atelectasis of the right lower lobe, and a small right pleural effusion.

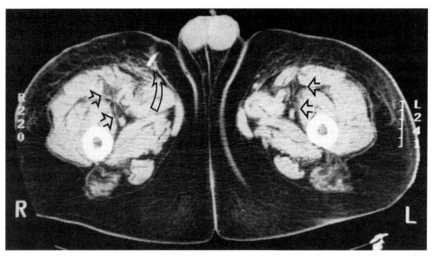

Figure 4.2.1. Computed tomographic image taken at the level of the upper thighs. A right femoral arterial catheter is visible (curved arrow). Minimal soft tissue edema is present over the left and right anteromedial thigh (small open arrows).

Blood, urine and sputum cultures were obtained and the patient started on broad-spectrum antimicrobial agents. Heparin therapy was considered but a cardio-pulmonary profile obtained after insertion of a pulmonary artery catheter did not support a diagnosis of massive pulmonary thromboembolism (Table 4.2.1).

In view of the hemodynamic data, Gram stain of an aspirate of the left leg at mid-calf level was performed that showed many polymorphonuclear leukocytes and Gram-negative rods compatible with a diagnosis of necrotizing fasciitis. The patient underwent urgent incision and drainage of the left lower extremity with fasciotomies of the medial and lateral aspects of the leg and foot. Microscopic

Table 4.2.1. Initial cardiopulmonary data[*]

Arterial pressure	120/50 mmHg
Heart rate	109/minute
Pulmonary artery systolic pressure/pulmonary artery diastolic pressure	38/18 mmHg
Mean pulmonary artery pressure	25 mmHg
Pulmonary artery occlusion pressure	12 mmHg
Right atrial pressure	10 mmHg
Cardiac index	$4.0 \, \text{L min}^{-1} \text{m}^{-2}$
Systemic vascular resistance index	$1100 \, \text{dyn-sec cm}^{-5}$
S_aO_2[†]	98%
S_vO_2[†]	78%

[*] On dopamine $14 \, \mu g \, kg^{-1} \, min^{-1}$ and norepinephrine $0.1 \, \mu g \, kg^{-1} \, min^{-1}$.
[†] On an F_iO_2 of 1.0.

findings of tissue removed at operation confirmed focally degenerated muscle, and adipose and fibrous tissue with necrosis and acute inflammation, which were culture-positive for *Pseudomonas aeruginosa*. The patient's hemodynamic status remained unchanged on pressor therapy. On the fifth day, a catheter tip was culture-positive for *Candida albicans* although blood cultures remained sterile.

Trap

The physicians were lulled into an initial non-aggressive posture by the lack of generalized signs of sepsis on presentation including fever and hypotension. In this afebrile patient, the acute onset of leg pain in association with rapid development of lower extremity edema, respiratory symptoms and severe hypoxemia suggested massive pulmonary thromboembolism. Although right heart catheterization excluded this and instead suggested underlying sepsis, the possibility of venous thrombosis remained. Recognition of necrotizing fasciitis was delayed because striking cutaneous changes or crepitus were lacking, and three separate radiologic studies failed to demonstrate gas in the tissues. Necrotizing fasciitis of the extremity has protean manifestations.[1] Delayed recognition and incomplete debridement are two chief causes of therapeutic failure.[2,3]

Trick

Elderly patients and those receiving corticosteroids have blunted thermoregulatory responses to sepsis. A high index of suspicion is therefore necessary in those presenting to the ICU with hemodynamic instability. Whenever possible, simple aspiration of involved areas may rapidly establish the diagnosis of necrotizing fasciitis and other serious soft tissue infections, guiding therapy in the critical first few hours after presentation. However, outcome from any form of sepsis is poor in patients with significant pre-existing liver dysfunction.[4] This results from multiple defects in host defense[5-7] and hepatocellular dysfunction persisting despite resuscitation.[8] In this context chronic steroid use increased the likelihood of disseminated candidiasis, despite the lack of positive blood cultures. In such immunosuppressed patients, a low threshold for initiating antifungal therapy is warranted when shock does not respond to antibacterial chemotherapy.

Follow-up

Despite aggressive therapy including dialysis for acute renal failure, the patient remained pressor-dependent and died seven days later of multiple organ failure. Post-mortem examination revealed cholestasis and submassive hepatic necrosis, cardiomegaly with biventricular dilatation and, unexpectedly, disseminated candidiasis involving the heart, lungs, liver and spleen.

References

1 Janevicius RV, Hann SE and Batt MD. Necrotizing fasciitis. *Surgery in Gynecology and Obstetrics* (1982) **154**: 97–102.

2 Wang K-C and Shih C-H. Necrotizing fasciitis of the extremities. *Journal of Trauma* (1992) **32**: 179–182.

3 Scully RE, Mark EJ, McNeely WF and McNeely BU. Case 41–1994. *New England Journal of Medicine* (1994) **331**: 1362–1368.

4 Matuschak GM, Rinaldo JE, Pinsky MR and Gavaler JS. Effects of end-stage liver failure on the incidence and resolution of the adult respiratory distress syndrome. *Journal of Critical Care* (1987) **2**: 162–173.

5 Matuschak GM. Liver–lung interactions during critical illness. *New Horizons* (1994) **2**: 488–504.

6 Chang S-W and Ohara N. Chronic biliary obstruction induces pulmonary intravascular phagocytosis and endotoxin sensitivity in rats. *Journal of Clinical Investigation* (1994) **94**: 2009–2019.

7 Matuschak GM, Mattingly M, Tredway TL and Lechner AJ. Liver–lung interactions during *E. coli* endotoxemia: TNF-α:leukotriene axis. *American Journal of Respiratory Critical Care Medicine* (1994) **149**: 41–49.

8 Wang P, Zheng FBA, Ayala A and Van Thiel DH. Hepatocellular dysfunction persists during early sepsis despite increased volume of crystalloid resuscitation. *Journal of Trauma* (1992) **32**: 389–397.

4.3 Left Ventricular Segmental Wall Motion Abnormality as a Feature of Septic Shock

Tarek A. Chidiac and Jeffrey E. Salon

History

A 45-year-old man with a history of chronic alcohol ingestion and 40 pack-years of smoking presented to the emergency department with hypotension, fever, shortness of breath and cough. He initially became ill one week before admission with generalized malaise, fever and cough. He continued smoking and drinking alcohol ([>6 oz] [200 mL] per day). On the day of his admission he became severely dyspneic and the paramedics were called. On admission his vital signs were: blood pressure 80/40 mmHg, heart rate 150/minute, temperature 38.3°C [101°F] and respirations 40/minute. Because of marked respiratory distress, his trachea was intubated and his lungs ventilated urgently.

Physical examination after intubation showed (peripheral) cyanosis, agitation and cold skin. There was no jugular venous distension. Examination of the lungs and heart showed bilateral diffuse inspiratory crackles and a loud second heart sound. Abdominal examination was normal.

Complete blood count showed neutrophilia with a left shift. The electrocardiogram showed non-specific ST–T wave changes and a sinus tachycardia. The chest radiograph showed diffuse bilateral infiltrates, with consolidation of the right upper lobe. The heart appeared enlarged. Gram stain of the sputum demonstrated >25 polymorphonuclear cells, <25 epithelial cells per high-power field, with many Gram-negative bacilli. Arterial blood gas analysis showed a P_aO_2 of 55 mmHg [7.3 kPa] with an F_IO_2 of 1.

Because the initial presentation could reflect acute ventricular dysfunction, a pulmonary artery catheter was inserted. Vascular pressures and cardiac output determination were highly variable because of marked respiratory efforts. Thus, a transesophageal echocardiogram was performed to assess left ventricular function. The bedside echocardiogram demonstrated left ventricular segmental wall motion abnormalities involving the inferoposterior wall. There was no dilation of any cavity nor were there any valvular abnormalities. The ejection fraction was 35%.

A diagnosis of septic shock and ARDS secondary to a Gram-negative pneumonia was made. However, the chest radiograph and echocardiographic findings consistent with left ventricular dysfunction were difficult to explain; the low ejection fraction with the segmental wall motion dysfunction suggested an additional cardiac event, possibly an acute myocardial infarction. Thus, vigorous fluid resuscitation was withheld for fear that it would worsen the already poor pulmonary gas exchange by promoting further pulmonary edema formation. A cardiology consultation was considered for possible salvage cardiac catheterization/angioplasty.

The patient's urine output decreased progressively over the first two hours after admission. Dobutamine $5\,\mathrm{mg\,kg^{-1}\,min^{-1}}$ was transiently started but had to be stopped because it caused profound hypotension.

Trap

There was a failure to recognize segmental wall motion abnormality as a feature of septic shock, and therefore treat the cardiovascular instability with intravascular fluid resuscitation.

Trick

Although pulmonary catheter pressure wave form analysis can be difficult to interpret in dyspneic patients, measures of mixed venous oxygen saturation are not. Low output states are characterized by an increased $(A–V)O_2$ content difference, whereas the converse is often true in hyperdynamic sepsis. However, if sepsis is also hypodynamic it, too, will resemble cardiogenic shock. In this patient, after tracheal intubation the C_aO_2 was $18\,\mathrm{mL\,dL^{-1}}$ and the S_vO_2 was 78%. Following the cardiovascular collapse induced by dobutamine S_vO_2 decreased to 48%, subsequently returning to 70%. This trend was noted by the physicians caring for this man. They used clinical information to defend a trial of vigorous fluid resuscitation which resulted in an immediate improvement in mean arterial pressure, without worsening gas exchange.

Segmental wall motion dysfunction is a well-recognized feature of septic shock, even in the absence of coronary artery disease and segmental myocardiopathy.[1,2] Previous reports of myocardial dysfunction during septic shock have focused on a circulating myocardial depressant substance, cytokines or other mechanisms.[3–6] This dysfunction has been described as a global suppression of myocardial performance.[7,8] Recent studies have shown that myocardial dysfunction in septic shock may be segmental.[1,2]

Table 4.3.1 summarizes other causes of regional wall motion abnormalities. While regional wall motion dysfunction remains difficult to explain, abnormalities in the distribution of myocardial blood flow during septic shock with or without the interference of local factors may be the major causes.[1,2,14]

Table 4.3.1. Causes of regional wall motion abnormalities

Cause	Reference
Coronary artery disease/infarction	9, 10
Focal myocardiopathy notably myocarditis	11, 12
Left mural thrombi	12
Coronary artery embolization	12
Left bundle branch block	12
Intraventricular conduction delay	12
Abnormalities in right ventricular contraction	12, 13

Follow-up

In this patient fluid and pressor (dopamine) therapy were used to keep a mean arterial pressure above 60 mmHg and a pulmonary artery occlusion pressure between 10 and 15 mmHg. Broad-spectrum antibiotic therapy was started (third generation cephalosporin and aminoglycoside). Serial cardiac enzymes were normal. Blood pressure improved over a 12-hour period, and he was weaned from vasopressor support and his trachea extubated later.

Sputum and blood cultures grew *Klebsiella pneumoniae*. A repeat echocardiogram showed a normal ejection fraction with no segmental wall motion abnormalities. A persantine thallium scan performed before discharge showed no evidence of coronary artery disease.

References

1 Ellrodt AG, Riedinger MS, Kimchi A, Berman DS, Maddahi J, Swan HJC and Murata GH. Left ventricular performance in septic shock: reversible segmental and global abnormalities. *American Heart Journal* (1985) **110**(2): 402–409.
2 Chidiac TA and Salon JE. Left ventricular segmental wall motion abnormality in septic shock. *Critical Care Medicine* (1995); **23**(3): 594–598.
3 Cunnion RE and Parrillo JE. Myocardial dysfunction in sepsis. *Critical Care Clinics* (1989) **5**(1): 99–118.
4 Reilly JM, Cunnion RE, Burch-Whitman C, Parker MM, Shelhammer JH and Parrillo JE. A circulating myocardial depressant substance is associated with cardiac dysfunction and peripheral hypoperfusion (lactic acidemia) in patients with septic shock. *Chest* (1989) **97**(6): 1072–1080.
5 Giroir BP, Johnson JH, Brown T, Allen GL and Beutler B. The tissue distribution of tumor necrosis factor biosynthesis during endotoxemia. *Journal of Clinical Investigation* (1992) **90**: 693–698.
6 Silverman HJ, Penaranda R, Orens JB and Lee NH. Impaired β-adrenergic receptor stimulation of cyclic adenosine monophosphate in human septic shock: association with myocardial hyporesponsiveness of catecholamines. *Critical Care Medicine* (1993) **21**: 31–39.
7 Parrillo JE, Parker MM, Natanson C, Suffredini AF, Danner RL, Cunnion RE and Ognibene FP. Septic shock in humans. Advances in the understanding of pathogenesis, cardiovascular dysfunction, and therapy. *Annals of Internal Medicine* (1990) **113**: 227–242.
8 Parker MM, Suffredini AF, Natanson C, Ognibene FP, Shelhamer JH and Parrillo JE. Responses of left ventricular function in survivors and nonsurvivors of septic shock. *Journal of Critical Care* (1989) **4**: 19–25.
9 Goldman MR and Boucher CA. Value of radionuclide imaging techniques in assessing cardiomyopathy. *American Journal of Cardiology* (1980) **46**: 1232–1236.
10 Bulkley BH, Hutchins GM, Bailey I, Strauss HW and Pitt B. Thallium-201 imaging and gated cardiac blood pool scans in patients with ischemic and idiopathic congestive cardiomyopathy: a clinical and pathologic study. *Circulation* (1977) **55**: 752–760.
11 Diaz RA, Nihoyannopoulos P, Athanassopoulos G and Oakley CM. Usefulness of echocardiography to differentiate dilated cardiomyopathy from coronary-induced congestive heart failure. *American Journal of Cardiology* (1991) **68**: 753–60.
12 Glamann DB, Lange RA, Corbett JR and Hillis LD. Utility of various radionuclide

techniques for distinguishing ischemic from nonischemic dilated cardiomyopathy. *Archives of Internal Medicine* (1992) **152**: 769–772.

13 Hagan AD, Francis GS, Sahn DJ, Karliner KS, Friedman WF and O'Rourke RA. Ultrasound evaluation of systolic anterior septal motion in patients with and without right ventricular volume overload. *Circulation* (1974) **50**: 248–254.

14 Cunnion RE, Schaer GL, Parker MM, Natanson C and Parrillo JE. The coronary circulation in human septic shock. *Circulation* (1986) **73**: 637–644.

5 Liver Failure

5.1 Spontaneous Bacterial Peritonitis
Graeme J.M. Alexander

History

A 64-year-old female patient was admitted to the high dependency unit with a 10-year history of chronic liver disease. A diagnosis of primary biliary cirrhosis had been made on the basis of a liver biopsy and the presence of antimitochondrial antibody. Follow-up in the clinic had shown no significant clinical evidence of chronic liver disease until one year previously when she first developed ascites. This had been readily controlled with sodium restriction and a small dose of spironolactone.

In the month leading up to the admission, the ascites had become more prominent and she had been complaining for the previous week of intermittent mid-epigastric discomfort. She had commented that she had been passing less urine. At the time of admission her history was almost impossible to elicit.

Clinical examination revealed a woman in grade II coma with a hepatic flap and bilateral extensor plantar reflexes. She was unable to provide a history and was unable to co-operate with clinical examination. Pulse was 74/minute and regular. Temperature was 35.2°C [95.4°F], blood pressure 90/60 mmHg. She was jaundiced, without lymphadenopathy. The thyroid was not palpable. The parotid gland was easily felt. Examination of the chest was normal and examination of the cardiovascular system revealed no further abnormalities. Examination of the abdomen showed her to have modest ascites as a result of which neither the liver nor spleen could be felt with confidence. There was no peripheral edema although she did have some sacral edema. Completion of the neurological examination revealed no evidence of a focal lesion.

Her laboratory investigations were: hemoglobin $12.8\,g\,dL^{-1}$, white blood cell count $7.4 \times 10^9\,L^{-1}$, 72% neutrophils, 22% lymphocytes, platelets $82 \times 10^9\,L^{-1}$, prothrombin time 15 s, bilirubin $74\,\mu mol\,L^{-1}$ [$4.4\,mg\,dL^{-1}$], albumin $33\,g\,L^{-1}$, alkaline phosphatase $983\,U\,L^{-1}$, alanine aminotransferase $125\,U\,L^{-1}$ (<50), gamma-glutamyl transpeptidase $600\,U\,L^{-1}$, sodium $130\,mmol\,L^{-1}$, potassium $5.0\,mmol\,L^{-1}$, urea $8.0\,mmolL^{-1}$ [BUN $48\,mEq\,L^{-1}$], creatinine $145\,\mu mol\,L^{-1}$ [$1.9\,mg\,dL^{-1}$].

A central line was inserted and she was shown to be hypovolemic with a central venous pressure of $1\,cmH_2O$. She was resuscitated with 4.5% human serum albumin on which regimen she remained oliguric with a urine output of 400 mL in 24 hours. The urinary sodium was $8\,mmol\,L^{-1}$.

An ascitic tap was performed and was not blood-stained. No organisms were seen and on the subsequent culture no organisms were identified. The ascitic fluid contained 450 white cells/mm^3 of which 95% were neutrophils; the protein content was $18\,g\,L^{-1}$. An ultrasound examination was performed which showed hepatomegaly, reversed blood flow in a patent portal vein and an enlarged spleen at 12 cm with moderate ascites. No focal lesion was seen.

The serum alpha feta protein was not elevated. The immunoglobulins showed elevation of IgM, IgG and IgA; she was antimitochondrial antibody positive, and her TSH was elevated at $11\,\mathrm{mU\,L^{-1}}$ (normal 0.4–$4.0\,\mathrm{mUL^{-1}}$) with a reduced T_4 of $9\,\mathrm{pmol\,L^{-1}}$. The resident staff attributed the hypothermia and coma to hypothyroidism.

Traps

This patient did not have hypothyroidism but spontaneous bacterial peritonitis. The major difficulty in the diagnosis of spontaneous bacterial peritonitis is simply the failure to consider the diagnosis. Every patient who has ascites with clinical deterioration of any sort should have an ascitic tap. It is common in patients with severe liver disease and betokens a poor prognosis. Its recognition is critical. The diagnosis is often missed because the conventional clinical signs indicative of underlying sepsis are often absent, i.e. white cell count, temperature, etc. In addition, the failure to identify organisms in the majority of cases on microscopy and on culture dissuades many from the diagnosis.

In this patient the hypothermia was attributed to hypothyroidism. This is a common association of primary biliary cirrhosis. Nevertheless, it would be unusual in the extreme for someone with this degree of hypothyroidism – which is mild – to become hypothermic. Hypothermia is almost certainly a feature of the cirrhosis and of the superimposed sepsis.

A further common error in the management of such patients is in the use of inappropriate antibiotics. The cause of spontaneous bacterial peritonitis is usually a Gram-negative aerobic organism or staphylococcus infection because of translocation. Anaerobic infection is extraordinarily rare. Nevertheless, many such patients will receive metronidazole, which is inappropriate.

Tricks

Spontaneous bacterial peritonitis is a medical emergency with a high mortality. It occurs because of the immune deficiency that is characteristic of patients with cirrhosis. The capacity for ascitic fluid from patients with cirrhosis to opsonize organisms is reduced. The ascitic fluid protein concentration was atypical for hepatocellular carcinoma or other malignancy. The diagnosis of spontaneous bacterial peritonitis should be considered in *any* patient with liver disease with ascites, and particularly in those who have resistant ascites, abdominal pain or clinical deterioration. Although it is often assumed that such patients will be pyrexial with an elevated white cell count and invariably have abdominal discomfort, these features are often absent and the basis for the diagnosis is an elevated white cell count in ascitic fluid. Runyon has defined bacterial peritonitis in the ascitic fluid as the presence of more than $500\,\mathrm{mL^{-1}}$ leukocytes or more than

$250 \, mL^{-1}$ neutrophils. Culture of ascitic fluid is frequently negative even in the presence of spontaneous bacterial peritonitis; indeed, culture of blood may be more valuable. The reasons for a failure to identify organisms in blood include the failure to collect ascitic fluid into broth and to proceed immediately to incubation.

Because of the high mortality associated with spontaneous bacterial peritonitis, any patient who suffers it should at least be considered for a liver transplantation although it is unwise to proceed in the presence of active sepsis. At this age this patient would be a good candidate and delay could only result in a worsening of her prognosis subsequent to transplantation.

There is considerable evidence that somebody who has suffered an episode of spontaneous bacterial peritonitis should thereafter receive prophylaxis, and current clinical trials suggest that either cotrimoxazole or norfloxacin/ciprofloxacin given long term would be suitable agents.

Evidence that this patient was likely to have infected ascites included the observation that her synthetic liver function was well preserved with a relatively normal prothrombin time and albumin and, in addition, the absence of peripheral edema. Synthetic function is usually well preserved in primary biliary cirrhosis even in the presence of severe disease. Based on albumin and prothrombin times alone one can gain a false impression of the severity of this disease.

Follow-up

A clinical diagnosis of spontaneous bacterial peritonitis was made on the basis of the white cell count. She was treated with a course of cefotaxime and azlocillin for seven days. After 48 hours the patient began to recover her normal well-being and became mentally alert. After seven days antibiotics were stopped and she was discharged home after a further five days. At that stage she was to be reviewed in clinic and an assessment made for the need for liver transplantation.

Bibliography

1 Gines P, Rimola A, Planas R, *et al*. Norfloxacin prevents spontaneous bacterial peritonitis recurrence in cirrhosis: results of a double blind placebo controlled trial. *Hepatology* (1990) **12**: 716.
2 Hoefs JC, Canawati HN, Spaico FL, *et al*. Spontaneous bacterial peritonitis. *Hepatology* (1982) **2**: 399.
3 Hoefs JC. Diagnostic paracentesis. A potent clinical tool. *Gastroenterology* (1990) **98**: 230.
4 Pelletier G, Salmon D, Ink O, *et al*. Culture-negative neutrocytic ascites: a less severe variant of spontaneous bacterial peritonitis. *Hepatology* (1990) **10**: 327.
5 Runyon BA. Patients with deficient ascitic fluid opsonic activity are predisposed to spontaneous bacterial peritonitis. *Hepatology* (1988) **18**: 632.
6 Tito L, Rimola A, Gines P, *et al*. Recurrence of spontaneous bacterial peritonitis in cirrhosis: frequency and predictive factors. *Hepatology* (1988) **8**: 27.

5.2 Acute Liver Failure due to Paracetamol Overdose

Graeme J.M. Alexander

History

A 28-year-old male patient working full-time as a salesman had presented to the emergency department on the first occasion 24 hours previously. At that point he had told the casualty officer that because of a failed relationship he had taken 20 tablets (10 g) of paracetamol 48 hours previously. At the time he had taken the tablets he had been suicidal but when he attended casualty he had a strong desire to live and expressed regret at his actions. Serum paracetamol assay had been requested; no paracetamol was detected and the patient was reassured and referred to the psychiatrists as an outpatient.

Seventy-two hours after taking the paracetamol he was admitted to a general medical ward. He was confused with slurred speech, but it was still possible to obtain a history from the patient. He denied ever having been ill previously but he had been receiving phenytoin 300 mg daily since the age of eight when he had suffered a series of *grand mal* epileptic fits. He did not drink alcohol regularly or to excess but he had taken an unquantified amount of alcohol with the paracetamol overdose.

On examination there was no hepatic flap and his peripheral reflexes were normal in character with flexor plantar responses. There was no neurological deficit. He was mildly jaundiced without any other stigmata of chronic liver disease. The liver was palpable and tender but the spleen could not be felt. There was no ascites and no peripheral edema. He was mildly pyrexial, 37.4°C [99.3°F], had a tachycardia, pulse of 106/minute and his blood pressure was 140/85 mmHg. He was not tachypneic and the examination of the chest and cardiovascular system was otherwise normal.

Relevant investigations revealed a creatinine of 360 μmol L^{-1} [4.7 mg dL^{-1}] with a urea of 6 mmol L^{-1} [BUN 36 mg dL^{-1}], normal sodium, potassium and he had a plasma pH of 7.25 [H$^+$ 55 nmol L^{-1}]. Prothrombin time (PT) was 122 s and did not correct following the administration of vitamin K intravenously. His albumin was normal at 36 g L^{-1} and the bilirubin was elevated at 70 μmol L^{-1} [4.1 mg dL^{-1}]. The alanine aminotransferase was 500 IU L^{-1}: 10 times normal. The alkaline phosphatase was normal. The hemoglobin was 12.0 g dL^{-1}, platelet count 35 × 10^9 L^{-1} and the white blood cell count 8.0 × 10^9 L^{-1}; 66% of the cells were neutrophils. Blood sugar was 57.6 mg dL^{-1} [3.2 mmol L^{-1}] and he was given a bolus of 50% dextrose on each occasion this fell below [3.5 mmol L^{-1}] thereafter. Serum phosphate was 0.4 mmol L^{-1} [1.2 mg dL^{-1}] and this was corrected.

He was started on N-acetylcysteine. A central line was inserted revealing marked hypovolemia with a central venous pressure of –1 cmH$_2$O. He was resuscitated with human serum albumin, but he did not pass urine and no urine could be obtained subsequently for the measurement of urinary electrolytes or culture. Chest radiograph was normal. His pH was 7.35 [H^+ 45 nmol L^{-1}] after resuscitation.

A psychiatric opinion was sought urgently; regrettably, by the time the patient was reviewed his clinical condition had deteriorated and psychiatric assessment was not possible. However, because of his deterioration in mental status he was reviewed jointly by the physicians and surgeons and a decision made to list the patient for transplantation; he had expressed regret at his impulsive action. Concomitant pancreatitis, a common complication, was excluded by estimate of serum amylase. His blood group was found to be O+.

Four hours after admission to the general medical ward he was in grade III coma and the nurse attending the patient noticed that he was developing extensor posturing and grinding his teeth. He was therefore electively ventilated although at that stage there was no evidence of hypoxia and there had been no immediate threat to his airway. His temperature had remained elevated since admission and he was started on cefotaxime and azlocillin. Continuous veno-venous hemodiafiltration was started and a pulmonary artery catheter was inserted with the aim of keeping his pulmonary artery occlusion pressure between 5 and 10 mmHg. He remained oliguric.

Twelve hours after his admission to the intensive care unit he became significantly pyrexial with a temperature of 38.5°C and flucloxacillin was added to the regimen. At this stage he had begun to develop episodes of systolic hypertension lasting a few minutes at a time, with the systolic blood pressure increasing to between 200 and 230 mmHg. In view of this, an extradural intracranial pressure (ICP) monitor was inserted. At this point the prothrombin time was 200 s but his platelet count had improved to 64 × $10^9 L^{-1}$.

He remained on continuous veno-venous hemodiafiltration with heparin cover, and episodes of cerebral edema were treated first with 20% mannitol given in 50–100 mL boluses. On each occasion that mannitol was prescribed, 300 mL of fluid was withdrawn by hemodiafiltration. The patient's position was 30° from the horizontal, head-up and he was nursed still, without stimuli. Tracheal suction was only performed when essential. It was always preceded by nebulized lidocaine [lignocaine] to prevent increases in ICP. The patient was not turned on any occasion. The urinary catheter was removed because he was anuric. Routine cultures were performed daily of blood and sputum when available.

Twenty-four hours after admission to the intensive care unit the evidence was of intracranial hypertension was worsening. Initially when the pressure monitor had been inserted, each increase in ICP had been accompanied by an increase in the systolic blood pressure such that the cerebral perfusion pressure had remained unaltered. However, at this stage episodes of intracranial hypertension were not accompanied by an increase in systolic blood pressure such that each episode of intracranial hypertension was compromising cerebral perfusion pressure. In addition mannitol, which had been administered on seven occasions to this stage (without change in osmolality) was no longer effective. He was therefore treated with a thiopentone infusion.

Traps

Many mistakes are made in the management of patients following a paracetamol overdose. There is an over-reliance on nomograms which indicate the relationship between the plasma level of paracetamol and the time from overdose. Patients who have taken overdoses may be unreliable. In addition, ingestion of alcohol may delay absorption of paracetamol into the bloodstream.

Further, there are important effects of enzyme induction. Phenytoin augments the metabolism of paracetamol through toxic pathways to create the noxious metabolite NAPQI (*N*-Acetylparabenzoquinonimine). This is also true in alcoholics. Other enzyme inducers have a similar effect. This means that it is possible to develop liver failure on smaller doses of paracetamol and indeed to develop liver damage at levels that in other patients would not be harmful according to the nomogram.

It is another common misconception that paracetamol persists in the blood and tissues of patients who have taken a paracetamol overdose. It is not; it is cleared rapidly. It is the metabolism through the noxious pathway that is critical. Early administration of *N*-acetylcysteine to all patients except those categorically *not* at risk is recommended. In addition, it should routinely be used in all those with acute liver failure where it has been shown to have proven value.

A further trap is in assessment. It is essential to attempt to correct the PT with vitamin K before making a decision about transplantation. Sometimes the PT will correct and liver failure may not be the only cause of coma. Another absolute indication for transplantation, psychological factors permitting, is the presence of acidosis but this should be estimated after resuscitation. Persistent acidosis after resuscitation carries a very grim prognosis indeed.

The criteria used to identify those at risk are occasionally used incorrectly. Once a patient develops renal impairment, a PT of >100 s and grade III hepatic coma, the risk of death without transplant greatly exceeds that with a transplant. Even if the PT improves (and it usually will) and falls below 100 s, the risk of death has not changed for that patient.

The classic signs of bacterial and fungal infection are absent in this immunocompromised group and they are therefore often missed. The only approach to diagnosing infection is routine culture, with early intervention with antimicrobial agents at the slightest hint of sepsis. Chest, urine and lines are all common sources of infection. Staphylococcal and Gram-negative infection are most commonly identified; fungal infection complicates about a third of those with hepatic and renal failure.

Intracranial pressure monitoring appears fraught with danger but in experienced hands it is a reliable and useful tool. It would be difficult now to imagine taking such a patient to theater for transplantation without this being available. Prior to transplantation the use of ICP monitoring increases the number of times in which therapy for intracranial hypertension is given and in combination with therapy buys probably between 10 and 24 hours. Mannitol is safe to use and has been shown to increase cerebral blood flow. However, osmolality must be checked and it will be necessary to remove fluid on each occasion that mannitol is given. If it is not effective there is little point in continuing it and at this stage the only remaining therapy is thiopentone. In other respects failure to pay attention to important factors such as position, stimulation, blood pressure and oxygenation is lethal.

Another trap for the unwary is in the postoperative period following liver transplantation. Even in the presence of early graft function the patient remains at risk of intracranial hypertension for about 24 hours after the procedure. Patients have died from intracranial hypertension at this stage and it is probably here as much as during the operation that ICP measurement remains beneficial.

Tricks

A patient with a prothrombin time over 100 s, grade III hepatic coma and renal impairment has an extremely poor prognosis and requires to be recognized at an early stage so that transplantation can be recommended where pertinent. Hepatic coma is one of the indications for transplantation and because of this great care must be taken to ensure that other causes of coma are excluded. Thus plasma glucose and serum phosphate need to be checked regularly and corrected. Both are very common and hypophosphatemia is especially common with paracetamol overdose. Most centers attempt psychiatric assessment before listing but this is not always possible in the time available. It is essential to make an assessment of long-term psychiatric outcome at the earliest possible opportunity recognizing that a later, more formal assessment may not be possible. N-Acetylcysteine has been shown to increase survival in patients with acute liver failure caused by paracetamol poisoning even when given 36 hours after the overdose and at a stage when paracetamol has already been metabolized.

It is essential to recognize that patients deteriorate rapidly. Patients should not wait until they are in frank respiratory failure needing emergency tracheal intubation. In the context of intracranial hypertension emergency tracheal intubation is likely to be disastrous. An early move to ventilatory support is therefore recommended, as in this patient. First-line therapy for intracranial hypertension is the use of mannitol. Clearly, in a patient with renal impairment it is essential in addition to remove water and to check and maintain osmolality. It cannot be emphasized too strongly that the maintenance of blood pressure and oxygenation are critical.

Bacterial infection is particularly common in patients with acute liver failure. The white cell count and temperature are not good indicators of infection. It must be sought by cultures taken according to a protocol. The commonest organism grown is *Staphylococcus aureus* which may be grown from blood lines or chest and, although broad-spectrum cover is required immediately after tracheal intubation, the majority of infections are likely to be *Staphylococcus aureus*. In a patient who has renal impairment, fungal infection is also common. This is particularly true once thiopentone has been used because this causes a severe functional impairment of the macrophages and polymorphs, and prophylactic antifungal agents are probably recommended at this stage although not yet proven by clinical trial.

The decision to insert an ICP monitor is not an easy one. Understandably, many neurosurgeons are anxious about dealing with patients who are frequently thrombocytopenic – a common feature of paracetamol overdose – and have prolonged clotting times. In practice, the majority of the bleeds occur in the patients who are thrombocytopenic. This patient's platelet count had recovered by the time the ICP monitor was inserted and although the PT was not corrected in this particular patient many centers will correct the PT before any procedures are undertaken. In practice, such patients do not bleed as a result of the prolonged PT.

In this situation where the decision to transplant had already been made, however, it would have been more excusable to use fresh frozen plasma to correct the PT before inserting an ICP monitor. In a patient in whom the decision has not already been made, the PT is critical in making a decision, and to modify this unnecessarily makes the decision to proceed to transplant even harder and will inevitably cause delay.

Recognition that the cerebral pressure is being compromised because it is no longer possible to protect the cerebral circulation by reflex hypertension is an important point in the clinical course. Once this point arrives there is little time available before death or definitive therapy (transplantation) and it is essential that patients go to theater in the best possible condition.

Follow-up

Fortuitously a donor liver became available. The patient was able to undergo an orthotopic liver transplant six hours after starting thiopentone, which was continued during the procedure.

After the operation he had two further episodes of intracranial hypertension 4 and 8 h postoperatively but thereafter there was no further compromise and, after a protracted illness complicated by sepsis and prolonged weaning period from ventilation, the patient was eventually discharged. Six months after medical discharge he was discharged from the psychiatric clinic.

Bibliography

1 Forbes A, Alexander G, O'Grady J, Keays R, Gullan R, Dawling S and Williams R. Thiopental infusion in the treatment of intracranial hypertension complicating fulminant hepatic failure. *Hepatology* (1989) **3**: 306–310.
2 Harrison P, Wendon J, Gimson A, Alexander G and Williams R. Improvement by acetylcysteine of haemodynamics and oxygen transport in fulminant hepatic failure. *New England Journal of Medicine* (1991) **324**: 1852–1857.
3 Keays R, Alexander G and Williams R. The safety and value of extradural intracranial pressure monitors in fulminant hepatic failure. *Journal of Hepatology* (1993) **18**: 205–209.
4 Keays R, Harrison P, Wendon J, Forbes A, Gove C, Alexander G and Williams R. Intravenous acetylcysteine in paracetamol induced fulminant hepatic failure: a prospective controlled trial. *British Medical Journal* (1991) **303**: 1026–1029.
5 Keays R, Potter D, O'Grady J, Peachey T, Alexander G and Williams R. Intracranial

and cerebral perfusion pressure changes before, during and immediately after orthotopic liver transplantation for fulminant hepatic failure. *Quarterly Journal of Medicine* (1991) **79**: 425–433.

6 O'Grady J, Alexander G, Hayllar K and Williams R. Early indicators of prognosis in fulminant hepatic failure. *Gastroenterology* (1989) **97**: 439–445.

7 Rolando N, Harvey F, Brahm J, Philpott-Howard J, Alexander G and Williams R. Fungal infection: a common, unrecognised complication of acute liver failure. *Journal of Hepatology* (1991) **12**: 1–9.

8 Rolando N, Harvey F, Brahm J, Philpott-Howard J, Alexander G, Gimson A, Casewell M, Fagan E and Williams R. Prospective study of bacterial infection in acute liver failure: an analysis of fifty patients. *Hepatology* (1990) **11**: 49–53.

5.3 Hypotension Complicating Chronic Liver Disease
Graeme J.M. Alexander

History

A 35-year-old male publican with a long history of alcohol abuse was found semi-conscious by his wife. He was admitted directly to the intensive care unit. There, because of hypoxemia, he was immediately ventilated.

On review, the patient was not anemic but was deeply jaundiced with numerous stigmata of chronic liver disease including palmar erythema, spider nevi, parotid enlargement, hepatosplenomegaly, modest ascites and peripheral edema. His pulse was 85/minute, temperature 38.2°C [100.8°F] and the blood pressure 90/60 mmHg after resuscitation. There were no additional heart sounds but there were widespread crackles throughout both lung fields. A nasogastric tube had been inserted at the time of admission and the gastric aspirate was vast containing fluid which was positive on occult blood testing.

Investigations at this time showed: hemoglobin $8.2\,g\,dL^{-1}$, white blood cell count of $22.3 \times 10^9\,L^{-1}$, 90% neutrophils, platelet $65 \times 10^9\,L^{-1}$, urea $19\,mmol\,L^{-1}$ [$114\,mg\,dL^{-1}$] (increasing on day 2 to $23\,mmol\,L^{-1}$ [$138\,mg\,dL^{-1}$]). Blood chemistry: creatinine $176\,\mu mol\,L^{-1}$ [$2.3\,mg\,dL^{-1}$], urinary sodium $4\,mmol\,L^{-1}$, urine volume $400\,mL$ in the first 24 hours, bilirubin $195\,\mu mol\,L^{-1}$ [$11.5\,mg\,dL^{-1}$], alanine aminotransferase (ALT) $132\,U\,L^{-1}$, albumin $28\,g\,L^{-1}$, alkaline phosphatase $115\,U\,L^{-1}$, plasma sodium $128\,mmol\,L^{-1}$, serum alpha feta protein normal. Plasma potassium was $4.3\,mmol\,L^{-1}$, prothrombin time (PT) 23 s. An ascitic tap was negative for cells, negative on culture and blood culture was negative.

A chest radiograph showed diffuse bilateral infiltrates consistent with an infectious process. Ultrasound of the abdomen showed a hyperechoic liver with hepatofugal flow, splenomegaly and moderate ascites. The kidney size was normal.

A diagnosis of acute alcoholic hepatitis was made and in view of the high bilirubin and prolonged PT he was started on prednisolone 40 mg daily. There was a suspicion that he had had a gastrointestinal hemorrhage and that this formed the basis of his acute deterioration, hypotension and encephalopathy. Supporting this diagnosis were the reduced hemoglobin and the increased blood urea, disproportionate to the elevation of serum creatinine. He was therefore started on an H_2-blocker and underwent a diagnostic endoscopy. This showed a small amount of blood within the stomach and multiple gastric erosions and small varices which had probably not bled.

In view of the increased temperature, broad-spectrum antibiotics were started. In addition, metronidazole was prescribed for a presumed aspiration pneumonia. However, ascitic fluid remained negative on culture, blood cultures were consistently negative and the white blood cell count remained elevated over the next four days. He remained pyrexial over that same period, but no cultures at any stage proved positive.

Traps

The features used to identify infection (increased white blood cell count, pyrexia and change in hemodynamic status) are unreliable in both acute and chronic liver disease and particularly in alcoholic liver disease, probably because of the very high cytokine levels in alcoholic hepatitis. However, on a practical level missing infection is more dangerous than treating infection when it is not present and it is preferable to use antimicrobial therapy.

A decision to proceed to transplantation also needs to be made at an early stage. Combined use of PT and bilirubin identifies those at risk of death. Those with evidence of evolving multiorgan failure have little chance of survival. In addition, recognition of a significant risk of alcohol abuse subsequent to transplantation should discourage referral. Factors of note include social and professional stability.

Tricks

Alcoholic hepatitis is a common, often unrecognized, complication of alcohol abuse characterized by an increased bilirubin, pyrexia and an elevated white blood cell count. The latter is probably caused by high levels of circulating interleukin 8. Characteristically, the ALT is only modestly elevated and many assume that in the absence of an elevated ALT liver damage cannot be severe. A combination of an elevated bilirubin and a prolonged PT suggest a poor prognosis with alcoholic hepatitis and in the presence of overt sepsis and other infections (such as in this case, aspiration pneumonia) the prognosis is very poor. Corticosteroids are recommended and have been shown to be effective by meta-analysis. However, patients with diabetes, active bleeding and active sepsis were excluded from the clinical trials and treating such patients with corticosteroids while logical, is not yet supported by clinical trials.

The diagnosis of an acute gastrointestinal bleed can sometimes be a very difficult one to make. Many patients with alcoholic liver disease have alcoholic gastritis and have increased incidence of a peptic ulcer. The presence of gastritis or peptic ulceration does not necessarily mean that that is the cause of the deterioration and an endoscopy is essential if bleeding is being considered as a realistic diagnosis. If the patient had had evidence of bleeding then direct injection into the site of a bleeding ulcer or of bleeding varices would have been appropriate. Hypotension and tachycardia are a feature of the underlying liver disease and cannot be assumed to be a reflection of gastrointestinal bleeding.

Sepsis in any form of chronic liver failure is common and alcoholics have poor immune function and are predisposed to bacterial infections. However, the high white blood cell count and the pyrexia are features of underlying alcoholic hepatitis and, again, in this group it is almost impossible to differentiate between clinical sepsis and uncomplicated alcoholic hepatitis. In that situation regular cultures are essential.

This particular patient also suffered from probable hepatorenal failure. On admission he was hypotensive, with a low urinary sodium, but after correction of hypovolemia the low urinary sodium persisted.

Distinguishing between the various causes of hypotension complicating chronic liver disease can be surprisingly difficult. Sepsis and gastrointestinal bleeding commonly occur together and such patients are likely to have the underlying hemodynamic change characteristic of cirrhosis (tachycardia, hypotension and a low systemic vascular resistance). The value of accurate hemodynamic monitoring cannot be stressed enough and routine use of pulmonary artery catheterization in this group is usually rewarding and is particularly valuable in protecting renal function. Alcohol may, in addition, cause cardiomyopathy which can make management especially difficult.

Follow-up

After ventilation he developed acute respiratory distress syndrome and died four days after admission.

Bibliography

1 Bird G, Sheron N, Goka J, Alexander G and Williams R. Increased plasma tumour necrosis factor in severe alcoholic hepatitis. *Annals of Internal Medicine* (1990) **112**: 917–920.

2 Carithers RL, Herlong HF, Diehl AM, *et al.* Methylprednisolone therapy in patients with severe alcoholic hepatitis. A randomised multicentre trial. *Annals of Internal Medicine* (1989) **110**: 685.

3 Imperiale TF and McCullough AJ. Do corticosteroids reduce mortality from alcoholic hepatitis? A meta analysis of the randomised trials. *Annals of Internal Medicine* (1990) **113**: 299.

4 Ramond M, Poynard T, Rueff B, *et al.* A randomised trial of prednisolone in patients with severe acute alcoholic hepatitis. *New England Journal of Medicine* (1992) **326**: 507.

5 Sheron N, Bird G, Goka J, Alexander G and Williams R. Elevated plasma interleukin-6 levels and increased severity and mortality in alcoholic hepatitis. *Clinical Experiments in Immunology* (1991) **84**: 449–453.

5.4 Hemorrhage in a Cirrhotic
Graeme J.M. Alexander

History

A 58-year-old Indian woman presented one month before with her first variceal hemorrhage. At this time a cryptogenic cirrhosis was diagnosed. Following treatment with Octreotide she had undergone a course of injection sclerotherapy. Despite this, she continued to bleed and had therefore been considered for an emergency shunt procedure transjugular intrahepatic portosystemic (TIPSS). This involves placing a stent percutaneously, usually linking a hepatic vein to a branch of the right portal vein. A Doppler ultrasound performed after this procedure showed hepatopetal flow through the shunt. Ten days later she had had a further small upper gastrointestinal hemorrhage and at endoscopy she was shown to have severe esophageal ulceration at the site of injection sclerotherapy. This was treated with omeprazole and sucralfate. She was subsequently discharged three weeks after the initial hemorrhage.

At that stage there was no ascites and no encephalopathy. Her liver function tests had shown a prolongation of the prothrombin time (PT) to 28 s during the acute stage of the illness settling to 20 s at the time of discharge, and a bilirubin during the acute illness had increased to 8.8 mg dL^{-1} [150 µmol L^{-1}] and had decreased to 2.9 mg dL^{-1} [50 µmol L^{-1}] by the time of discharge. The plasma concentration of albumin was between 22 and 28 g L^{-1} throughout her initial stay. The other liver enzymes were normal. Serum alpha feta protein (AFP) was normal and the ultrasound performed to examine the shunt had revealed no evidence of a focal lesion within the liver.

She was subsequently readmitted one month after the first hemorrhage. On admission she was hypotensive with a blood pressure of 80/55 mmHg, with a pulse of 110/minute, apyrexial and was confused in grade II coma. There was a marked hepatic flap. She was cyanosed. Examination of the chest showed the cardiovascular system to be otherwise normal. The abdomen had a modest amount of ascites. The liver could still be felt and there had been no change in the size; the spleen was enlarged. There was no peripheral edema, however. Rectal examination revealed no evidence of melaena. She was oliguric.

Laboratory investigations showed: hemoglobin 10.9 g dL^{-1}, white blood cell count 1.8 × 10^9 L^{-1}, 65% neutrophils. The platelet count was 35 × 10^9 L^{-1}. The PT was prolonged at 33 s. The serum albumin concentration was 26 g L^{-1}, bilirubin 85 µmol L^{-1} [5 mmol L^{-1}]. ALT, AST and alkaline phosphatase were normal. AFP <10 ng L^{-1}, sodium 134 mmol L^{-1}, potassium 4.2 mmol L^{-1}, urea 2.8 mmol L^{-1}, [BUN 16.8 mg dL^{-1}], creatinine 145 µmol L^{-1} [1.88 mg dL^{-1}], urinary sodium <10 mmol L^{-1}.

A chest radiograph and urine culture were normal.

The differential diagnosis at this stage included a further gastrointestinal hemorrhage either from varices (because of poor shunt function), or sepsis, and hepatic encephalopathy unrelated to either of these events.

Immediate treatment included the insertion of a central line. This showed that she was hypovolemic. Her volume status was restored to normal with 4.5% human serum albumin. Although there was no evidence of clinical sepsis, she was treated with broad-spectrum antibiotics. After resuscitation she remained oliguric and encephalopathic.

Although the platelet count had been low and the prothrombin time elevated on the initial admission, on this occasion a search for disseminated intravascular coagulation was undertaken. This revealed that her fibrinogen was $0.3\,\text{g}\,\text{L}^{-1}$ (low) lower than on her initial admission $(0.87\,\text{g}\,\text{L}^{-1})$ and she had markedly elevated fibrinogen degradation products.

Traps

This patient should have been considered for liver transplantation at an earlier stage. The insertion of a TIPSS stent shunt can be a life-saving procedure. However, this patient had evidence of severe decompensation around the time of the gastrointestinal hemorrhage and it was most unlikely that she was going to survive long term without a liver transplant being performed. The TIPSS should therefore have been considered as a temporising procedure rather than a definitive treatment procedure in itself. The most important point to make about stent shunt procedures is to assess the overall state of the patient in other respects. The presence of a prolonged PT and the development of jaundice at the time of the hemorrhage indicates that there was very little hepatic reserve.

An important decision to make the second time the patient is reviewed is whether to proceed with the stent and so attempt to recannulate the existing stent. In the presence of DIC this would be regarded as extremely risky. The more direct option would be to proceed to liver transplantation at the earliest opportunity.

Tricks

It is almost impossible to make a diagnosis of sepsis on clinical criteria alone. In this patient the low white cell count could have been a reflection of severe sepsis and the disseminated intravascular coagulation would certainly have accounted in part for the low platelet count and the increased PT. However, she was always apyrexial. An ascitic tap was performed that showed no white cells and blood cultures remained persistently negative. It is not inappropriate, however, to treat for sepsis in someone as ill as this, but on this occasion no infection was identified.

There was no evidence of electrolyte imbalance on admission although there was renal impairment with oliguria. This failed to respond to resuscitation and indeed even the addition of dopamine at a low dose had no effect on her urine output. The likely cause for her oliguria was hepatorenal failure. In this situation an expectant policy can be employed. If she had had a gastrointestinal hemorrhage underlying this particular admission then a component of acute tubular necrosis would have been more likely; again, an expectant policy can be employed in most of these cases. The absence of a defined electrolyte abnormality on routine urea and electrolyte estimation does not exclude more subtle abnormalities, and serum magnesium and phosphate should be sought in all cases. In this particular patient the serum magnesium was marginally reduced as was the serum zinc. Both these findings are fairly typical for severe liver disease. Phosphate was in the normal range.

The more likely cause of encephalopathy arising *de novo* in this particular setting is the presence of portocaval shunting. The use of expandable stents means that the diameter of the stent can be increased to ensure adequate flow and the stents can be inserted at as narrow a diameter as possible at the early stages. The greater the diameter the more likely the encephalopathy is to occur. However, in this situation an alternative explanation can be offered. The presence of DIC in the absence of sepsis is one of the well-recognized features that complicate occlusion of the shunt.

Critical to both these diagnoses was the performance of Doppler ultrasound. This revealed that the stent shunt was no longer patent.

Follow-up

The patient underwent liver transplantation with a very satisfactory outcome.

Bibliography

1 Blei AT. Vasopressin analogues in portal hypertension: different molecules but similar questions. *Hepatology* (1986) **6**: 146.
2 Bosch J, Groszmann RJ, Garcia-Pagan JC, *et al*. Addition of transdermal nitroglycerin to vasopressin infusion in the treatment of variceal hemorrhage: a placebo controlled trial. *Hematology* (1989) **10**: 962.
3 Burroughs AK, McCormick PA, Hughes MD, *et al*. Randomised, double blind, placebo controlled trial of somatostatin for variceal bleeding. Emergency control and prevention of early variceal rebleeding. *Gastroenterology* (1990) **99**: 1388.
4 Goff JS, Reveille RM and van Stiegmann GV. Endoscopic sclerotherapy versus endoscopic variceal ligation: oesophageal symptoms, complications and motility. *American Journal of Gastroenterology* (1988) **83**: 1240.
5 Ring EJ, Lake JR, Roberts JP, *et al*. Using transjugular intrahepatic portosystemic shunts to control variceal bleeding before transplantation. *Annals of Internal Medicine* (1992) **116**: 304.

5.5 Water, Electrolyte and Acid–Base Balance in Hepatic Cirrhosis

John A. Kellum and David J. Kramer

History

A 56-year-old male with alcoholic cirrhosis was admitted to the intensive care unit (ICU) with hypotension and a metabolic acidosis. Two months before this, he presented to his internist with a tense abdomen and decreased urine output. An abdominal ultrasound showed massive ascites and a small cirrhotic liver. Mild hydronephrosis of the right kidney was also noted. A diagnostic paracentesis was performed and 1 liter of clear fluid was removed. Bacterial cultures were sterile. Following this, the patient was placed on furosemide [frusemide] 40 mg orally every 12 hours and spironolactone 50 mg orally every 12 hours. The patient returned to his internist one month later with lethargy and confusion. A serum ammonia level was measured at 43 μmol L^{-1}, so the patient was started on lactulose 30 mL orally every 8 hours.

One week before admission, the patient presented to the emergency department with worsening symptoms as well as decreasing appetite and urine output. He continued to have tense ascites. A repeat diagnostic paracentesis showed no change in the fluid characteristics and repeat cultures were negative. Serum electrolytes revealed the following: sodium 119 mEq L^{-1}, potassium 4.0 mEq L^{-1}, chloride 87 mEq L^{-1}, and bicarbonate 20 mEq L^{-1}.

The patient was admitted to the hospital. A physical examination revealed a supine arterial blood pressure of 100/50 mmHg, heart rate of 108/minute and temperature of 37.3°C [99.1°F]. He was mildly encephalopathic. The lungs were clear, and examination of the heart was normal. There was no jugular venous distension and the abdomen was firm and protuberant. A fluid wave was easily demonstrable. Spider angiomata were present on the chest, back and abdomen. There was mild peripheral edema.

Additional laboratory data included a BUN of 74 mg dL^{-1} [12.3 mmol L^{-1}] and creatinine of 1.9 mg dL^{-1} [145 μmol L^{-1}]. The white blood cell count was 8.9 × 10^3 L^{-1}, and the hemoglobin and hematocrit were 8.8 g dL^{-1} and 30%. Liver function studies showed an alanine aminotransferase of 55 U L^{-1}, aspartate aminotransferase of 80 U L^{-1}, alkaline phosphatase of 135 mU mL^{-1} and a total bilirubin of 3.4 mg dL^{-1} [57.8 μmol L^{-1}]. The serum albumin was 2.2 g dL^{-1} [22 g L^{-1}] and the prothrombin time (PT) was 14.2 s.

Because of the presence of massive ascites and peripheral edema, the patient's hyponatremia was judged to be dilutional and his furosemide was increased to 80 mg IV twice daily. Free water restriction was also instituted. The urine output did not increase substantially and on the third hospital day the electrolytes were relatively unchanged (sodium 120 mEq L^{-1}, potassium 3.3 mEq L^{-1}, chloride 88 mEq L^{-1}, bicarbonate 20 mEq L^{-1}). The peripheral edema had resolved, however. A repeat abdominal ultrasound showed worsening hydronephrosis on the right and new, mild hydronephrosis on the left. A decision was made to carry out large-volume paracentesis to reduce the pressure in the pelvis and reduce the hydronephrosis. After replacement of potassium with 40 mEq IV over 2 hours, paracentesis was performed and 7 L of ascites fluid was removed over a 3-hour period.

Following paracentesis, the patient's blood pressure was 76/38 mmHg, pulse of 123/minute. One liter of 0.9% saline was given IV over 20 minutes with little change in blood pressure. A second liter of saline was given over the next hour when the patient's heart rate increased to 160/minute and the blood pressure decreased to 50/30 mmHg. An ECG showed ventricular tachycardia which was treated successfully with electrocardioversion. A third liter of saline and lidocaine [lignocaine] 100 mg IV bolus and oxygen 4 L min^{-1} by nasal cannula were started and the patient was transferred to the ICU.

On arrival in the ICU, the patient's blood pressure was 70/35 mmHg, pulse of 132/minute. A fourth liter of saline was given and an arterial blood gas was pH 7.22 [H$^+$ 60 nmol L^{-1}], P_aCO_2 30 mmHg [4 kPa], P_aO_2 118 mmHg [15.7 kPa]. The blood pressure was still low at 85/40 mmHg, so dopamine was begun at 10 µg kg^{-1} min^{-1}. The metabolic acidosis was attributed to hypoperfusion, secondary to shock, and additional volume was given to a total of 6 L of saline. Serum electrolytes were then measured (sodium 127 mEq L^{-1}, potassium 3.5 mEq L^{-1}, chloride 100 mEq L^{-1} bicarbonate 14 mEq L^{-1}). An arterial blood gas showed a pH of 7.19 [H$^+$ 65 nmol L^{-1}]. The patient's trachea was intubated, and he was begun on a continuous infusion of sodium bicarbonate 150 mEq L^{-1} at 200 mL h^{-1} for 'refractory' acidosis. With these measures the patient's pH and bicarbonate levels returned to normal. However, his serum sodium concentration reached 141 mEq L^{-1} over the next 24 hours.

Traps

Controversy exists about the intravascular volume status of patients with cirrhosis. The presence of ascites and peripheral edema show an increased total body water and sodium. Indeed, disordered free water excretion has been described by Bichet *et al.* However, typically there are low filling pressures, low urine output and sodium retention. In addition, plasma concentrations and vasoactive hormones, such as angiotensin and norepinephrine [noradrenaline] are elevated, and the prostaglandin balance favors vasoconstriction (e.g. urinary PGF_2 is elevated relative to PGE_1). This evidence suggests that despite increased total body water and sodium, intravascular volume (effective circulating volume) is decreased. These physiologic derangements begin with portal hypertension and are exacerbated by hypoalbuminemia. Diuretics further decrease the effective circulating volume and may worsen azotemia. Deranged free water handling, secondary to antidiuretic hormone excess because of thirst, and increased free water intake result in more severe hyponatremia.

Large-volume paracentesis is the treatment of choice for tense ascites.

However, prior treatment with diuretics, which further reduce intravascular volume, increases the risk of circulatory collapse and acute tubular injury to the kidney. The abrupt release of tense ascites is similar to undoing MAST (military anti-shock trousers). There is a prompt decrease in systemic vascular resistance and hypotension results. This can be avoided by volume loading before or with paracentesis. Alternatively, fluid may be removed more slowly.

The acidosis in this case was mostly caused by saline resuscitation. As a result of the reduced albumin and hemoglobin concentrations, the buffering capacity of the blood is markedly reduced. As a consequence, patients are particularly susceptible to 'dilutional' or 'rehydration' acidosis. This non-anion gap metabolic acidosis occurs as a result of fluid administration that is acidic relative to blood (0.9% saline has a pH <7.0 [H^+ 100 mmol L^{-1}]). Usually, massive doses (several liters) are needed to significantly lower the pH. However, in situations such as this, where the buffering capacity is reduced, dilutional acidosis may occur more readily. A simple explanation for this is that the bicarbonate is diluted by the addition of fluids that are non-bicarbonate containing. A more precise explanation, however, is that the relative concentrations of sodium and chloride, the two major extracellular ions, are changed by the addition of saline. This relative increase in the chloride concentration tends to promote greater water dissociation and hence an increased free hydrogen ion concentration.

The frequent assumption that the acidosis represents under-resuscitation and tissue hypoxia is invalid in this patient. Lactic acidosis invariably produces an increase in the anion gap. However, a note of caution should be made here. Hypoalbuminemia is frequently associated with a decreased anion gap. Therefore, a normal anion gap acidosis might still represent increased (unmeasured) anions in this patient population. The mild hypotension seen in these patients will frequently fail to respond to volume until massive quantities are used. If crystalloid is used (particularly saline), dilutional acidosis may result. The acidosis itself may also have contributed to the hemodynamic instability.

The arrhythmia this patient experienced was secondary to magnesium deficiency. Alcoholic patients and those treated with loop diuretics are at particular risk. However, this population is also at risk for development of dilated cardiomyopathy and ventricular tachycardia is a frequent manifestation. The differential diagnosis would also include decreased coronary artery perfusion, even though this patient had no history of coronary artery disease.

Tricks

Large-volume paracentesis should be used as the primary therapy for symptomatic ascites. Patients (especially those without peripheral edema) should be given colloid solutions to replace intravascular volume as the ascites is drained[1].

Patients with end-stage liver disease have a primary excess in aldosterone. They have low intravascular volume and elevated renin/angiotensin levels[8]. This occurs despite total body water and total body sodium overload. Treatment with spironolactone (especially in addition to a loop diuretic) will produce a state of *intravascular* water and sodium depletion. It will usually reduce ascites, but only in addition to these effects. Spironolactone will produce a mild non-anion gap metabolic acidosis and may mask the 'contraction alkalosis' which is mediated by aldosterone[2,4,5].

Resuscitation in hypoalbuminemic patients with large volumes of 0.9% saline will be fraught with difficulties. The acidosis can be avoided by selecting smaller volumes of colloid solutions, such as 5% albumin, or by using lactated Ringer's solution (even in patients with liver disease). Lactated Ringer's causes less acidosis because lactate makes up part of the anion load instead of chloride and lactate is quickly metabolized, even in patients with cirrhosis. In any case, one should not assume that the metabolic acidosis is from lactate or other sources secondary to hypoperfusion[7].

Magnesium replacement is particularly important. Even if the serum magnesium level is normal, total body magnesium can be deficient. Empiric treatment with magnesium is generally a safer approach. Magnesium 40–112 mg dL^{-1}, [8–16 mmol L^{-1}] [2–4 g of MgSO$_4$] can be given safely over 2 hours intravenously. Patients with renal failure may require smaller doses[6].

Large sodium shifts can occur with sodium bicarbonate. They are less likely to occur with use of colloid or lactated Ringer's solutions. Careful monitoring of the sodium concentration is advisable in any case as rapid shifts may result in significant neurologic injury (central pontine myelinolysis)[3].

Follow-up

The patient eventually returned to his prehospital condition. However, he was put at substantial risk for renal failure, from the sudden decrease in circulating volume. It is worth noting, however, that his renal function did improve after his ill-fated paracentesis. This is commonly seen and secondary to the improvement in renal perfusion that occurs following relief of tense ascites.

He was also put at risk for central pontine damage from the rapid sodium fluxes (119 to 141 mEq L^{-1} in 24 hours).

References

1 Gines P, *et al.* Comparison of paracentesis and diuretics in the treatment of cirrhotics with tense acites. Results of a randomized study. *Gastroenterology* (1987) **93**: 234–241.

2 Narins RG, *et al.* Diagnostic strategies in disorders of fluid, electrolyte, and acid–base homeostasis. *American Journal of Medicine* (1982) **72**: 496.

3 Sterns RH. Severe symptomatic hyponatremia: treatment and outcome. A study of 64 cases. *Annals of Internal Medicine* (1987) **107**: 656.

4 Bichet D, Szatalowky V, Chaimovitis C and Schrier RW. Role of vasopressin in abnormal water excretion in cirrhotic patients. *Annals of Internal Medicine* (1982) **96**: 413.

5 Rosoff L, *et al.* Studies of renin and aldosterone in cirrhotic patients with ascites. *Gastroenterology* (1975) **69**: 698.

6 Pin L and Jacob E. Magnesium deficiency in liver cirrhosis. *Quarterly Journal of Medicine* (1972) **41**: 291.
7 Adrogue HJ, *et al.* Plasma acid–base patterns in diabetic ketoacidosis. *New England Journal of Medicine* (1982) **307**: 1603.
8 Wong PY, Talamo RC and Williams GH. Kallikrein-kinin and reninangiotensin systems in functional renal failure of cirrhosis of the liver. *Gastroenterology* (1977) **73**: 1114.

6 Renal Failure

6.1 Maintaining Renal Perfusion Pressure
Rinaldo Bellomo

History

A 29-year-old man was admitted to hospital through the emergency room after a motor vehicle accident. He had a blood pressure of 110/60 mmHg, a pulse rate of 115/minute, and a respiratory rate of 28/minute. His Glasgow coma scale was 12. A chest radiograph showed fractures of the lateral aspects of the 6th, 7th and 8th left ribs. Abdominal examination was suggestive of an acute abdomen and a peritoneal lavage was positive for blood. After resuscitation in the emergency room, which included tracheal intubation, insertion of an arterial line, and an urgent head CT scan (showing no gross intracranial pathology), the patient was taken to the operating room. After removal of a ruptured spleen and repair of two liver lacerations he was returned to the intensive care unit He remained intubated, was sedated and had a pulmonary artery catheter in place.

Twenty-four hours after admission his mental state had improved, but he remained on mechanical ventilation for worsening hypoxemia and his chest radiograph showed changes suggestive of right lower lobe, superior segment pneumonia and diffuse bilateral infiltrates consistent with acute lung injury. His abdomen was noted to be distended. He had a fever of 39°C [102.2°F], a moderately elevated partial thromboplastin time of 45 seconds and an INR of 2.1. One unit of packed red blood cells was needed over 12 hours to maintain a hematocrit of 29%. His cardiac index was $3.9 \, L \, min^{-1} \, min^{-2}$, right atrial pressure 12 mmHg and pulmonary artery occlusion pressure (PAOP) 16 mmHg. Systemic blood pressure was 100/40 mmHg. Urinary output, which had been $75 \, mL \, h^{-1}$ 6 hours before, had decreased to $10 \, mL \, h^{-1}$ for the last 2 hours. Dopamine $2 \, \mu g \, kg^{-1} \, min^{-1}$ was started. Over the following 4 hours there were no appreciable changes in hemodynamic variables and in urinary output. A 500 mL challenge of IV colloids was given over 30 minutes. His right atrial pressure transiently increased to 14 mmHg and his PAOP to 19 mmHg, with an increase in his cardiac index to $4.3 \, L \, min^{-1} \, m^{-2}$. Despite these changes, his blood pressure remained essentially unchanged and his urinary output increased only slightly to $13 \, mL \, h^{-1}$. His P_aO_2, which was 75 mmHg [10 kPa] on an F_IO_2 of 0.6, decreased to 64 mmHg [8.5 kPa].

Trap

There was an underestimation of the appropriate perfusion pressure for the maintenance of adequate renal functioning in the presence of sepsis, early renal failure and increased intra-abdominal pressure (IAP). There was also excessive reliance on the time-honoured use of an unproven strategy (low-dose dopamine).

Administration of a short-term measure (fluid bolus, with adverse effect on lung function) to deal with a persistent problem (sepsis and hypotension), is not advisable.

Trick

Adequate renal perfusion pressure (at least 80 mmHg)[1,2] should be restored by increasing mean arterial pressure (MAP) as necessary. In this septic patient, this would probably have needed an alpha agonist, such as norepinephrine [noradrenaline], which should have been infused and titrated to achieve a target MAP of 80–90 mmHg.[3,4] This would have been necessary as, in this patient, there was both a loss of renal blood flow autoregulation and vasoconstriction, with increased renal vascular resistance.[5–7] Under these conditions, the maintenance of adequate perfusion pressure is vital.

In this kind of patient, both development of an ileus and possible persistent blood loss into the abdominal cavity may account for increased IAP. This, by itself, would significantly impede renal perfusion.[8] In this situation, true renal perfusion pressure may be equal to MAP–IAP so that, even with a MAP of 80 mmHg, if the IAP is 20 mmHg, renal perfusion may remain insufficient to maintain excretory renal function.

IAP can easily be estimated using intravesical (bladder) pressure measurements by means of a Foley catheter.[9] In some patients, abdominal decompression may become necessary.[8,9]

In these situations, precious time is often lost implementing maneuvers for which there is no good proof of benefit in this context (low-dose dopamine)[10,11] or giving fluid boluses in patients who have no evidence of intravascular volume depletion. Furthermore, the additional administration of fluids in patients with acute lung injury may induce worsening hypoxemia.

Follow-up

In this patient, an infusion of norepinephrine was initiated and titrated to achieve a MAP of 85 mmHg. Cardiac index increased to $4.4\,L^{-1}\,min^{-2}\,m^{-2}$ and urinary output increased to $25\,mL\,h^{-1}$. Measurement of intravesical pressure revealed an IAP of 20 mmHg. A decision was made to decompress the abdomen. The distended intestine was decompressed and clot and serosanguinous fluid were also removed.

After these maneuvers, urinary output returned to $80\,mL\,h^{-1}$ and the mean blood pressure remained stable on $4\,\mu g\,min^{-1}$ of norepinephrine. The patient eventually survived to be discharged from hospital and renal function was normal (Figure 6.1.1).

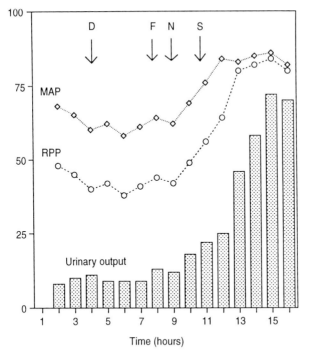

Figure 6.1.1. Graph showing the effect of various maneuvers on the urinary output of this patient. **MAP**, Mean arterial pressure; **RPP**, estimated renal perfusion pressure (both in mmHg). Various therapeutic interventions and their timing are indicated by arrows: **D**, start of low-dose dopamine infusion; **F**, administration of fluids; **N**, start of a norepinephrine infusion; **S**, surgical decompression. As can be seen, urinary output increased in association with increase in renal perfusion pressure.

References

1 Shipley RE and Study RS. Changes in renal blood flow, extraction of inulin, glomerular filtration rate, tissue pressure, and urine flow with acute alterations in renal artery pressure. *American Journal of Physiology* (1951) **167**: 676–688.

2 Stone AM and Stahl WM. Renal effects of haemorrhage in normal man. *Annals of Surgery* (1970) **172**: 825–836.

3 Hesselvik JF and Bridin B. Low-dose norepinephrine in patients with septic shock and oliguria. Effects on afterload, urine flow, and oxygen transport. *Critical Care Medicine* (1989) **17**: 179–180.

4 Redl-Wenzel EM, Armbruster C, Edelmann G, *et al.* The effects of norepinephrine on hemodynamics and renal function in severe septic shock. *Intensive Care Medicine* (1993) **19**: 151–154.

5 Stein JH and Sorkin MI. Pathophysiology of a vasomotor and nephrotoxic model of acute renal failure in the dog. *Kidney International* (1976) **10**: S86–S93.

6 Miller WL, Thomas RA, Berne RM and Rubio R. Adenosine production in the ischaemic kidney. *Circulation Research* (1978) **43**: 390–397.

7 Shibouta Y, Suzuki N, Shino A, *et al.* Pathophysiological role of endothelin in acute renal failure. *Life Science* (1990) **46**: 1611–1618.

8 Richards WO, Scovill W, Shin B and Reed W. Acute renal failure associated with increased intraabdominal pressure. *Annals of Surgery* (1983) **197**: 183–187.

9 Kron IL, Harman PK and Nolan SP. The measurement of intraabdominal pressure as a criterion for abdominal re-exploration. *Annals of Surgery* (1984) **199**: 28–30.

10 Duke GJ and Bersten AD. Dopamine and renal salvage in the critically ill patient. *Anaesthesiology in Intensive Care* (1992) **20**: 277–302.

11 Szerlip HM. Renal-dose dopamine: face and faction. *Annals of Internal Medicine* (1991) **115**: 153–154.

Specific Gravity, Osmolality, Tonicity and the Control of Serum Sodium

Rinaldo Bellomo

History

A 42-year-old man successfully received an orthotopic liver transplant for end-stage liver disease secondary to chronic active hepatitis and was admitted to the intensive care unit for postoperative care. After an initial period of stability, his course was complicated by the development of allograft rejection on day 9 and by the subsequent development of right lower lobe *Acinetobacter anitratus* pneumonia on day 11 (diagnosed by bronchoalveolar lavage with quantitative bacterial cultures). On day 13 he remained sedated with his trachea intubated, and dependent on mechanical ventilation. His circulatory condition was stable, without the need for vasopressor drugs. He was receiving antibiotics (tobramycin and ceftazidime) for his chest infection, and his temperature was 38.2°C [100.8°F]. His immunosuppression had been increased, from FK506 at 3 mg/day and prednisolone at 20 mg/day, by the addition of daily IV boluses of 500 mg of methylprednisolone. Because of rejection, his fluid therapy consisted of parenteral nutrition only, in the form of 2 liters of a solution containing 1 liter of 10% amino acids and 1 liter of 25% dextrose. He was also receiving 500 mL of a 20% lipid emulsion. The electrolyte content of his parenteral nutrition solution was as follows: sodium 75 mmol L^{-1}, chloride 105 mmol L^{-1}, potassium 50 mmol L^{-1}, phosphate 6.5 mg dL^{-1} [20 mmol L^{-1}] and magnesium 3.2 mg dL^{-1} [8 mmol L^{-1}]. During review of his morning laboratory data on day 14, he was noted to have a serum BUN of 70 mg dL^{-1} [25 mmol L^{-1}] despite a urine output of 5 L, a serum glucose of 270 mg dL^{-1} [15 mmol L^{-1}], a serum potassium of 3.1 mmol L^{-1} and a serum sodium of 158 mmol L^{-1}. Testing of his urine revealed a normal specific gravity and a urinary osmolality of 400 mosmol L^{-1}. It was felt that his urinary concentrating ability was adequate.

Over the next 24 hours, sodium was removed from the parenteral solution and an additional 10 g of potassium given intravenously. The following morning, the patient remained on mechanical ventilation and maintained his cardiovascular stability. His chest radiograph showed resolving pneumonia and a small right-sided pleural effusion. His temperature remained elevated at 38.4°C [101.1°F]. His serum sodium was 165 mmol L^{-1} and the patient was noticed to be 'twitchy'. One hour later, the patient experienced a short-lived *grand mal* seizure.

Trap

Assessment of urinary osmolality and specific gravity in a catabolic patient is not a useful guide to the patient's ability to retain free water. In patients such as these, the higher-than-expected osmalility is caused by the urinary excretion of solutes like urea which has no effect on the tonicity (effective osmolality)[1] of serum because of its equal distribution across cell membranes. The use of urinary osmolality or specific gravity will lead to the incorrect estimation of free water losses and inadequate free water replacement. This, in turn, will cause an increase in serum sodium with its associated morbidity (confusion, seizures and coma).

Trick

The correct approach to the problem of hypernatremia is based on the calculation of electrolyte-free water losses.[1,2] This is because it is electrolyte-free water loss that determines the change in serum tonicity (the physiologically effective osmolality responsible for the amount of intracellular hydration). If more electrolyte-free water is lost than received, the patient's serum sodium (the marker of the patient's total body water status) will inevitably increase,[3] intracellular hydration decrease and major changes in cerebral function will take place.

This case can be used as an example. With a body of weight of 80 kg, this patient's estimated total body water is 48 L (60% of body weight). With a serum sodium of 165 mmol L^{-1} (the effect of hyperglycemia[4] is not being taken into account for the sake of simplicity and because of its minimal relative importance in this case) and the normal serum sodium being 140 mmol L^{-1}, his present total body water is equal to:

48 liters × 140/165

i.e. 40.7 L. This means that the patient in question has an estimated free water deficit of 7.3 L. This deficit needs to be replaced if the patient is to return to a normal serum sodium and total body water. In addition, there will be ongoing water losses such as about 1 liter of free water from insensible losses caused by his fever[5] and urinary losses. In order to know his urinary free water losses his urinary sodium concentration must be known (potassium losses are typically replaced at near isotonic concentration to avoid hypokalemia).[6] If this man is excreting 5 L of urine per day with a urinary sodium concentration of 30 mmol L^{-1}, he will lose 150 mmol of sodium each day which, in 1 liter of urine water is the equivalent of 1 liter of isotonic saline. The remaining 4 L, therefore, will be made of 'electrolyte-free water' and will add to his previous total body of water deficit of more than 7 L. If sodium-free parenteral nutrition fluids only are administered (2.5 L), over the ensuing 24 hours his sodium will rise further as the free water deficit is increased to nearly 10 L! (predicted serum sodium of 175 mmol L^{-1}). If urinary free water loss remains approximately the same, a target serum sodium of 152 mmol L^{-1} within 24 hours (to avoid cerebral edema)[7] can be achieved by replacing ongoing losses (5 liters − 2.5 liters of nutritional fluids = 2.5 liters of free water) and replacing part of the present deficit according to the formula:

48 liters × 152/165 = 44.2

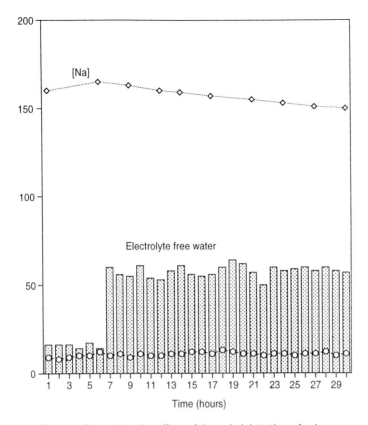

Figure 6.2.1. Diagram illustrating the effect of the administration of a large amount of electrolyte-free water (5% dextrose solution expressed as a fraction (1/6) of its hourly infusion rate) on the patient's serum sodium (**Na**) expressed in milliequivalents) and central venous pressure (dots at base of illustration, expressed in mmHg). A smooth decrease in serum sodium was achieved without evidence of intravascular volume overload once the appropriate infusion rate was chosen (at 7 hours on the graph).

i.e. 3.8 L (48–44.2) of free water are needed. The above calculations imply that this man needs an additional 3.8 + 2.5 L (6.3 L) of free water to achieve the desired serum sodium level. There is often concern about the circulatory effect of administering 6 L of 5% dextrose. Because only 1/12 of this will be expected to remain in the intravascular space, however, its hemodynamic effect should be similar to the infusion of 500 mL of colloid solution over 24 hours.

Follow-up

The patient was immediately started on 5% dextrose infusion with a rate of 250 mL h^{-1}. Because of the additional glucose load (300 g/day) his glucose concentration in the nutritional fluid was changed to 10% and he was started on an insulin infusion at $4\,units\,h^{-1}$. His serum sodium began to decrease and continued to do so (Figure 6.2.1). Twenty-four hours later, his serum sodium was $150\,mmol\,L^{-1}$ (Figure 6.2.1) and no further seizures took place. During this period of time his central venous pressure increased from 9 to 11 mmHg. His serum sodium was corrected back to normal within a further 48 hours and he suffered no ill effects. He was discharged from the intensive care unit 12 days later with a serum sodium of $138\,mmol\,L^{-1}$, his pneumonia having responded to antibiotics and his rejection episode having come under control.

References

1 Palevsky P. Water and tonicity homeostasis. In: Carlson RW, Geheb MA (eds) *Principles and Practice of Medical Intensive Care*. Philadelphia, W.B. Saunders, pp 1168–1179, 1993.
2 Rose BD. New approach to disturbances in the plasma sodium concentration. *American Journal of Medicine* (1986) **81**: 1033–1040.
3 Edelman IS, Leibman J and O'Meara MP. Interrelations between serum sodium concentration, serum osmolarity and total exchangeable sodium, total exchangeable potassium and total body water. *Journal of Clinical Investigation* (1958) **37**: 1236–1256.
4 Katz M. Hyperglycemia-induced hyponatremia: calculation of expected serum sodium depression. *New England Journal of Medicine* (1973) **289**: 843–844.
5 Baumber CD and Clark RG. Insensible water loss in surgical patients. *British Journal of Surgery* (1974) **61**: 53–57.
6 Laragh JH. The effect of potassium chloride on hyponatremia. *Journal of Clinical Investigation* (1954) **33**: 807–818.
7 Brennan S and Ayus JC. Acute versus chronic hypernatremia: how fast to correct ECF volume? *Journal of Critical Illness* (1990) **5**: 330–335.

6.3 The Need to Tailor Artificial Renal Support
Rinaldo Bellomo

History

A 17-year-old man was transferred to the intensive care unit (ICU) of a teaching institution from another hospital for urgent hemodialysis. His initial admission had taken place after a motor vehicle accident four days earlier. The only injuries sustained at the time were a closed head injury, a broken left clavicle and left-sided pulmonary contusion with a broken left 3rd rib. His Glasgow coma score on admission to the emergency room was 9. A CT scan performed at the time showed two small subdural hematomas and small intracranial hemorrhages. His trachea was intubated to protect his airway and he was admitted to the local ICU.

Neurosurgical opinion was sought and the subdural hematomas were treated conservatively. He developed a right-sided basal infiltrate, a high fever and hypotension despite the vigorous administration of IV fluids. Sepsis from his chest was thought to be the most likely cause. His urinary output decreased over a few hours and he became anuric. An ultrasound of his kidneys showed no evidence of obstruction. Because of his hypotension, he was started on a dopamine infusion at a rate of $12 \, \mu g \, kg^{-1} \, min^{-1}$. During the following two days his septic state had slightly improved. *Escherichia coli* was isolated from his sputum and blood and it was found to be sensitive to the antibiotics he was receiving.

His neurological function did not improve and the BUN increased to $123 \, mg \, dL^{-1}$ [$43.9 \, mmol \, L^{-1}$]. This increase in BUN was thought to be contributing to the coma. A repeat CT scan showed persistent subdural hematomas with no change in size, but evidence of moderate cerebral edema. Because of the possible need for invasive neurosurgical monitoring as well as dialysis he was transferred to a tertiary institution.

On arrival he was hypotensive (mean blood pressure of 59 mmHg) febrile ($T = 39°C$ [$102.2°F$]) and with a tachycardia. A pulse oximeter showed an arterial oxygen saturation of 94%, while on mechanical ventilation with an $F_{I}O_2$ of 0.5 and $10 \, cmH_2O$ of PEEP. An arterial and central venous catheter were in place.

On examination he opened his eyes on painful stimuli and was able to respond with semi-purposeful movements accompanied by groan-like sounds. There were no focal neurological signs. Asterixis was present.

A decision was made to place an intracranial pressure monitor. His intracranial pressure (ICP) was recorded at 18 mmHg and remained stable over the following 3 hours. A dual lumen hemodialysis catheter was inserted and hemodialysis was started with a blood flow of $200 \, mL \, min^{-1}$ and a dialysate flow of $300 \, mL \, min^{-1}$. After 15 minutes of hemodialysis, he was noted to be twitchy and his ICP was recorded at 22 mmHg. After 30 minutes of hemodialysis his ICP had increased to 25 mmHg and his mean blood pressure had decreased from 72 to 65 mmHg, requiring an increase in the dopamine infusion rate. After 35 minutes of hemodialysis the patient started having *grand mal* seizures and his intracranial pressure increased to 43 mmHg (Figure 6.3.1).

Trap

Errors were made in waiting until the development of a markedly elevated BUN before starting renal replacement therapy and in using inappropriate 'standard' renal replacement therapy. The method used in this patient is known to induce cerebral edema in patients with uremia[1-3] as well as triggering the disequilibrium syndrome.[1]

Trick

Critical care physicians need to be aware that in uremic patients, particularly in those with a high plasma BUN >80 mg dL^{-1} [28.6 mmol L^{-1}], starting hemodialysis is associated with a significant risk of developing the disequilibrium syndrome.[1]

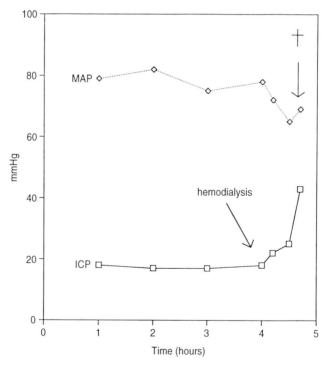

Figure 6.3.1. Diagram illustrating the relationship of the patient's intracranial pressure (**ICP**) and mean arterial pressure (**MAP**) with the onset of hemodialytic therapy (as indicated by the arrow). Hemodialysis was rapidly associated with the onset of intracranial hypertension and systemic hypotension resulting in the patient's death (cross).

This syndrome is characterized by neurological dysfunction and the possible development of seizures. In a patient with established cerebral edema, marginal cerebral perfusion pressure and clinical evidence of metabolic encephalopathy, the development of *grand mal* seizures with a sudden increase in ICP can be fatal. In these patients, it is better to provide early renal replacement therapy rather than waiting for the establishment of clinical evidence of uremia. The renal replacement treatment of choice in this patient was continuous hemofiltration, which allows full control of uremia with no adverse effects on intracranial pressure.[4,5] There are no reports of disequilibrium syndrome when continuous hemofiltration is used as renal replacement therapy. This may be because osmotic equilibration is achieved gently and large intra- to extracellular osmolality shifts are avoided. In addition, unlike hemodialysis,[6] hemofiltration does not diminish cerebral perfusion pressure at a time when its maintenance is paramount.

Follow-up

Thirty seconds after the onset of *grand mal* seizures, the patient developed an asystolic cardiac arrest. Cardiopulmonary resuscitation was started immediately but was unsuccessful. A post-mortem examination of the brain revealed diffuse mild to moderate petechial damage to the cortex and severe diffuse cerebral edema.

References

1 Arieff AI. Dialysis disequilibrium syndrome: current concepts on pathogenesis and prevention. *Kidney International* (1994) **45**: 629–635.
2 LaGreca G, Dettori P, Biasioli S, Fabris A, Feriani M, Pinna V, Pisani E and Rono C. Brain density studies during dialysis. *Lancet* (1980) **2**: 258.
3 Davenport A, Finn R and Goldsmith HJ. Management of patients with renal failure complicated by cerebral edema. *Blood Purification* (1989) **7**: 203–209.
4 Davenport E, Will EJ and Davison AM. Early changes in intracranial pressure during hemofiltration treatment in patients with grade 4 hepatic encephalopathy and acute oliguric renal failure. *Nephrology, Dialysis and Transplant* (1990) **5**: 192–198.
5 Davenport A, Will EJ and Davison AM. Continuous vs intermittent forms of hemofiltration and/or dialysis in the management of acute renal failure in patients with defective cerebral autoregulation at risk of cerebral edema. *Contributions to Nephrology* (1991) **1**: 225–233.
6 Baldamus CA, Ernst W, Frei U and Koch KM. Sympathetic and hemodynamic response to volume removal during different forms of renal replacement therapy. *Nephron* (1981) **31**: 324–332.

6.4 The Importance of Adequate Nutrition during Acute Renal Failure
Rinaldo Bellomo

History

A 67-year-old man with a history of a previous myocardial infarction and diminished ventricular function (left ventricular ejection fraction of 37%) and chronic renal impairment (serum BUN of $567\,mg\,dL^{-1}$ [$20\,mmol\,L^{-1}$) was admitted to the intensive care unit (ICU) of a nearby hospital following emergency laparotomy for suspected colonic perforation and septic shock. At the time of surgery a perforation of the sigmoid colon was found in association with severe diverticular disease. This segment of colon was removed. Extensive peritoneal soiling was treated by peritoneal lavage and a double-barrel colostomy was fashioned before the abdomen was closed.

On arrival in the ICU he needed mechanical ventilation with an F_IO_2 of 0.6 to achieve a P_aO_2 of 75 mmHg [10 kPa]. His chest radiograph showed bilateral pulmonary infiltrates and his circulatory status was consistent with the presence of sepsis (cardiac index of $3.1\,L\,min^{-1}\,m^{-2}$, right atrial pressure of 13 mmHg and a mean arterial pressure of 72 mmHg on a dopamine infusion of $5\,\mu g\,kg^{-1}\,min^{-1}$). He was oliguric (urinary output of $25\,mL\,h^{-1}$) and had a fever of 39°C [102.2°F]. In the next 24 hours, his oliguria progressed to anuria and on day 3 after admission intermittent hemodialysis was started.

During the next 2 weeks, anuria persisted and hemodialysis was continued. In this man, hemodialysis was frequently associated with hemodynamic instability (decrease in blood pressure and arterial oxygen desaturation) so that the treating physicians chose to use it as little as possible (Figure 6.4.1). In order to avoid uncontrolled uremia, protein intake was limited to $0.5\,g\,kg^{-1}$ per day. Caloric intake was kept constant at $35\,kcal\,kg^{-1}$ per day. Over a period of 2 weeks the patient's condition had gradually improved, the lungs were improving and the patient appeared ready for weaning, despite persistent renal failure. Repeated attempts to wean him off the ventilator, however, failed and he was transferred to a university hospital for further management.

On arrival, the patient's trachea was intubated. Ventilation was by synchronized intermittent mandatory ventilation with a tidal volume of 800 mL and a respiratory rate of 10/minute. His arterial oxygen saturation was 95% on an F_IO_2 of 0.35. His chest radiograph showed evidence of mild pulmonary congestion. Vascular access had been obtained using a dual lumen hemodialysis catheter and a central venous line. His right atrial pressure was 12 mmHg. He was afebrile with a blood pressure of 120/75 mmHg and a heart rate of 95/minute, without the infusion of any inotropes. Physical examination was remarkable because of marked muscle wasting with loss of pectoral and intercostal muscle bulk and marked thinning of deltoids and quadriceps. There was significant loss

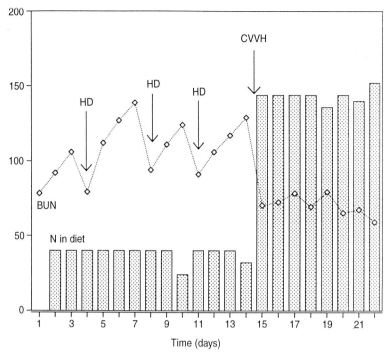

Figure 6.4.1. Diagram illustrating the level of azotemic control during intermittent hemodialysis (**HD**) and a low protein diet (days 1–14) and the favorable change in blood urea nitrogen induced by the initiation of continuous veno-venous hemodialysis (**CVVH**). With the latter technique, despite a tripling in daily protein intake, control of azotemia was clearly superior.

of muscle strength. His total body nitrogen was assessed by the technique of *in vitro* neutron activation[1] and found to be 56% of predicted. His total body nitrogen deficit (normal minus current value) was estimated at more than 150 g (approximately 1 kg of protein). His serum BUN on arrival was 129 mg dL^{-1} [46 mmol L^{-1}]. His serum albumin and transferrin were low. It was felt that respiratory muscle weakness played an important role in his inability to wean.

Trap

This man was both inadequately dialyzed and inadequately fed. In patients with a fragile circulatory state and myocardial dysfunction, it is common for intermittent hemodialysis to cause hypotension and lead to arterial oxygen desaturation.[2] This, in turn, leads clinicians to limit its application for fear of inducing further renal ischemia, arrhythmias or myocardial damage. In this setting, uremia becomes difficult to control and attempts may be made to diminish the rate of rise in serum BUN by limiting protein intake.[3,4] In septic, highly catabolic patients the results of this approach can be disastrous, as this patient shows, with an adverse impact on the function of organs other than the kidney.[5,6]

Trick

In this kind of patient, the correct form of renal support is continuous hemofiltration or hemodiafiltration.[7] With continuous hemofiltration techniques, uremia is gradually and steadily controlled on a 24-hourly basis, without any hemodynamic instability. This allows aggressive, nitrogen-rich nutritional support to be implemented without the fear of uncontrolled uremia and/or of fluid overload.[8–10]

In this way, malnutrition, hypotension and uremia are all prevented. Patients with acute renal failure and sepsis or catabolic states have the same nutritional requirements as similar patients without renal failure. They are entitled to receive the same degree of nutritional support as all other critically ill patients. If this nutritional goal cannot be met with intermittent hemodialysis, the appropriate renal replacement therapy (continuous hemofiltration) should be started.

Follow-up

The patient was started on continuous veno-venous hemofiltration (CVVH)[10] via his dual lumen catheter using a peristaltic pump to maintain blood flow at $150\,mL\,min^{-1}$. His serum BUN decreased from 112 to $70\,mg\,dL^{-1}$ [18.7 to $11.7\,mmol\,L^{-1}$] (Figure 6.4.1) over a period of 24 hours without any hemodynamic instability. A negative fluid balance of 1.8 L was achieved over a period of 24 hours and his pulmonary congestion improved. His diet was changed to one containing $1.8\,g$ protein kg^{-1} per day. His daily nitrogen balance was measured on two separate occasions and found to be positive by 6 and 12 g, respectively. Six days later, his muscle bulk and strength appeared to have significantly increased. He was successfully weaned off the ventilator on the eighth day after transfer.

References

1 Hill GL, King RFG and Smith RC. Multi-element analysis of the living body by neutron activation analysis application to critically ill patients receiving intravenous nutrition. *British Journal of Surgery* (1970) **66**: 868–872.

2 Keshaviah P and Shapiro FL. A critical examination of dialysis-induced hypotension. *American Journal of Kidney Diseases* (1982) **2**: 290–293.

3 Borah MF, Schoenfeld PY, Gotch FA, Sargent JA, Wolfson M and Humphries MH. Nitrogen balance during intermittent dialysis therapy of uremia. *Kidney International* (1978) **14**: 491–497.

4 Bouffard Y, Viale JP, Annat G and Delafosse B, Guillame G and Motin J. Energy

expenditure in the acute renal failure patient mechanically ventilated. *Intensive Care Medicine* (1987) **13**: 401–404.

5 Kelly SM, Rosa A, Field M, Couglin M, Shizgal HM and Macklem PT. Inspiratory muscle strength and body composition in patients receiving total parenteral nutrition therapy. *American Reveiw of Respiratory Diseases* (1984) **130**: 33–37.

6 Larca L and Greenbaum DM. Effectiveness of intensive nutritional regimes in patients who fail to wean from mechanical ventilation. *Critical Care Medicine* (1992) **10**: 297–300.

7 Bellomo R. Acute renal replacement therapy. In: Dobb GJ (ed.) *Current Topics in Intensive Care*. London, W.B. Saunders, pp 162–179, 1994.

8 Chima CS, Meyer L, Hummell C, Bosworth C, Heytar R and Paganini E. Protein catabolic rate in patients with acute renal failure on continuous arteriovenous hemofiltration and total parenteral nutrition. *Journal of the American Society of Nephrology* (1993) **8**: 1516–1521.

9 Bellomo R, Martin H, Parkin G, Love J, Kearley Y and Boyce N. Continuous arteriovenous hemodiafiltration in the critically ill: influence on major nutrient balances. *Intensive Care Medicine* (1991) **17**: 399–402.

10 Canaud B, Garred LJ, Christol JP, Anbas S, Beraud JJ and Mion C. Pump-assisted continuous venovenous hemofiltration for treating acute uremia. *Kidney International* (1988) **33**: S154–S156.

7 Hematological Failure

7.1 Thrombocytopenia
T. Baglin

History

A 37-year-old female with established Budd–Chiari syndrome was referred for liver transplantation. Impaired hepatic synthetic function and portal hypertension with splenomegaly and ascites were present. Before surgery the alanine aminotransferase (ALT) was $198\,U\,L^{-1}$ (normal $<50\,U\,L^{-1}$), bilirubin $202\,\mu mol\,L^{-1}$ [$11.9\,mg\,dL^{-1}$] (normal $<17\,\mu mol\,L^{-1}$ [$1.0\,mg\,dL^{-1}$]), prothrombin time (PT) 26 s (normal <16 s), partial thromboplastin time (PTT) 51 s (normal <46 s), hemoglobin $10.3\,g\,dL^{-1}$, neutrophils $2.1 \times 10^9\,L^{-1}$ and platelets $76 \times 10^9\,L^{-1}$. Immediately before transplantation, 5 units of fresh frozen plasma and 10 units of random donor platelets were infused. Surgery was performed with a continuous infusion of fresh frozen plasma and a further 5 units of random donor platelets. Intraoperative blood loss was 7.2 L and heterologous red cell transfusion was given to maintain a hemoglobin of $10.0\,g\,dL^{-1}$. Orthotopic liver transplantation, with elective splenectomy was performed. After operation, cyclosporine [cyclosporin] and azathioprine were given to prevent graft rejection, and intravenous heparin was given to prevent hepatic vessel thrombosis.

Recovery was uneventful and by day 4 both ALT and bilirubin were gradually decreasing to $76\,U\,L^{-1}$ and $65\,\mu mol\,L^{-1}$ [$3.8\,mg\,dL^{-1}$], respectively. Prothrombin time was 17 s and heparin at $1000\,U\,h^{-1}$ was maintaining a PTT of approximately twice normal. Hemoglobin was $12.2\,g\,dL^{-1}$ with a white blood cell count of $14.6 \times 10^9\,L^{-1}$ ($9.3 \times 10^9\,L^{-1}$ neutrophils). The platelet count was $130 \times 10^9\,L^{-1}$. On day 7, despite continued improvement in hepatic function, her platelet count decreased precipitously to $61 \times 10^9\,L^{-1}$ and by the following day it was $30 \times 10^9\,L^{-1}$. There was protracted bleeding from venepuncture sites and mild macroscopic hematuria. The house staff treated this with an infusion of 6 units of platelets. The bleeding did not stop.

Traps

The likely cause of hemorrhage in this patient was the combination of thrombocytopenia and heparin administration rather than either alone. Spontaneous hemorrhage is unusual with a platelet count of $30 \times 10^9\,L^{-1}$ but bleeding may be prolonged after surgery or venepuncture. Whilst therapeutic heparinization rarely results in spontaneous bleeding, the combination of anticoagulation and a low platelet count can cause significant hemorrhage. Platelet clumping can occur in blood samples taken into EDTA for blood count analysis leading to a spurious diagnosis of thrombocytopenia. It is essential to examine a blood film as this phenomenon is readily apparent and is of no clinical significance. Careful examination of red cells is essential as red cell fragmentation is a subjective observation and easily missed if not looked for specifically. The presence of fragmentation and severe thrombocytopenia is indicative of a severe consumptive coagulopathy with microvascular thrombosis. It can also occur with cyclosporine therapy and cyclosporine may have to be stopped.

Tricks

Coagulation studies should be performed to determine if there is evidence of disseminated intravascular coagulation (DIC) and to exclude excessive anti-coagulation caused by heparin, both of which may contribute to bleeding. If DIC is present the possibility of bacterial sepsis should be considered as this is a common cause with bacterial endotoxin and cell membrane lipid causing activation of coagulation. Blood cultures should be taken and if there is fever or shock broad-spectrum antibiotic therapy should be started. Liver function tests should be reviewed to determine if there is evidence of acute rejection as failing liver function can quickly lead to a deficiency of coagulation factors and eventually a consumptive coagulopathy and thrombocytopenia.

Thrombocytopenia without evidence of red cell fragmentation was confirmed by examination of the blood film. The coagulation screen revealed a PT of 13 s, a PTT of 50 s and fibrin degradation products of $4 \, mg \, L^{-1}$ (normal $<0.5 \, mg \, L^{-1}$). A bone marrow aspirate was also performed and showed plentiful platelet precursors indicating that thrombocytopenia was the result of platelet destruction in the circulation rather than inadequate production by the bone marrow. The ALT was $50 \, U \, L^{-1}$, the cyclosporine level was therapeutic at $213 \, \mu mol \, L^{-1}$ $[77 \, mg \, L^{-1}]$.

Thrombocytopenia is common in critically ill patients and this patient showed the potential complex nature of thrombocytopenia in such patients and the difficulty often faced in establishing the diagnosis and understanding the cause.

Patients with liver disease are frequently thrombocytopenic and while this is often attributed to hypersplenism there are probably many causes. There may be reduced marrow platelet production. Peripheral consumption caused by activation of the coagulation system with thrombin-induced platelet aggregation or aggregation of platelets by immune complexes may also be involved.

This particular patient had marked splenomegaly caused by portal hypertension and it was likely that the moderate thrombocytopenia before operation was caused by hypersplenism. After surgery the platelet count became normal because of removal of the spleen.

Dilutional thrombocytopenia can occur in the context of massive blood transfusion and indeed this patient had almost a complete blood volume replacement at the time of surgery. However, the severe thrombocytopenia several days later could not be explained on this basis because massive transfusion was not needed postoperatively.

Surgery is associated with thrombin generation and probably increased platelet turnover. However, the typical response to surgery is increased marrow platelet production and in the absence of dilutional thrombocytopenia a resultant postoperative increase in platelet count is typical.

Disseminated intravascular coagulation caused by sepsis should be considered in any critically ill patient, particularly those with existing or pre-existing liver disease. In this condition intravascular thrombin generation leads to consumption of both coagulation factors and platelets with secondary fibrinolysis releasing fibrin degradation products from intravascular thrombi. Thrombocytopenia of less than $100 \times 10^9 L^{-1}$ caused by disseminated intravascular coagulation is usually associated with prolongation of the PT and PTT and an increase in fibrin degradation products to $>16 \, mg \, L^{-1}$. However, one should remember that fibrin degradation products are usually elevated postoperatively, but not to this level. Furthermore, as they are removed by the liver, circulating levels may be high in the absence of overt DIC when there is impaired liver function as a consequence of delayed clearance. In this patient the PT was normal, the PTT was prolonged and caused by giving heparin. The mild elevation of fibrin degradation products was compatible with postoperative recovery after liver transplantation. In addition, this patient did not have clinical disseminated intravascular coagulation and there was no evidence of microangiopathic hemolysis which frequently accompanies this complication.

Sepsis may cause DIC but occasionally severe thrombocytopenia in the absence of coagulation changes may occur in septic patients. Viral infections such as cytomegalovirus can cause thrombocytopenia in immune-suppressed patients and should also be considered.

Azathioprine is both immune suppressive and myelosuppressive and patients on such therapy may develop severe thrombocytopenia. The generalized myelosuppressive effect of azathioprine makes patients anemic and neutropenic as well. It usually follows giving azathioprine for several weeks. Short-term administration of azathioprine would not be expected to produce significant myelosuppression and certainly not isolated thrombocytopenia. In this patient bone marrow examination confirmed the presence of a cellular marrow with visible platelet production thus excluding azathioprine-induced myelosuppression.

Cyclosporine can cause an idiosyncratic consumptive thrombocytopenia analogous to classical thrombotic thrombocytopenic purpura (TTP). The mechanism of action is unknown but patients typically have red cell fragmentation and other manifestations of the TTP syndrome such as fever, neurological disturbance and renal impairment. It can occur with therapeutic levels of cyclosporine.

Thrombocytopenia is an almost universal finding after liver transplantation and there is typically a progressive decrease in platelet count with a nadir at day 6. The nadir closely correlates with elevation of ALT and may be a reflection of acute graft rejection. There was no evidence of graft rejection in this patient, however, and whilst subclinical rejection can occur without elevation of ALT the degree of thrombocytopenia in this patient was profound and cannot be readily explained by subclinical acute graft rejection.

Bone marrow examination indicated that platelet production was probably normal and therefore the thrombocytopenia in this patient was more likely to have been caused by peripheral platelet consumption or destruction. The precipitous decrease in platelet count in the absence of overt sepsis, DIC or in this case hypersplenism raised the possibility of heparin-induced thrombocytopenia. This diagnosis was subsequently confirmed by showing aggregation of normal platelets in the presence of the patient's serum and heparin *in vitro*. This is a well-recognized complication of heparin therapy and probably occurs more frequently than is currently appreciated. The disorder is caused by the development of heparin-dependent IgG antibodies which bind platelet-bound heparin through specific antigen binding. The antibody Fc region then either binds complement or Fc-receptors on the platelet membrane causing platelet activation with consequent *in vivo* aggregation and in some instances thrombus formation. Thrombocytopenia probably occurs much more frequently than overt thrombosis, but when thrombosis does occur the mortality rate is high. The reported incidence varies between 0.5 and 5.0% but a high index of suspicion is needed to recognize the syndrome. It can be confirmed by *in vitro* platelet aggregation studies.

Follow-up

In this patient the heparin was stopped and the patient given warfarin with resolution of thrombocytopenia within 48 hours of stopping the heparin.

This patient was receiving heparin as prophylaxis for hepatic vessel thrombosis, but in patients receiving heparin as treatment for established thrombosis it may be necessary to give other antithrombotic therapy while the anticoagulant effect of warfarin is being achieved. Such agents include new heparinoids and direct thrombin inhibitors, such as hirudin and prostacyclin.

Bibliography

1 Machin SJ. Acquired disorders of haemostasis. In: Hoffbrand AV and Lewis SM (eds) *Postgraduate Haematology*. London, Heinemann, pp 655–671, 1989.
2 McCaughan GW, Herkes R, Powers B, Richard K, Gallagher ND, Thompson JF and Sheil AG. Thrombocytopenia post liver transplantation. *Journal of Hepatology* (1992) **16**: 16–22.
3 Chong BH. Heparin-induced thrombocytopenia. *Blood Reviews* (1988) **2**: 108–114.
4 Magnani HN. Heparin-induced thrombocytopenia (HIT): an overview of 230 patients treated with Orgaran (Org 10172). *Thrombosis and Haemostasis* (1993) **70**: 554–561.

7.2 Postoperative Bleeding
T. Baglin

History

A 46-year-old male with long-standing alcoholic cirrhosis was admitted with end-stage hepatic failure for liver transplantation. Before surgery the prothrombin time (PT) was 22 s with a partial thromboplastin time (PTT) of 48 s, a fibrinogen of $1.5 \, g \, dL^{-1}$ and a platelet count of $104 \times 10^9 \, L^{-1}$. Six units of fresh frozen plasma were given before liver transplantation with a further 6 units given over 3–4 hours during the course of transplantation. Intraoperative blood loss was 4.3 L and heterologous red cell transfusion was given to maintain a hemoglobin of $10.0 \, g \, dL^{-1}$. As the abdomen was closed there was a slight ooze from the surface of the diaphragm, but the surgeon did not consider this to be excessive and the abdominal wound was closed with a drain *in situ*. At the end of the procedure the patient was well perfused with a pulse of 76/minute and blood pressure of 135/75 mmHg.

The patient was transferred to the intensive care unit. Blood stained fluid was obtained from the abdominal drain and this continued over the next 3 hours at a rate of $400 \, mL \, h^{-1}$. The pulse gradually increased to 110/minute and blood pressure decreased to 100/60 mmHg despite the transfusion of 2 units of packed red cells.

The hemoglobin was $8.0 \, g \, dL^{-1}$, PT 32 s, PTT 65 s, fibrinogen $1.2 \, g \, dL^{-1}$ and platelet count $70 \times 10^9 \, L^{-1}$. Ten units of fresh frozen plasma and 2 units of packed red cells were given, but two hours later there was evidence of further bleeding with $450 \, mL \, h^{-1}$ of blood-stained fluid coming from the abdominal drain.

Tricks

The first step in the evaluation and management is to resuscitate the patient and establish the cause of hemorrhage. The blood volume should be increased to maintain tissue perfusion, rather than a normal hemoglobin concentration. The hemoglobin concentration must be measured as a further index of hemorrhage as some blood loss may be concealed, as suggested in this case by the cardiovascular changes. Whilst these procedures are instituted the cause of continued hemorrhage should be assessed.

A surgical cause is the first consideration but this was a planned elective procedure and there was no obvious source of significant hemorrhage when the surgery was finished. The second most likely explanation for the postoperative hemorrhage is an acquired disorder of hemostasis. This may be because the patient was given a drug which interferes with hemostasis, such as preoperative aspirin or the use of an excessive amount of heparin, for example in flushes for arterial and venous catheters. Liver disease and the process of liver transplantation are associated with various abnormalities of hemostasis and these must all be considered (see below).

The final cause of postoperative bleeding is a pre-existing hereditary hemorrhagic disorder. Mild hemophilia, von Willebrand's disease and a variety of platelet defects would not be detected on routine perioperative coagulation testing and it is essential that a clear history be obtained from a relative if this has not already been obtained from the patient before operation. It is unlikely that any significant pre-existing coagulopathy is present if there is no history of excessive hemorrhage at the time of previous surgery or dental extraction.

The patient should be examined for evidence of a systemic coagulopathy by inspecting venepuncture sites, cannula insertion sites, the tracheal tube and the abdominal wound. In this patient there was no excessive hemorrhage from any site, other than the abdominal drain. In this patient the hemostatic system should be reassessed with a PT, PTT, fibrinogen level, XDPs and platelet count.

Traps

Further coagulation tests were ordered and the patient was re-examined. There was a slight ooze from a venous cannula site, as well as from the abdominal drain. The laboratory tests showed a PT of 17 s, a PTT of 42 s, fibrinogen 1.2 g dL^{-1}, fibrin degradation products (XDPs) 4 mg L^{-1} and platelets 84 x 10^9 L^{-1}.

In addition, the serum creatinine was measured as severe renal impairment with uremia could have caused a major defect of platelet function for which the primary treatment is dialysis. The creatinine was 1.7 mg dL^{-1} [133 μmol L^{-1}] (normal 1.6 mg dL^{-1} [<120 μmols L^{-1}).

A further 10 units of fresh frozen plasma, 6 units of cryoprecipitate and 6 units of platelets were transfused but the patient continued to bleed from the abdominal drain. A request for whole blood was sent to the blood transfusion laboratory, but this product was not available.

It should be remembered that bleeding is prolonged by anaemia and in a bleeding patient progressive anaemia may contribute to the bleeding tendency. There is no explanation for the relationship between bleeding time and hematocrit but it may relate to platelet-endothelial interaction at high shear rates with less interaction at low hematocrits.

The most common cause for excessive postoperative bleeding is local hemostatic failure caused by bleeding points. Systemic coagulopathy is a rare cause of postoperative bleeding.

In this particular patient there was no clinical evidence of a pre-existing coagulopathy. No drugs had been given that impair hemostasis. Protracted blood loss was isolated to a single site, i.e. the drain, with no blood loss from venepuncture sites apart from on one occasion, from cannulae or the abdominal wound. A mild coagulopathy was documented with prolongation of the PT and PTT but this was corrected by giving fresh frozen plasma. The patient continued to bleed and a hyperfibrinolytic state was excluded by a normal clot lysis time at more than 300 minutes. At this stage the patient should have been returned immediately to theater as primary surgical bleeding is the most likely explanation.

Postoperative bleeding is a common clinical problem. Whilst there was no obvious bleeding vessel when the abdomen was closed, this explanation must always remain a consideration in a patient bleeding after operation. All the evidence in this patient supported surgical bleeding and exploration should probably have taken place sooner. Continued hemorrhage in such patients may lead to a secondary coagulopathy which exacerbates blood loss and may delay definitive treatment even further as hemorrhage is then attributed to failure of the hemostatic system. These patients may then suffer life-threatening hemorrhage because of delayed corrective surgery. An early appraisal of this situation can lead to the correct diagnosis and treatment.

There are many causes of acquired disorders of hemostasis after major surgery, including deficiency of coagulation factors and platelets either because of dilution after massive blood loss and transfusion, or because of consumption in association with sepsis or poor tissue perfusion. Occasionally, patients develop disseminated intravascular coagulation (DIC) due to underlying malignant disease, postoperative sepsis, tissue damage or hypoxia. The development of DIC will lead to end-organ damage due to microvascular thrombosis with subsequent further impairment of tissue perfusion and progressive coagulopathy and bleeding. Maintenance of tissue perfusion is critical. If DIC does develop then the underlying disorder must be corrected. Supportive blood component therapy may reduce the bleeding manifestations. The use of heparin in such patients is likely to exacerbate bleeding and all efforts should be made to maintain tissue perfusion and treat sepsis with appropriate antibiotics. In this patient there was no evidence of DIC, sepsis or malignancy.

Hyperfibrinolysis is usually secondary to DIC and contributes to the bleeding seen in this syndrome. Occasionally it can occur in the absence of DIC, so-called 'primary fibrinolysis', as in liver transplant patients or occasionally those with carcinoma of the prostate. There was no supportive evidence for systemic hyperfibrinolysis in this patient with a level of XDPs of $4\,mg\,L^{-1}$ and a normal clot lysis time. XDPs are typically elevated after operation because of breakdown of clots and small-vessel thrombi at wound sites, but levels are only moderately elevated. XDPs are cleared by the liver and in patients with liver disease XDPs are further elevated owing to delayed clearance. Following liver transplantation it is common to see some elevation of XDPs without DIC or hyperfibrinolysis. In this patient the level of XDPs was consistent with the postoperative state and did not support a diagnosis of hyperfibrinolysis.

The liver has a central role in the regulation of the hemostatic system and surgery in patients with liver disease may result in a major disturbance of coagulation and hemorrhage. In conjunction with the endothelium and bone marrow it is responsible for maintaining hemostasis in an equilibrium such that generation of thrombin and plasmin is minimal within the circulation. However, it can be readily amplified when the integrity of blood vessels is compromised. Liver disease is often associated with a variety of abnormalities of hemostasis including decreased and abnormal protein synthesis, intravascular consumption of hemostatic factors, delayed clearance of activated products and hyperfibrinolysis. The nature of the abnormalities is dependent on the underlying liver disease, the severity of disease and the speed of onset of impairment of liver function. These abnormalities can lead to both excessive hemorrhage and thrombosis. Therapeutic manipulation of the hemostatic system with blood components and pharmacological agents is frequently needed to stop and prevent hemorrhage and thrombosis in patients with liver disease. Patients receiving liver transplants have additional specific alterations in hemostasis and management of these patients can be particularly difficult. General surgery is often associated with fibrinolytic shutdown but in patients receiving liver transplants a severe primary hyperfibrinolytic syndrome may occur. This is most apparent during the anhepatic phase as the liver is the primary clearance site for tissue plasminogen activator (tPA) and liver transplantation can result in high levels of circulating tPA. This syndrome is characterized by widespread bleeding, very high XDPs and a short clot lysis time (often <60 minutes).

This patient had neither a severe deficiency of clotting factors or platelets, nor evidence of pathological fibrinolytic activity. In an attempt to correct the coagulopathy, this patient was transfused with fresh frozen plasma, cryoprecipitate and random donor platelets. It is often not possible to completely correct a prolonged PT and PTT with the use of fresh frozen plasma without whole plasma volume exchange. Correction of the PT to 3–4 s beyond the control and correction of the PTT to near-normal is usually associated with the bleeding stopping when it is caused by coagulation factor deficiency. In this patient the continued blood loss from a single site when the PT was 17 s (normal <16 s), the PTT 42 s (normal <42 s) and the platelet count $84 \times 10^9 L^{-1}$ should immediately suggest a local cause for hemorrhage, such as a bleeding vessel. It was not necessary to infuse cryoprecipitate as a source of fibrinogen as normal hemostasis can be achieved with a fibrinogen level $<1 \, g \, dL^{-1}$. Transfusion of platelets was not necessary as thrombocytopenia to this degree would not usually be associated with excessive hemorrhage. A platelet count of $>60 \times 10^9 L^{-1}$ is sufficient to stop bleeding when platelet function is normal. There was no reason to suspect defective platelet function in this patient.

Whole blood is of no therapeutic value and should not be used. Whole blood is essentially red cells in old plasma. The plasma and platelets are not hemostatic and individual components including red cells, platelets and fresh frozen plasma should be given as individual components to patients who are deficient in these factors. Fresh whole blood offers no advantage over individual components and would not be readily available because of the time delay involved in collection, processing and particularly the viral testing that is now mandatory before transfusion.

In conclusion, the management of postoperative bleeding requires full evaluation through history, examination and laboratory assessment of hemostasis, a fundamental understanding of the hemostatic system and the appropriate use of blood component therapy.

Follow-up

When the bleeding failed to stop the patient was returned to the operating room. At laparotomy 2 L of intra-abdominal blood were drained and a bleeding vessel identified and sutured. The patient returned to the intensive care unit where his condition then remained stable without excessive blood loss.

Bibliography

1 White GC, Marder VJ, Colman RW, Hirsh J and Salzman EW. Approach to the bleeding patient. In: Colman, Hirsh, Marder, Salzman (eds). *Hemostasis and Thrombosis*. Philadelphia, J.B. Lippincott, pp 1134–1147, 1994.
2 Rapaport SI. Preoperative hemostatic evaluations: which tests, if any? *Blood* (1983) **61**: 229.
3 Kitchens CS. Approach to the bleeding patient. *Hematology and Oncology Clinics of North America* (1992) **6**: 983–990.

7.3 Progressive Rapid Anemia in a Previously Resuscitated Patient
T. Baglin

History

A 53-year-old female with a three-year history of menorrhagia was admitted for elective hysterectomy under general anesthesia. On admission her hemoglobin was $9.0 \, g \, dL^{-1}$ with a mean corpuscular volume (MCV) of 75 fl. She was receiving ferrous sulfate 200 mg/day orally but no other medication. She had three healthy children and there was no other significant medical history. In view of her anemia, surgery was postponed 72 hours and she was given a 3-unit transfusion of packed red cells. On the day of surgery she was assessed in theater for induction of anesthesia. She was found to be unwell with a fever of $39°C$ [$102.2°F$], pulse 105/minute, blood pressure 105/60 mmHg. There was no apparent vaginal blood loss or hemorrhage elsewhere. An intravenous infusion of crystalloid was started and the patient transferred to the intensive therapy unit for resuscitation and diagnosis. On arrival at the unit the patient was noted to have macroscopic hematuria.

Following infusion of 1.5 L of crystalloid over 60 minutes there was a reduction in pulse rate to 90/minute and an increase in blood pressure to 115/60 mmHg. Investigations revealed a hemoglobin of $6.2 \, g \, dL^{-1}$ with a normal prothrombin time (PT) at 13 s and a partial thromboplastin time (PTT) at 36 s. Creatinine was normal at $97 \, \mu mol \, L^{-1}$ [$1.26 \, mg \, dL^{-1}$]. Red cells were not present on urine microscopy.

Because of the hematuria, an urgent cystoscopy was organized to see if the bladder was the cause of her continuing blood loss. Four units of red cells were cross-matched for transfusion but three were incompatible and the cystoscopy was cancelled.

Trap

The most likely cause of tachycardia and hypotension in a patient with a hemorrhagic history is blood loss. In this case there was no evidence of hemorrhage from the uterus which was the site of previous chronic blood loss. Initially, there was no evidence of hemorrhage elsewhere but subsequently macroscopic hematuria was noted. This unusual site of blood loss should suggest either contamination from vaginal blood loss or, in the absence of known bladder pathology, the possibility of a coagulopathy. Hematuria as a result of coagulopathy would usually be accompanied by blood loss at other sites including venepuncture.

Trick

The most likely diagnosis is a delayed hemolytic transfusion reaction with intravascular hemolysis causing hemoglobinuria. A blood sample should be taken for a direct antiglobulin test, determination of specificity of the antibody responsible for incompatibility and serum bilirubin measurement. The patient should be transfused with selected antigen-negative red cell units.

In view of the history of menorrhagia, the moderate hypochromic anemia present on admission is most likely the result of iron deficiency. The need for elective transfusion before surgery is questionable in a 53-year-old woman who was fit and well without hypovolemia. As the hemoglobin concentration is a determinant of arterial oxygen concentration, red cell transfusion is frequently used to improve oxygen delivery. However, animal experiments show that tissue oxygen extraction is maintained with an 80% reduction in red cell mass, so long as blood volume and blood flow are maintained. Furthermore, in critically ill patients impaired tissue oxygen extraction is corrected by volume resuscitation alone and subsequent red cell transfusion may not result in any improvement in tissue oxygen metabolism. Thus, for tissue oxygen delivery maintenance of blood volume and flow may be more important than maintaining the red cell mass and hence circulating hemoglobin. Traditionally, patients have received elective transfusion of red cells before surgery with a hemoglobin of $<10 \, g \, dL^{-1}$ but more latterly it has been suggested that the threshold for transfusion should be $<7 \, g \, dL^{-1}$ in otherwise well patients. In one study in which patients declined blood transfusions for religious reasons there was no increase in mortality in patients with a hemoglobin of $>8 \, g \, dL^{-1}$ but a high mortality in those with a hemoglobin of $<6 \, g \, dL^{-1}$. In view of the numerous potential complications, transfusion of red cells before operation should be reserved for those patients with a very low hemoglobin or for those who have compromised cardiorespiratory function.

As a consequence of transfusion this patient developed a severe delayed hemolytic transfusion. The development of red cell incompatibility and hemoglobinuria should immediately indicate the diagnosis. Hemolytic transfusion reactions may be immediate or delayed. Immediate reactions tend to be more severe and are either caused by the presence of naturally occurring antibodies (e.g. anti-A, anti-B) or immune antibodies as a consequence of previous alloimmunization at the time of previous transfusion or transplacental transfer of red cells. Antibodies to antigens of the ABO system are complement activating IgM antibodies causing immediate intravascular hemolytic reactions which may be fatal.

More than 90% of ABO mismatched transfusions occur as a result of clinical error rather than serological errors in the transfusion laboratory. These are usually the result of either sending a sample with the wrong points of identification or transfusing red cells to the wrong patient. Both errors are easily avoided: in the first case by labeling samples for compatibility testing at the time of blood sampling and checking identification points against the patient's identity band; and in the second case by checking the patient's details on the red cell transfusion bag against the patient's identity band and the patient's notes immediately before transfusion. Immediate reactions caused by immune antibodies arising from previous exposure are usually the result of non-complement activating IgG antibodies and reactions are typically milder than with naturally occurring antibodies to the ABO system.

Delayed reactions occur in individuals who have typically been previously immunized to a foreign red cell antigen, but in whom antibody concentration is insufficient to be detected on compatibility testing. On further exposure to the antigen at the time of transfusion a secondary immune response results in a high titer of antibody and rapid destruction of the transfused red cells. Delayed reactions occur after about 1 : 500 transfusions and whilst not usually fatal may cause significant morbidity. Jaundice occurs 1–2 days after the onset of hemolysis and renal impairment is exceptional in contrast to immediate reactions. Red cell destruction is typically extravascular with antibodies against the rhesus system most commonly responsible. These antibodies do not activate complement and antibody-coated red cells are removed by macrophages as they pass through the spleen. The manifestations of the reaction were unusual in this patient as the hemoglobinuria was suggestive of intravascular rather than extravascular hemolysis. This strongly suggests a delayed reaction caused by an antibody against the Kidd system (anti-Jκ). These antibodies are unusual in that they may activate complement and may be present in high titers before disappearing and subsequently increasing rapidly after antigen re-exposure. It is noteworthy that whilst there was no previous transfusion history the patient had three children and in view of the rapidity of the delayed hemolysis this strongly suggests previous alloimmunization. On admission, compatibility testing revealed no atypical antibody but following the reaction the direct antiglobulin test was strongly positive and an anti-Jκ$_a$ antibody was confirmed in the patient's serum. In this case clinical findings were caused by complement activation with hypotension and tachycardia.

Follow-up

The hysterectomy was postponed and she was sent home still anemic, five days later. Her family doctor gave her iron and vitamin supplements and her hemoglobin increased to 11 g dL^{-1}. The menorrhagia continued and three months later she had an uneventful hysterectomy, without the need for blood transfusion.

Bibliography

1 Office of Medical Applications of Research. National Institutes of Health: perioperative red cell transfusion. *Journal of the American Medical Association* (1988) **260**: 1700.
2 Cane RD. Hemoglobin: how much is enough? *Critical Care Medicine* (1990) **18**: 1046–1047.
3 Dietrich KA, Conrad SA, Herbert CA, Levy GL and Romero MD. Cardiovascular and metabolic response to red blood cell transfusion in critically ill volume resuscitated non-surgical patients. *Critical Care Medicine* (1990) **18**: 940–944.

4 Carson JL, Spence RK, Poses RM and Bonavita G. Severity of anaemia and operative
   mortality and morbidity. *Lancet* (1988) 727–728.
5 Contriros M (ed.) *ABC of Transfusion*. London, British Medical Journal, 1990.

7.4 Leukopenia of Sepsis
T. Baglin

History

A 55-year-old male vagrant was found unconscious. On examination he responded to painful stimuli and smelt strongly of alcohol. He was admitted to the intensive care unit because of concern about maintenance of his airway. He had a fever of 39.5°C [103.1°F]. His pulse rate was 88/minute and completely irregular with a blood pressure of 145/90 mmHg. The jugular venous pressure was not elevated, normal first and second heart sounds were present with a 1/6 ejection systolic murmur in the aortic area. Widespread wheezes and bilateral basal crackles were present. His liver was palpable 3 cm below the costal margin in the mid-clavicular line and his spleen was palpable 5 cm below the left costal margin. There was no palpable lymphadenopathy.

A chest radiograph showed bilateral basal shadowing. His hemoglobin was $9.2\,\mathrm{g\,dL^{-1}}$ with a mean corpuscular volume (MCV) of 103 fl, a white cell count of $1.0 \times 10^9\,\mathrm{L^{-1}}$ with 50% neutrophils and 40% lymphocytes, platelets $27 \times 10^9\,\mathrm{L^{-1}}$, prothrombin time (PT) 17 s and partial thromboplastin time (PTT) 35 s.

The resident staff, on seeing his low white cell count in the presence of a severe pneumonia, rang the transfusion laboratory to ask about white cell donation and transfusion. They also started intravenous antibiotics with azlocillin 200 mg 12 hourly and benzylpenicillin 1.2 g 6 hourly.

Traps

Whilst there is no relative neutropenia or lymphopenia, this patient clearly had an absolute deficiency of both. It is always necessary to calculate absolute numbers of blood cells otherwise misdiagnosis can result. For example, a patient with chronic lymphocytic leukemia and a white cell count of $50 \times 10^9\,\mathrm{L^{-1}}$ may only have 10% neutrophils but this is a normal neutrophil count at $5 \times 10^9\,\mathrm{L^{-1}}$ and the patient is not neutropenic. Alternatively, even a patient with neutrophils of 90% will be neutropenic once the total white cell count decreases below $1.5 \times 10^9\,\mathrm{L^{-1}}$. This patient was both neutropenic ($0.5 \times 10^9\,\mathrm{L^{-1}}$) and lymphopenic ($0.4 \times 10^9\,\mathrm{L^{-1}}$) and in the setting of sepsis it is necessary to determine whether this predisposed to infection or whether it was a result of the infection.

Lymphopenia is extremely common in any acutely ill patient, but this observation in the peripheral blood does not indicate an absolute total deficiency of the body lymphoid mass and the patient is not at risk of additional infection as a direct consequence of lymphopenia. There is therefore no need to investigate this aspect further unless there is the possibility of pre-existing lymphopenia with immunodeficiency.

An important cause of lymphopenia is the acquired immune deficiency syndrome associated with HIV infection. Antibody serology should be determined in patients from high risk groups with disease compatible with this syndrome. In AIDS the lymphopenia is associated with a reduction in the total body lymphoid mass and is caused by a reduction in CD4 positive lymphocytes initially with other lymphocyte subpopulations affected later. Other patients who suffer from total body lymphoid deficiency and immunodeficiency are those receiving long-term immunosuppressive therapy.

Tricks

Neutropenia may be associated with defective production, such as when the bone marrow myeloid mass is deficient. Alternatively, excess adhesion of neutrophils to vessel walls (margination) or consumption or destruction in the circulation may cause neutropenia. The risk of secondary bacterial infection increases exponentially when the peripheral blood neutrophil count decreases below $0.5 \times 10^9 \mathrm{L}^{-1}$. However, the greatest risk is in patients who are neutropenic because of high-dose cytotoxic therapy as the gastrointestinal mucosa is also compromised and there is no barrier to the entry of organisms from the gastrointestinal tract.

Neutropenia may also arise from defective bone marrow production as in bone marrow aplasia, primary marrow disorders such as leukemia or infiltration of the bone marrow by carcinoma, lymphoma or fibrosis. Alternatively, peripheral neutrophil margination/consumption/destruction may occur as a consequence of hypersplenism, immune complex formation, presence of antineutrophil antibodies or overwhelming infection with endotoxin-producing organisms. Regardless of the cause, bacterial infection can be fatal within a few hours and these patients should receive immediate empirical antibiotic therapy to cover both Gram-positive and Gram-negative organisms. In patients with indwelling arterial or venous catheters it is prudent to use an antibiotic with activity against penicillin-resistant *Staphylococcus epidermidis*, such as vancomycin, instead of benzylpenicillin. This patient had no indwelling catheters and was not known to have been on antibiotics before so the choice of antibiotics was appropriate. Failure to implement immediate intravenous antibiotic therapy could result in rapid death. Once started, the cause of neutropenia can then be determined.

In this case there was a strong suspicion of chronic alcohol abuse. The hepatosplenomegaly would be consistent with chronic liver disease and a high MCV can result from direct marrow toxicity caused by alcohol. However, hepatosplenomegaly could also have been caused by infection or a primary hematological disorder. Therefore, bone marrow examination was necessary to determine whether marrow failure was responsible for the pancytopenia. This was performed and showed an active marrow indicating peripheral margination, consumption or destruction of neutrophils. Megaloblastic change was present caused by folate deficiency which undoubtedly compromised the productive capacity of the marrow and predisposed the patient to neutropenia associated with overwhelming pneumococcal infection.

A variety of infections can cause neutropenia, especially certain bacterial infections such as typhoid and paratyphoid. They often produce a transient neutrophilia during the bacteremic phase followed by neutropenia. Moderate neutropenia is also common in bacillary dysentery and brucellosis. Acute systemic viral infections, including influenza, infectious hepatitis, infectious mononucleosis and rickettsial infections, may cause neutropenia lasting 4–5 days. During this time toxic granulation is often prominent. Bone marrow examination is variable with occasional evidence of myelosuppression in some patients whilst in others the marrow is hypercellular as in this patient. Overwhelming bacterial infection causing neutropenia is usually associated with a predominance of neutrophil bands and metamyelocytes in the marrow. This is because of the premature release of mature neutrophils and does not represent defective maturation as the term 'maturation arrest' used to describe these appearances suggests.

Normally, the bone marrow contains a store of neutrophil precursors which can be rapidly mobilized during infection allowing a rapid increase in the neutrophil count whilst there is a proliferation of the neutrophil stem cells over several days in order to replenish the granulocyte pool. Thus, amplification and neutrophil release are able to combat infection. During prolonged viremia or sustained streptococcal infection neutrophil reserves may become exhausted and even amplified proliferation may be outweighed by destruction. This is unusual in healthy, young adults but is much more common in the newborn and elderly and in anyone receiving myelosuppressive drugs or toxins such as alcohol. A further possibility in a malnourished alcoholic is disseminated tuberculosis, which can be rapidly fatal.

In this patient with pneumococcal infection, severe neutropenia suggested that the infection had been present for some days. The mechanism of the neutropenia is not yet fully understood and whilst folate deficiency undoubtedly compromised the marrow response in this patient severe neutropenia can occur in the absence of marrow impairment. In septic patients there is a rapid increase of tumor necrosis factor (TNF)-alpha in the circulation which appears to initiate migration of neutrophils into the extravascular space. In response to TNF there is a dramatic increase in adhesion receptor expression on the surface of neutrophils and endothelium leading to anchorage of neutrophils on the endothelium and subsequent passage through spaces between endothelial cells into the extravascular tissue. There is increasing evidence that this process is a primary mediator for acute lung injury associated with sepsis. Thus, TNF blockade attenuates upregulation of the adhesion receptors preventing neutropenia and pulmonary dysfunction. In keeping with this finding is the observation that pretreatment of animals with monoclonal antibodies to the adhesion molecules on the neutrophil surface prevents neutrophil sequestration in endotoxin-induced neutropenia. Thus, endotoxin neutralization, TNF inhibition or receptor blockade have been suggested as potential strategies for the attenuation of pulmonary damage associated with septic shock. However, septic shock is complicated and it remains to be seen if such ideas have a useful clinical value.

Studies of the neutropenia of sepsis may give important insight into mechanisms of pulmonary dysfunction in critically ill patients, and treatment aimed at modifying neutrophil responses may be useful.

Follow-up

In this particular patient the lymphopenia was attributed to acute illness and an HIV antibody test was not performed. A blood film was examined which confirmed neutropenia with toxic granulation suggesting neutropenia secondary to infection. A bone marrow aspirate revealed a hypercellular marrow with production of all elements, but with left-shifted myelopoiesis (i.e. an absence of full maturation). Megaloblastic features were seen and a sample was obtained for measurement of B_{12} and folate levels. Blood cultures were obtained and sputum was examined by Gram staining and sent for bacterial culture. Broad-spectrum antibiotic therapy was started empirically with intravenous benzylpenicillin 1.2 g 6 hourly and ciprofloxacillin 200 mg 12 hourly. Both vitamin B_{12} (1 mg) and folinic acid (15 mg) were given intramuscularly and intravenously, respectively. Renal and liver function tests were performed.

The temperature resolved within 48 hours of starting antibiotics with a concomitant increase in neutrophil count to $24 \times 10^9 \, L^{-1}$ before decreasing 10 days later to $7.8 \times 10^9 \, L^{-1}$. The Gram stain had shown some positive diplococci but no acid-fast bacilli, and blood and sputum cultures subsequently confirmed the presence of *Streptococcus pneumoniae*. The chest radiograph shadowing resolved over the next 4 weeks. There was no clinical or radiographic evidence of empyema and mycobacterium cultures were negative 6 weeks after admission. The platelet count increased to $140 \times 10^9 \, L^{-1}$ during the admission and the hemoglobin increased to $11.0 \, g \, dL^{-1}$ with normalization of the MCV. Folate deficiency was confirmed as was cirrhosis with hepatosplenomegaly.

Pneumovax should be administered to reduce the risk of infection in the future with other strains of pneumococcus in this high risk patient.

Bibliography

1 Windsor AC, Walsh CJ, Mullen PG, Cook DJ, Fisher BJ, Blocher CR, Leeper-Woodford SK, Sugarman HJ and Fowler AA. Tumor necrosis factor-alpha blockade prevents neutrophil CD18 receptor upregulation and attenuates acute lung injury in porcine sepsis without inhibition of neutrophil oxygen radical generation. *Journal of Clinical Investigation* (1993) **91**: 1459–1468.
2 Burch RM, Noronha-Blob L, Lowe VC and Sullivan JP. Mice treated with a leumedin or antibody to Mac-1 to inhibit leukocyte sequestration survive endotoxin challenge. *Journal of Immunology* (1993) **150**: 3397–3403.
3 Windsor AC, Mullen PG, Walsh CJ, Fisher BJ, Blocher CR, Jesmok G, Fowler AA and Sugarman HJ. Delayed tumour necrosis factor alpha blockade attenuates pulmonary dysfunction and metabolic acidosis associated with experimental Gram-negative sepsis. *Archives of Surgery* (1994) **129**: 80–89.

7.5 Postoperative Hemorrhage in a Patient Receiving Aspirin

T. Baglin

History

A 42-year-old 70 kg male with a three-year history of angina and diffuse coronary arteriosclerosis underwent coronary artery bypass grafting to three vessels using autologous saphenous vein. Before surgery he was receiving aspirin 150 mg daily and slow release nifedipine 20 mg twice daily. The procedure was performed using extracorporeal bypass with full heparinisation. The bypass circuit was primed with 6000 units of heparin and a bolus of intravenous heparin 300 units kg^{-1} was given to the patient. Two minutes later an activated clotting time (ACT) was 500 s and the ACT was monitored at 30-minute intervals throughout the procedure. A bypass flow rate of 2.4 L min^{-1} was maintained with a minimally occlusive roller pump. Systemic hypothermia to 30°C [86°F] was maintained during aortic occlusion with the mean arterial blood pressure maintained at 60 mmHg. Surgery lasted 1 hour and the ACT did not decrease below 400 s. No further heparin was given. The patient was warmed to 37°C, weaned from bypass and heparin reversed with protamine sulfate 200 mg. Following transfer to the intensive care unit, intermittent positive-pressure ventilation was maintained. On arrival at the intensive care unit there was excessive blood loss from the drain. A coagulation screen revealed a prothrombin time (PT) of 13 s, a partial thromboplastin time (PTT) of 54 s (normal <45 s) and a platelet count of 145 × 10^9 L^{-1}. The patient continued to bleed excessively from a chest drain.

A bleeding time was performed and was normal at 8.5 min (normal range 4–9 min). Platelet transfusion was therefore withheld and in view of the long PTT 4 units of fresh frozen plasma (FFP) were given. The patient continued to bleed excessively through the chest drain.

Trap

In this patient the postoperative PT was normal, thrombocytopenia was minimal and the prolonged PTT was most probably caused by incomplete heparin neutralization by protamine sulfate. There was therefore no appreciable abnormality of hemostasis resulting directly from this short duration of extracorporeal circulation. Giving FFP is of no value.

Tricks

This case raises several points for discussion:

1. What is the effect of the extracorporeal circulation on hemostasis?
2. What is the effect of aspirin on blood loss in cardiac surgery?
3. How should heparin therapy be managed?
4. What is the value of the bleeding time?
5. Can blood loss in cardiac surgery patients be modified by agents such as DDAVP® or aprotinin?

During bypass, blood is in contact with a large area ($3\,m^2$) of plastic in the circuit. This surface can activate the coagulation, fibrinolytic, complement and inflammatory cascades. Furthermore, plasma proteins are adsorbed on to the artificial surface and platelets are secondarily 'contact-activated' leading to thrombocytopenia and impaired platelet function. The proteins are progressively denatured resulting in increased plasma viscosity and further impairment of platelet function. This effect is greater with bubble rather than membrane oxygenators but differences between the two are minimal with procedures lasting less than 3 hours.

The ability of the bypass circuit to activate the coagulation system necessitates the use of high-dose anticoagulation. This is traditionally achieved with heparin given to maintain the whole blood clotting time in excess of 400 s. This is easily achieved with 6000 units of heparin to prime the circuit and a bolus of 300 units kg^{-1} given to the patient. If the ACT falls below 400 s, a further bolus of 300 units kg^{-1} is given. When surgery is finished the heparin is neutralized by protamine sulfate at a dose of 1 mg per 100 units of heparin administered. This patient received 27 000 units of heparin necessitating 270 mg of protamine sulfate. Only 200 mg was administered initially. The correct treatment is to give more protamine sulfate and not infuse FFP. Heparin exerts its anticoagulant effect by binding to the naturally occurring anticoagulant protein antithrombin III and increasing its anticoagulant properties approximately 2000-fold. Thus, administration of FFP does not reverse the heparin effect as it does the anticoagulant effect of warfarin where coagulation factors are deficient.

The bleeding time is occasionally useful in identifying patients with congenital platelet dysfunction. However, it does not correlate with bleeding at surgery in normal patients. Thus, patients receiving aspirin may bleed excessively at surgery without any prolongation of the bleeding time. This procedure is therefore of little if any value in the routine management of cardiac surgery patients. Aspirin irreversibly acetylates platelet cyclo-oxygenase, an enzyme required for thromboxane formation. This is an important secondary activator required for optimal platelet function. As acetylation is irreversible, the antiplatelet effect of aspirin is maintained for the duration of the platelet life and only when new platelets, formed in the absence of aspirin, enter the circulation is the aspirin defect lost. In contrast, non-steroidal anti-inflammatory drugs are competitive inhibitors of cyclo-oxygenase and the milder antiplatelet effect resulting after ingestion of these drugs is short-lived, lasting only as long as the half-life of the drug. Patients are therefore often asked to stop aspirin several days before surgery. The bleeding time cannot be used to accurately quantitate the aspirin effect and reversal requires transfusion of platelets that have not been exposed to aspirin. An empirical approach is therefore often employed in which patients who have received aspirin within 5 days of surgery and are bleeding postoperatively despite adequate heparin neutralization are transfused with donor platelets (approximately 1 unit per 10 kg).

Since the recognition that giving the synthetic analog of vasopressin – DDAVP (desmopressin) – elevates von Willebrand protein levels and reduces surgical blood loss in patients with a variety of hereditary coagulation and platelet defects, several studies have now evaluated its effect in cardiac surgery patients. In general, DDAVP does not reduce blood loss in either adults or children, but does in patients who have previously received aspirin. It may be useful, therefore, to administer DDAVP ($0.3 \,\mu g \, kg^{-1}$ intravenously or subcutaneously) preoperatively to patients who have continued to take aspirin. Whilst there are as yet no clinical reports of its efficacy when given to treat hemorrhage in such patients it may be reasonable to try this before platelet transfusion, if it has not already been given before operation.

Finally, the serine protease inhibitor, aprotinin, has been found to reduce blood loss during a variety of surgical procedures. By chance in the 1980s it was found that aprotinin greatly reduced blood loss in cardiac surgery patients even in patients with no apparent impairment of hemostasis. Aprotinin is a 6.5 kDK polypeptide extracted from cattle and available as vials of 100 000 or 500 000 kallikrein inhibitor units (Trasylol®, Bayer). Its mode of action is uncertain as it inhibits many serine proteases, but inhibition of the fibrinolytic effector molecule plasmin may account largely for its hemostatic property. The circuit is primed with 2 000 000 units and the patient receives a bolus of 2 000 000 units followed by 500 000 units h^{-1} until 1 hour after bypass. This reduces blood loss by more than 50% and obviates the need for blood transfusion in many patients. In patients having re-operations, blood loss may be reduced from more than 1 L to less than 250 mL and septic patients, e.g. infected heart valves, also benefit from this effect. Patients receiving aspirin have also been studied. Reduction in blood loss is dramatic with reductions from more than 1.5 L to less than 250 mL.

Follow-up

The patient was given another 100 mg of protamine and 20 µg of DDAVP. The bleeding stopped and the rest of his time in hospital was uneventful.

Bibliography

1 Lind SE. The bleeding time does not predict surgical bleeding. *Blood* (1991) **77**: 2547–2552.
2 Channing Rodgers RP and Levin J. A critical reappraisal of the bleeding time. *Seminars in Thrombosis and Hemostasis* (1990) **1**: 1–21.
3 Levy JH. Aspirin and bleeding after coronary artery bypass grafting. *Anaesthesiology and Analgesics* (1994) **79**: 1–3.
4 Sheridan DP, Card RT, Pinilla JC, Harding SM, Thomson DJ, Gauthier L and Drotar

D. Use of desmopressin acetate to reduce blood transfusion requirements during cardiac surgery in patients with acetylsalicylic-acid-induced platelet dysfunction. *Canadian Journal of Surgery* (1994) **37**: 33–36.

5 Royston D. The serine antiprotease aprotinin (Trasylol): a novel approach to reducing postoperative bleeding. *Blood Coagulation and Fibrinolysis* (1990) **1**: 55–69.

8 Neurological Dysfunction

8.1 Cerebral Vascular Accident in a Young Adult
Lisa L. Kirkland

History

A 44-year-old male school teacher was admitted to the intensive care unit with a diagnosis of acute stroke. His family said that he had been well before the event, except for a slight 'cold' with fatigue, generalized headache, myalgias and chills for about a week. On the morning of admission he collapsed while getting ready for work. His wife noted immediately that he was alert but unable to speak or move his right side. She was unaware of any past medical problems, but said he smoked one pack per day and his father died of a myocardial infarction at the age of 70 years. His wife also said that he was told he had a heart murmur as a teenager.

In the ICU, he was alert but made no attempt to speak. His vital signs were: blood pressure 150/80 mmHg, pulse 115/minute and regular, respiratory rate 20/minute and non-labored, oral temperature 38.7°C [101.7°F]. Examination of the head was unremarkable except for scattered petechia over the soft palate. There was no neck stiffness or venous distension, carotid pulsations were equal bilaterally and no bruits were heard. His chest was clear and on examination of the heart a II/VI systolic murmur was heard at the apex, with faint radiation to the axilla. There were no rubs or gallops. His abdomen and extremities were normal. The skin had a few petechial hemorrhages over the tibias. Neurological examination showed a right hemiparesis and hemiplegia with complete expressive aphasia. He was able to follow commands with his left side. The cranial nerves were intact.

Laboratory investigations were as follows: white blood cells $18 \times 10^9 \, L^{-1}$ ($18\,000 \, mm^{-3}$) with 85% neutrophils, 6% bands, 10% lymphocytes, hematocrit 36%. His blood chemistry was normal, as were coagulation studies and platelet count. Urinalysis showed no white blood cells, 20–50 red blood cells, no bacteria or casts and 1+ protein.

Computed tomography of the head showed no abnormalities.

A diagnosis of an acute ischemic embolic stroke was made. The patient was anticoagulated with heparin; carotid Doppler studies and a transthoracic echocardiogram were ordered.

Trap

Stroke is uncommon in the young adult. The trap is neglecting the differential diagnosis of stroke in this patient population. The inadequate diagnostic evaluation in this patient led to the starting of potentially harmful therapy (anticoagulation) without looking for other causes of stroke in which this treatment would be contraindicated.

Tricks

The differential diagnosis of cerebral vascular accident in young adults (less than 45 years of age), is as complex as that in older patients. While young patients have strokes caused by arteriosclerotic disease, it is much less common than in older adults. Other causes must be sought *before* anticoagulation is started.

Cerebrovascular accidents in young adults may be caused by athero-sclerosis, non-atherosclerotic vasculopathies, cardiac lesions and hematological disorders. However, less than a third of cases are caused by atherosclerotic lesions.[1]

One cause of cerebral ischemic infarction may be non-atherosclerotic vasculopathies, including arterial dissection, vasculitis, fibromuscular dysplasia and non-penetrating traumatic arterial disease. Carotid or vetebral artery dissection is a major cause of ischemic cerebral vascular accidents in young adults. Dissection should be considered even in the absence of cervical trauma or manipulation. While carotid Doppler blood flow studies are useful in detecting carotid artery dissection in blunt trauma, angiography is the diagnostic procedure of choice to detect carotid or vertebral dissection.

Other vascular events include subarachnoid hemorrhage from ruptured intracranial saccular aneurysm, which may be missed by computed tomography. Anticoagulating a patient with a subarachnoid hemorrhage may prove disastrous. Additional vascular causes of ischemic stroke include drug or alcohol ingestion; crack cocaine is increasingly linked to both ischemic and hemorrhagic stroke. Migraine may induce cerebral ischemia, but should not be considered the sole cause of stroke until other possibilities have been investigated.

Heart lesions that may cause stroke in young adults include embolism from rheumatic heart valves, prosthetic cardiac valves, infective endocarditis, mitral valve prolapse and a cardiomyopathy. Paradoxical embolism from deep venous thrombosis may also occur. Often, transthoracic echocardiography is inadequate to assess cardiac valves and chamber structure/function. Transesophageal echocardiography is better.

Hypercoagulable states are associated with ischemic stroke in young adults. Oral contraceptives have an uncertain association with stroke and should not be considered the sole cause.

CNS infections (including HIV) and vasculitides may cause stroke in young patients. Syphilis is increasing in the USA, and leutic arteritis is associated with arterial dissection.

This patient has risk factors for arteriosclerotic cardiovascular disease; however, there are several other indicators in the history, an examination and indicate that the cause of the stroke. A history of fatigue, 'cold' for one week, fever, leukocytosis with a shift, soft palate and tibial petechiae, hematuria and anemia associated with a history of mitral valve prolapse are classic signs for subacute bacterial endocarditis. Up to 30% of patients with endocarditis will experience a cerebral infarction after an embolus; 90% of these occur in the middle cerebral artery distribution, but infarcts in the anterior or posterior cerebral artery also occur. Up to a third of these patients will have cerebral infarction as their presenting event.[2] Other CNS complications of endocarditis include formation and rupture of mycotic aneurysms owing to specific emboli and focal vasculitis or other infections such as cerebral abscess, meningitis or meningeal encephalitis. Hemorrhage may also result from hemorrhagic change in an ischemic infarct. Thus, anticoagulation is controversial in infective endocarditis.[3] Retrospective studies in patients with both infected native and prosthetic valves emphasize antibiotic therapy as the treatment which most consistently reduces recurrence of cerebral embolic and hemorrhagic events in endocarditis. Patients who are anticoagulated generally have a higher incidence of hemorrhagic stroke, regardless of the adequacy of antibiotic therapy.[4] Furthermore, anticoagulation has not been shown to decrease the recurrence of embolic phenomena. In general, for anticoagulation bacterial endocarditis with or without ischemic stroke is not warranted without clear-cut indications such as prosthetic cardiac valves, particularly in young adults.[5,6]

Follow-up

In this patient, transesophageal echocardiography demonstrated mitral valve prolapse with vegetations on the valve. Multiple blood cultures were positive for *Streptococcus viridans*. A carotid Doppler study was normal. Anticoagulation was stopped. The patient received ceftriaxone which reduced the fever and by day 7 blood cultures were sterile. Although he later developed peripheral signs of embolization (splinter and subconjunctival hemorrhages, Osler's nodes) he did not experience further cerebral events. He regained partial function of his right arm, but his expressive aphasia persisted.

References

1 Toffol G, Swiontoniowski M. Stroke in young adults. *Postgraduate Medicine* (1992) **91**: 123–127.
2 Lerner P. Neurologic complications of infective endocarditis. *Medical Clinics of North America* (1985) **69**: 385–398.
3 Hart R, Kagan-Hallet K and Joerns S. Mechanisms of intracranial hemorrhage in infective endocarditis. *Stroke* (1987) **18**: 1048–1056.
4 Delahaye JP, Poncet P, Malquarti V, Beaune J, Gare JP and Mann JM. Cerebrovascular accidents in infective endocarditis: role of anticoagulation. *European Heart Journal* (1990) **11**: 1074–1078.
5 Hart RG, Foster JW, Luther MF and Kanter MC. Stroke in infective endocarditis. *Stroke* (1990) **21**: 695–700.
6 Paschalis C, Pugsley W and Harrison JR. Rate of cerebral embolic events in relation to antibiotic and anticoagulant therapy in patients with bacterial endocarditis. *European Neurology* (1990) **30**: 87–89.

8.2 Respiratory Assessment in Acute Neuromuscular Paralysis

Christopher Veremakis and Subhash Todi

History

A 35-year-old truck driver was admitted to hospital with complaints of progressive weakness in all the extremities. The weakness began in both legs the day before admission and progressed so that he was unable to stand without support by the next morning. The weakness was by then affecting his hands and he was unable to pick up objects. He also complained of tingling and numbness in his hands and legs. He denied any back pain, bladder or bowel problem, headache, nausea or vomiting. He had no complaints of shortness of breath, swallowing difficulty or visual problems.

Previously he had been in good health with no history of recent vaccination. He had a 'flu-like illness with mild gastrointestinal upset a few weeks earlier.

On examination he was a well-built, white male, not in any obvious discomfort. Vital signs were normal. Chest, cardiac and abdominal examination were normal. He was awake, alert and fully oriented. There was no neck stiffness and examination of the cranial nerves was within normal limits. Cough and gag reflexes were intact. There was generalized hypotonia, and all deep tendon reflexes were diminished. Plantar response was equivocal. Upper limb power was 2/5 and weaker distally; lower limb power was 1/5. He was able to sit upright without losing balance. There was mild hypoesthesia of hands and feet, but no major sensory loss.

His hematocrit was 42%; his white blood count, platelets, BUN and creatinine were normal. A lumbar puncture was performed which revealed clear fluid under normal pressure. Protein was slightly raised at $60 \, \text{mg} \, \text{dL}^{-1}$, sugar normal, cell count < 5 cells, all lymphocytes. EMG and nerve conduction studies were ordered.

The patient was given oxygen by nasal prongs, and monitored by a continuous pulse oximetry which revealed an S_aO_2 of 99%. The physician left an instruction to be informed if the patient complained of dyspnea, or the oxygen saturation was below 93%. Four hours later, at 02.00 hours, he was found unresponsive and apneic. The cardiac arrest team was called. He was hand-ventilated. The peripheral pulses could not be felt and he had very weak central pulse. Electrocardiographic monitoring showed a marked sinus bradycardia. After tracheal intubation and starting of cardiopulmonary resuscitation, an arterial blood gas showed a pH of 7.20 [H^+ 62], P_aCO_2 65 mmHg [8.7 kPa], P_aO_2 165 mmHg [22 kPa] on an F_IO_2 of 1.0. He was rapidly resuscitated and then placed on assist-control ventilation.

Trap

There was an inappropriate reliance of arterial oxygenation to detect hypopnea in a patient on supplemental oxygen. Apneic oxygenation is possible in this setting since the F_IO_2, at a fixed oxygen flow, will increase as minute ventilation decreases. Furthermore, failure to appreciate the rapidity with which polyneuritis may affect the respiratory muscle can be a life-threatening mistake.

Tricks

Although patients with acute polyneuritis may present with only limb weakness, they may develop a rapid ascending paralysis involving the intercostal muscles and the diaphragm over a period of a few hours.[1,2] Such patients may look quite well and have no complaint of shortness of breath, immediately before a fatal respiratory arrest.[2,3] Moreover signs of increased work of breathing and impending respiratory muscle fatigue, such as the use of accessory muscles of respiration, alternate use of intercostal and diaphragmatic breathing (respiratory alternans) or paradoxical inward abdominal motion during inspiration (abdominal paradox) may be missing because all muscles may be involved.[4] Therefore reliance on these features as a warning of serious respiratory compromise or as a guide for tracheal intubation may create a false sense of security, and place the patient at needless risk. An increasing respiratory rate is probably the only reliable sign of impending respiratory failure in these patients. However, even this sign is subject to a high degree of interobserver variability.[4]

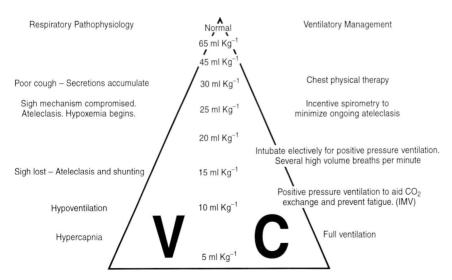

Figure 8.2.1. Relation between respiratory pathophysiology, vital capacity (**VC**) and ventilatory management in patients with respiratory distress.

Paralysis of the respiratory muscles and reduction in ventilatory capacity may be extremely subtle in onset. Only through careful monitoring can the need for supportive measures be properly appraised. Ventilatory function is best monitored by frequent direct measurements of pulmonary mechanics.[2] A vital capacity is easily performed at the bedside, is sensitive and reproducible, and causes no discomfort to the patient. Experience in large respiratory ICUs has produced guidelines based on vital capacity criteria regarding the need for tracheal intubations (Figure 8.2.1). These have been validated in many others.[3,5–7]

A normal forced vital capacity is $65 \, \text{mL kg}^{-1}$; a volume of $30 \, \text{mL kg}^{-1}$ is generally associated with a poor forced cough, and accumulation of secretions requiring careful observation, chest physiotherapy and incentive spirometry. At a level of $25 \, \text{mL kg}^{-1}$ the sigh mechanism is compromised and atelectasis occurs. At this level, atelectasis is usually miliary and not visible radiographically, but may cause a widening of the A–a gradient, with resulting hypoxemia.[7] Early application of supplemental oxygen as was employed in this patient may mask the progressive increase of the A–a gradient that indicates deteriorating respiratory mechanics. With a reduction of vital capacity to $15 \, \text{mL kg}^{-1}$ elective tracheal intubation should be considered. A deterioration to $7–10 \, \text{mL kg}^{-1}$ is associated with hypercarbia, respiratory acidosis and, if not promptly treated, will result in the need for emergency tracheal intubation with all the associated complications.[7]

The expiratory vital capacity should be measured with the patient sitting at 30–60 degrees, every 4 hours using a hand-held spirometer, with the nose clipped, taking special care to seal the lips around the mouthpiece, and exhorting the patient to maximal effort. The highest value of three trials should be recorded.[7]

These measurements need patient cooperation and effort, and intact power of facial muscles. However, if the pharyngeal and laryngeal muscles become involved, depressing normal airway protective mechanisms, elective tracheal intubation is recommended regardless of vital capacity measurements.[3]

Other circumstances in which monitoring serial vital capacity proves difficult is in the presence of pre-existing obstructive airway disease. In this situation, measuring maximal respiratory pressure on inspiration (i.e. Pi_{max}) and on expiration (Pe_{max}) may be useful.[8,9] In some series, Pe_{max} was the most sensitive indicator of weakness and became abnormal before changes in vital capacity.[3,10,11] These measurements can be made with simple pressure manometers, calibrated in centimeters of water. When Pe_{max} is reduced to less than $40 \, \text{cmH}_2\text{O}$ in an adult, cough is usually ineffective and the patient is unable to adequately clear secretion from the upper airways. A Pi_{max} of less than $20 \, \text{cmH}_2\text{O}$ generally correlates with a reduction in vital capacity to barely twice the tidal volume. This reflects severe weakness of inspiratory muscles and is also an indication for tracheal intubation.[3]

In summary, diligent measurements of pulmonary mechanics are necessary to avoid the disastrous respiratory consequences of acute polyneuritis.

Follow-up

After a prolonged course of ventilatory support, the patient recovered almost completely. He was left with some residual weakness in his legs. This was thought to be caused by his polyneuritis. His intellectual functions were normal indicating that he had not suffered any hypoxic injury to his brain.

References

1 Newsum JK, Smith RM and Croker D. Intubation for acute respiratory failure in Guillian–Barré syndrome. *Journal of the American Medical Association* (1979) **242**: 1650–1651.

2 Sunderrajan EV and Davenport J. The Guillain–Barre syndrome; pulmonary–neurologic correlations. *Medicine* (1985) **64**: 333–341.

3 O'Donohue WJ, Baker JP and Bell GM. Respiratory failure in neuromuscular disease–management in a respiratory intensive care unit. *Journal of the American Medical Association* (1976) **235**: 733–735.

4 Cohen CA, Zagelbaum G and Ditza G. Clinical manifestations of inspiratory muscle fatigue. *American Journal of Medicine* (1982) **73**: 308–316.

5 Griggs RC, Donhoe KM and Utell MJ. Evaluation of pulmonary function in neuromuscular disease. *Archives of Neurology* (1981) **38**: 9–12.

6 Ropper AH. Severe acute Guillian–Barre syndrome. *Neurology* (1986) **36**: 429–432.

7 Ropper AH and Kehne SM. Guillain–Barre syndrome: management of respiratory failure. *Neurology* (1985) **35**: 1662–1665.

8 Rahn H, Otis AB, Chadwick LE and Fenn WO. The pressure volume diagram of the thorax and lung. *American Journal of Physiology* (1946) **146**: 161–178.

9 Rinqvist T. The ventilatory capacity in healthy subjects: an analysis of causal factors with special references to the respiratory forces. *Scandinavian Journal of Clinical Laboratory Investigations* (1966) **18**(5): 179.

10 Black LF and Hyatt RE. Maximal respiratory pressures: normal values and relationship to age and sex. *American Review of Respiratory Diseases* (1969) **99**: 696–702.

11 Black LF and Hyatt RE. Maximal static respiratory pressures in generalised neuromuscular disease. *American Review of Respiratory Diseases* (1971) **103**: 641–650.

12 Moore P and James O. Guillain–Barre Syndrome: incidence, management and outcome of major complications. *Critical Care Medicine* (1981) **9**: 549–555.

13 Pontopiddan H, Geffin B and Lowenstein E. Acute respiratory failure in the adult. *New England Journal of Medicine* (1972) **287**: 743–752.

8.3 Polyneuropathy of Critical Illness
J.C. Farmer

History

A 32-year-old male was admitted to a medical intensive care unit with sepsis and emerging multiorgan failure. He was diagnosed with acute myelomonocytic leukemia 10 days before, and received induction chemotherapy shortly thereafter. He was febrile and pancytopenic for the three days before this ICU admission. On arrival he was hypotensive and required both fluids and vasopressor support. His trachea was intubated and he was placed on positive-pressure ventilation with $12\,cmH_2O$ of PEEP and an F_IO_2 of 0.80 for progressive hypoxemia, respiratory distress and bilateral pulmonary infiltrates. Unfortunately, his $P_aO_2 : F_IO_2$ ratio decreased to <200 and his proximal airway pressures exceeded $50\,cmH_2O$ because of both worsening lung disease and poor synchrony of his spontaneous respiratory pattern with the ventilator. To minimize airway pressures and reduce systemic oxygen consumption, continuous infusions of midazolam and vecuronium were begun after intravenous bolus doses of both. Over the next two days he developed severe bronchospasm and significant auto-PEEP that reduced his cardiac output (see Section 3). He had a variable, and at times adequate response, to inhaled beta agonists, but improved dramatically over several hours with the addition of intravenous methylprednisolone.

   The patient's problems included sepsis in an immunocompromised host, respiratory failure (pseudomonas pneumonia, bronchospasm and ARDS), oliguria and worsening azotemia (BUN: $51\,mg\,dL^{-1}$ [$8.5\,mmol\,L^{-1}$], creatinine: $2.2\,mg\,dL^{-1}$ [$168\,\mu mol\,L^{-1}$], pancytopenia (WBC: $0.5\,mm^{-3}$, hemoglobin: $7.2\,g\,dL^{-1}$, platelets: $12\,\mu L^{-1}$), altered mental status, disseminated intravenous coagulation and hyperbilirubinemia (direct: $4.8\,mg\,dL^{-1}$ [$82\,\mu mol\,L^{-1}$] with elevated hepatic transaminases (AST: $230\,IU$; ALT: $183\,IU$). He was continued on a third-generation cephalosporin and an aminoglycoside, adjusted for renal function. Erythromycin and vancomycin were added empirically on arrival to the ICU. Intravenous drug infusions given concomitantly included: dopamine $10\,\mu g\,kg^{-1}$ min–1, vecuronium $0.01\,mg\,kg^{-1}\,h^{-1}$ and midazolam $2\,mg^{-1}\,h^{-1}$. Peripheral nerve stimulation was performed every 6 hours to monitor the depth of muscle relaxation. It was maintained at a level of 1 out of 4 contractions, using a train of four stimulus to the adductor pollicus branch of the ulnar nerve.

Traps

Polyneuropathy of critical illness is a serious complication which prolongs ICU length of stay.[1] Several variables contribute to its development: (1) prolonged use of muscle relaxant drugs (usually non-depolarizing agents such as vecuronium and pancuronium); (2) concurrent use of aminoglycosides; (3) prolonged use of steroids; (4) other drugs (e.g. aminophylline); and (5) sepsis-induced multiorgan failure, particularly with renal and hepatic dysfunction.

Polyneuropathy of critical illness presents variably, but usually includes extremity weakness and often respiratory muscle weakness. In this patient, tracheostomy and prolonged mechanical ventilation were ultimately needed while awaiting the return of acceptable motor function. Muscle fiber necrosis occurs in a significant number of patients with polyneuropathy of critical illness; the cause is unknown. Clinically, this manifests as creatinine phosphokinase and aldolase elevations.

Tricks

A heightened awareness of the risk factor for developing polyneuropathy of critical illness is the best way to prevent its development. The typical patient is one with status asthmaticus who needs mechanical ventilation and additionally receives high-dose corticosteroids and muscle relaxant drugs. Sepsis and multiorgan failure are present in over half of the patients with this disorder. Aminoglycoside use is the next most common association. Other less common associations include: presence of a metabolic acidosis, elevated serum magnesium levels, female sex, renal failure, increased concentrations of the metabolite of vecuronium bromide (3-desacetylvecuronium).[2,3]

Use of a peripheral nerve stimulator may help monitor and prevent the accumulation of muscle relaxant drugs. However, polyneuropathy of critical illness has been described in patients who had an appropriate level of neuromuscular blockade throughout muscle relaxant administration. Myopathy and polyneuropathy of motor fibers were implicated as causal.[4]

Most patients who develop polyneuropathy of critical illness eventually return to their normal level of motor function. Unfortunately, the time interval to return varies from days to weeks to months. A minority of patients are left with residual motor function deficits, which are usually manifested as peripheral extremity weakness.

Therapy is primarily supportive. Ongoing mechanical ventilation and tracheostomy are often required. Prevention of complications associated with ventilator use is paramount. These include, but are not limited to: failure to recognize ventilator malfunctions, barotrauma and nosocomial pneumonia. Supplemental nutrition and attention to metabolic details are crucial to successful weaning from mechanical ventilation. Finally, physical therapy, occupational therapy, psychological support and prevention of deep venous thrombosis should be attended to as well.[5]

Follow-up

Over the next five days, the patient stabilized and his multiorgan dysfunction significantly resolved. Weaning from mechanical ventilation was begun. Unfortunately, all attempts at weaning failed during the next several days because of inadequate respiratory muscle function. A tracheostomy was performed, and the patient was gradually weaned from mechanical ventilation over the next 21 days.

References

1 Chad DA and Lacomis D. Critically ill patients with newly acquired weakness: the clinicopathological spectrum. *Annals of Neurology* (1994) **35**: 257–259.
2 Isenstein DA, Venner DS and Duggan J. Neuromuscular blockade in the intensive care unit. *Chest* (1992) **102**: 1258–1266.
3 Segredo V, Caldwell JE, Matthay MA, Sharma ML, Gruenke LD and Miller RD. Persistent paralysis after long-term administration of vecuronium. *New England Journal of Medicine* (1992) **327**: 524–528.
4 Coursin DB. Neuromuscular blockade: should patients be relaxed in the ICU? *Chest* (1992) **102**: 988–989.
5 Bolton FC. Polyneuropathy of critical illness. *Journal of Intensive Care Medicine* (1994) **9**: 132–138.

8.4 Focal Neurologic Presentation of Diffuse Metabolic Encephalopathy

Jeffrey E. Salon and Tarek A. Chidiac

History

A 67-year-old woman was found by her family on the floor of her bathroom. She was unrousable and her right side was flaccid. Paramedics were called and she was given naloxone 0.4 mg, thiamine 100 mg and 2.5cc 50% dextrose intravenously with only slight improvement of her mental status. She was given supplemental oxygen by mask.

Routine laboratory studies were taken on arrival in the emergency department. 5% Dextrose and 0.45% saline at $100\,mL\,h^{-1}$ were given into a peripheral vein. After stabilization of vital signs, she was transferred to the neurosurgical service of a large teaching hospital for a CT scan and management of her acute stroke.

At this hospital her CT scan was reviewed. No surgical lesion was found and she was sent to the intensive care unit for medical management. Her past medical history was significant in that she had long-standing hypertension treated with diuretics and an ACE-inhibitor, and type II diabetes for which she took oral hypoglycemic agents.

Physical examination revealed an obese, lethargic woman in no acute distress. Her heart rate was 110/minute and regular, respirations 20/minute, temperature 37.8°C [100.1°F] and blood pressure 170/105 mmHg. There was no sign of head injury, the pupils were equally round and reacted to light, and fundoscopic examination showed mild, copper-wire changes without papille-dema. Neck veins were flat and breath sounds were normal in all lung fields. The cardiac impulse was displaced 4 cm laterally and there was a II/VI systolic ejection murmur (SEM). The abdominal examination was normal and there was no peripheral edema.

The neurological examination demonstrated that the patient was easily rousable to noxious stimuli. She did not have doll's eyes movements and cranial nerves II–XII were grossly intact. Sensation to pain and pin-prick were intact, except for paresis of the right arm. Both plantar responses were downgoing.

Unenhanced CT of the head demonstrated no mass effect, mid-line shift or focal densities. Electrolytes from the other hospital's emergency department revealed an Na^+ $137\,mEq\,L^{-1}$, K^+ $3.3\,mEq\,L^{-1}$, Cl^- $105\,mEq\,L^{-1}$, HCO_3^- $24\,mEq\,L^{-1}$, glucose $61\,mg\,dL^{-1}$ [$3.4\,mmol\,L^{-1}$], BUN $31\,mg\,dL^{-1}$ [$5\,mmol\,L^{-1}$] Creatinine $1.9\,mg\,dL^{-1}$ [$145\,\mu mol\,L^{-1}$] (FBC, PT, PTT and hepatic enzymes were normal). Arterial blood gas analysis revealed a pH of 7.45 [H^+ $35\,nmol\,L^{-1}$], P_aCO_2 $31\,mmHg$ [$4.1\,kPa$] P_aO_2L $101\,mmHg$ [$13.5\,kPa$], 96% saturation while on $2\,L\,min^{-1}$ nasal oxygen.

Trap

Acute focal neurological deficits are usually the result of focal defects in cerebral circulation (embolic or ischemic) but they should not cause stupor or coma. Stupor or coma suggests either massive intracranial events (which were not seen by CT scan) or toxic-metabolic encephalopathy.

Trick

This patient's level of consciousness improved after the paramedics arrived and gave glucose, thiamine and naloxone. Unfortunately, no dextrostix measurement or blood was examined before she received these medications.[1] A low blood sugar after 50% dextrose in the face of improved mental status along with a history of oral hypoglycemic agents should lead to a thorough investigation of hypoglycemia as the cause of coma.

Although the focal neurological signs in this patient pointed toward a localized, organic lesion, consciousness should not be affected. To produce stupor or coma one of three sites must be damaged; these are (1) a diffuse bilateral injury in the cerebrocortical area; (2) the ascending reticular activating system; or (3) the brainstem.[2] Toxic or metabolic insults should be considered whenever there is a dramatic alteration of consciousness and intact pupillary reflexes. Metabolic coma most commonly results in symmetrical neurological signs, but this is not absolute.[2] Focal neurological deficits have been reported with diffuse metabolic abnormalities and certainly with hypoglycemia.[3]

Importantly, the common antidotes given in emergency situations usually have a duration of action much shorter than the toxin they are reversing. The half-life of opioids and their semisynthetic derivatives are much longer than that of naloxone (half-life 20–60 min)[4] while the hypoglycemic effects of oral hypoglycemic agents and their metabolites can last many days.[5] Both opioids and oral hypoglycemic agents can be detected by toxin screening. Transient improvement in the level of consciousness after the antidotes should prompt an investigation into metabolic causes of stupor and coma. A normal glucose of 61 mg dL^{-1} [3.38 mmol L^{-1}] in a diabetic with acute illness should be viewed with suspicion as a more typical response is hyperglycemia in response to the stress.[6] It is also important to note that the symptoms of hypoglycemia often occur at relatively normal levels in patients with a history of poorly controlled diabetes.[7]

Follow-up

Repeat electrolytes and an automated chemical profile were obtained. Toxicology screens were sent to a reference laboratory. Serum glucose was 19 mg dL^{-1} [1.05 mmol L^{-1}]. The patient was given another milliliter of 50% dextrose intravenously and the intravenous fluid was changed from 0.45% saline to 10% dextrose with KCl. Blood sugars were monitored every 15 minutes until her glucose increased slightly above the normal (kept between 175–199 mg dL^{-1}). This required an infusion of 20% dextrose by central vein for the next 6 hours.

Her sensorium cleared quickly while motor function returned to the right arm after the dextrose infusion was begun. She needed intravenous dextrose for nearly 72 hours to prevent hypoglycemia and did not need any diabetic medication until her fourth hospital day. Before discharge she was placed on a weight-reduction diet and received formal education in diabetic classes. Four months later she had lost weight and the oral hypoglycemic agents could be stopped.

References

1 Mills ML. Coma and altered consciousness. In: Harwood-Nuss A, Linden CH, Luten RC, Sternbach G, Wolfson AB (eds) *The Clinical Practice of Emergency Medicine.* Philadelphia, J.B. Lippincott, pp 15–17, 1991.

2 Plum F and Posner JB. *Diagnosis of Stupor and Coma,* 2nd edn. Philadelphia, F.A. Davis, p 7, 1972.

3 Malouf F and Brust JCM. Hypoglycemia: causes, neurological manifestations and outcome. *Annals of Neurology* (1985) **17**: 421–430.

4 Goldfrank LR and Bresnitz EA. Opioids. In: Goldfrank LR, Flomenbaum NE, Lewin NA, Weisman RS, Howland MA, Kulberg AG (eds) *Toxicologic Emergencies.* East Norwalk, CT, Appleton-Century-Crofts, p 406, 1986.

5 Kahn CR and Schecter Y. Insulin, oral hypoglycemic agents, and the pharmacology of the endocrine pancreas. In: Gilman AG, Rall TW, Nies AS, Taylor P (eds) *The Pharmacological Basis of Therapeutics,* 8th edn. Elmsford, NY, Pergamon Press, pp 1463–1495, 1990.

6 Bessey PQ, Downey RS and Monafo WW. Metabolic response to injury and critical illness. In: Civetta JM, Taylor RW, Kirby RR (eds) *Critical Care.* Philadelphia, J.B. Lippincott, pp 527–539, 1992.

7 Boyle PJ, Schwartz NS, Shah SD, Clutter WE and Cryer PE. Plasma glucose concentrations at the onset of hypoglycemia symptoms in patients with poorly controlled diabetes and in nondiabetics. *New England Journal of Medicine* (1988) **318**: 1487–1492.

8.5 The Importance of Free (Unbound) Anticonvulsants in Critically Ill Patients

Tarek A. Chidiac and Jeffrey E. Salon

History

A 35-year-old male, intravenous drug abuser with AIDS was transferred to the intensive care unit from the medical floor for worsening respiratory failure from a *Pneumocystis carinii* pneumonia. He had a history of *grand mal* epilepsy for which he received phenytoin 300 mg daily. His vital signs on admission to the unit were: temperature 38.5°C [101.3°F], respirations 35/minute, blood pressure 100/70 mmHg and heart rate 115/minute. Physical examination showed a poor nutritional status, severe respiratory distress and agitation. His lungs had bilateral crackles and his cardiovascular examination was unremarkable. There were no focal neurological deficits. Pulse oximetry on 40% oxygen by face mask was 82%. Because of the hypoxemia and respiratory distress, his trachea was urgently intubated and ventilatory support was started. He was being treated with trimethoprim/sulfamethoxazole for the pneumonia and was also receiving enteral feedings. His respiratory status gradually improved and he was successfully weaned from mechanical ventilation and his trachea extubated four days later.

On the fifth day, however, he became difficult to rouse. Vital signs were: temperature 37°C [98.6°F], heart rate 100/minute, blood pressure 140/80 mmHg and respirations 20/minute. His eyes showed bilateral horizontal nystagmus with normal pupillary reactions. The rest of his neurological examination was normal, except for intermittent dysarthria. A CT scan of the brain showed one 0.5 cm contrast-enhancing lesion in the basal ganglia of the right hemisphere. His phenytoin level was 18 μg mL^{-1} [71 mmol L^{-1}]. A presumptive diagnosis of CNS toxoplasmosis with cerebellar involvement was made. Pyrimethamine-clindamycin was started and an MRI of the brain was ordered.

Traps

This patient had developed phenytoin toxicity, which was initially missed because of underestimation of the importance of the concentration of the unbound fraction (free) phenytoin.[1] There was a failure to recognize the factors (hypoalbuminemia, sulfamethoxazole, etc.) that may contribute to increased phenytoin toxicity in critically ill patients.[1,2] There was also an overreliance on expensive tests (MRI) to pursue a rare diagnosis (cerebellar toxoplasmosis) when simple measures (such as stopping phenytoin) may clarify the issue. The failure to recognize phenytoin toxicity (especially in the face of some rather classic physical findings), reflects our reliance on technology over routine clinical management.

Tricks

Since the patient was recently started on sulfamethoxazole, an agent known to displace phenytoin from albumin-binding sites, one may either simply stop the phenytoin or document phenytoin toxicity by measuring serum albumin and free (unbound) plasma phenytoin levels.[1] Unbound plasma phenytoin and other free anticonvulsant levels (valproic acid, carbamazepine, phenobarbital) are responsible for both the therapeutic effect and the toxicity.[3]

In this patient many factors may have influenced the concentration of free plasma phenytoin. Phenytoin toxicity may be insidious and difficult to differentiate from neurological disorders.[4] Total plasma concentrations of 10–20 mg mL^{-1} [40–80 mmol L^{-1}] are usually effective to control the seizures.[5] While therapeutic unbound phenytoin is usually less than 10% (1–2 µg mL^{-1}) [4–8 mmol L^{-1}], in certain circumstances the free fraction may increase above 20% of the total concentration.[1,6]

At steady state, free phenytoin concentration in normal individuals correlates well with total plasma concentration and thus efficacy and/or toxicity.[1,4] Therefore, measurement of free plasma phenytoin concentration is not necessary when protein binding is not altered.[4] However, in special circumstances, protein binding may be disrupted and measuring free serum

Table 8.5.1. Circumstances associated with reduction of protein binding of phenytoin[1,2,4,5,9,14–16]

Mechanism	Clinical situation
Displacement from protein-binding sites	Concomitant therapy with: Diazepam Heparin Phenylbutazone Salicylates Valproate Sulfonylureas Antibiotics (nafcillin, ceftriaxone and sulfamethoxazole) High free fatty acid serum levels (pregnancy)
Hypoalbuminemia	Malnutrition (elderly, cancer) Liver failure Renal failure (nephrosis) Critical illness (sepsis, trauma, burn, etc.)
Dilutional hypoalbuminemia	Last trimester of pregnancy
Reduced affinity of albumin to phenytoin	Renal failure Critical illness (sepsis, trauma) Increased sampling temperature*

* When free concentrations are measured by high-performance liquid chromatography.

concentrations becomes essential for determining therapeutic efficacy and/
or toxicity. Table 8.5.1 summarizes the circumstances that result in
decreased protein binding of phenytoin. Factors that may alter total plasma
phenytoin concentration and other anticonvulsants are widely recognized
and are not reviewed here.[3] While variation of the free serum concentrations of antiepileptics with total serum concentrations is well known, other
less-well-recognized factors are discussed here.[3,5] In this patient, toxicity
was not manifest until the fifth day in the critical care unit. Fever and
enteral feeding are two factors that may reduce total plasma phenytoin
concentration.[7,8] After tracheal extubation, the enteral feeding was stopped
and the fever controlled. Both would increase the free fraction of phenytoin
in addition to that expected from hypoalbuminemia and sulfamethoxazole
therapy.[2,4] The lack of a reliable method to calculate free phenytoin
concentration in critically ill patients supports the necessity of quantifying
both free and total phenytoin concentrations.[9,10]

   Unbound plasma levels of other anticonvulsants (valproic acid, carbamazepine, phenobarbital) also need to be monitored in critically ill patients.[11,13]
Many methods have been employed for their determination. Fluorescence
polarization immunoassay is widely used[6] (Table 8.5.2). Table 8.5.3 summarizes
the clinical circumstances influencing solely free plasma concentrations of
valproic acid, carbamazepine and phenobarbital. Factors that may affect total
plasma concentrations of such anticonvulsants are reviewed elsewhere.[3,5]

Follow-up

In this patient an MRI showed no evidence of cerebellar lesions. The phenytoin
was stopped and signs of toxicity gradually disappeared. Later, the phenytoin was
reintroduced at a lower dose. Free phenytoin was measured and adjustment of the
phenytoin dosage was made to maintain a free phenytoin level between 1 and
$2\,\mu g\,mL^{-1}$ [4–8 mmol L^{-1}] during this patient's acute illness.[6] After an additional
four days, the patient's respiratory status had improved enough for him to be
discharged from the hospital.

Table 8.5.2. Reported optimal free and total plasma concentrations (C) of various
antiepileptic drugs as determined by fluorescence polarization immunoassay[6]

Drug	Total (C) ($\mu g\,mL^{-1}$)	Free (C) ($\mu g\,mL^{-1}$)
Phenytoin	10–20	1–2
Valproic acid	80–150	4–50
Carbamazepine	8–12	1.6–2.4
Phenobarbital	15–40	7.5–20

Table 8.5.3. Direct influence exerted on free antiepileptic drug concentrations in certain clinical circumstances[5,11,14,16,17–21]

Clinical situation	Valproic acid	Carbamazepine	Phenobarbital
Hypoalbuminemia	Increased	Increased	Increased
Co-medication*			
Phenytoin	No effect	Decreased	Not reported
Valproic acid	Not applicable	Increased	Not reported
Carbamazepine	No effect	Not applicable	Not reported
Phenobarbital	No effect	No effect	Not applicable
Pregnancy**	Increased	Increased	Not reported
Hepatic disease	Increased	Increased	Not reported
Renal disease	Increased	Not reported	Not reported
Increased sampling temperature†	Not reported	Increased	Increased
Increased free fatty acid concentrations (pregnancy, individual variability, fasting)	Increased	No effect	Not reported
Increased triglyceride concentrations	Not reported	Increased	Not reported

* Influence on total concentrations is not represented. Effect exerted via competitive protein binding.
** Two mechanisms may be involved: dilutional hypoalbuminemia (valproic acid, carbamazepine) and displacement of valproic acid from albumin by high plasma concentrations of free fatty acids.
† When free concentrations are measured by high-performance liquid chromatography.

References

1 Baird-Lambert J, Manglick MP, Wall M and Buchanan N. Identifying patients who might benefit from free phenytoin monitoring. *Therapeutic Drug Monitor* (1987) **9**: 134–138.

2 Dasgupta A, Dennen DA, Dear R and McLawhon RW. Displacement of phenytoin from serum protein carriers by antibiotics: studies with ceftriaxone, nafcillin, and sulfamethoxazole. *Clinical Chemistry* (1991) **37**: 98–100.

3 Rall TW and Schleifer LS. Drugs effective in the therapy of the epilepsies. In: Goodman Gilman A, Rall TW, Nies AS, Taylor P (eds). *The Pharmacological Basis of Therapeutics*, 8th edn. New York, Pergamon Press, pp 436–462, 1990.

4 Aronson JK, Hardman M and Reynolds DJM. Phenytoin. *British Medical Journal* (1992) **305**: 1215–1218.

5 Leppik IE. Metabolism of antiepileptic medication: newborn to elderly. *Epilepsia* (1992) **33**: S32–S40.

6 *Laboratory Reference Manual*. Cleveland, Ohio, ARUP, Cleveland Clinic Foundation, January 1994.

7 Leppik IE, Fisher J, Kriel R and Sawchuk RJ. Altered phenytoin clearance with febrile illness. *Neurology* (1986) **36**: 1367–1370.

8 Haley CJ and Nelson J. Phenytoin–enteral feeding interaction. *Annals of Pharmacotherapy* (1989) **23**: 796–798.

9 Griebel ML, Kearns Gl, Fiser DH, Woody RC and Turley CP. Phenytoin protein binding in pediatric patients with acute traumatic injury. *Critical Care Medicine* (1990) **18**: 385–391.

10 Beck DE, Farringer JA, Ravis WR and Robinson CA. Accuracy of three methods for predicting concentrations of free phenytoin. *Clinical Pharmacology* (1987) **6**: 888–894.

11 Ieiri I, Higuchi S, Hirata K, Yamada H and Aoyama T. Analysis of the factors

influencing antiepileptic drug concentrations – valproic acid. *Journal of Clinical Pharmacology and Therapeutics* (1990) **15**: 351–363.

12 Ichikou N, Ieiri I, Higuchi S, Hirata K, Yamada H and Aoyama T. Analysis of the factors influencing antiepileptic drug concentrations – carbamazepine. *Journal of Clinical Pharmacology and Therapeutics* (1990) **15**: 337–349.

13 Sadahiro N, Kodama S, Matsui T, Komatsu M and Matsuo T. Effect of serum albumin on free fractions of phenobarbital and valproic acid in patients with convulsive seizures. *Brain Development* (1985) **7**: 377–384.

14 Ratnaraj N, Goldberg VD and Hjelm M. Temperature effects on the estimation of free levels of phenytoin carbamazepine and phenobarbitone. *Therapeutic Drug Monitor* (1990) **12**: 465–472.

15 Umstead GS and Neumann KH. Correlation of free phenytoin to serum albumin in cancer patients. *Annals of Pharmacotherapy* (1990) **24**: 923–926.

16 Bardy AH, Hiilesmaa VK, Teramo K and Neuvonen PJ. Protein binding of antiepileptic drugs during pregnancy, labor, and puerperium. *Therapeutic Drug Monitor* (1990) **12**: 40–46.

17 Patel IH and Levy RH. Valproic acid binding to human serum albumin and determination of free fraction in the presence of anticonvulsants and free fatty acids. *Epilepsia* (1979) **20**: 85–90.

18 Bowdle TA, Patel IH, Levy RH and Wilensky AJ. The influence of free fatty acids on valproic acid plasma protein binding during fasting in normal humans. *European Journal of Clinical Pharmacology* (1982) **23**: 343–347.

19 Melten JW, Wittebrood AJ, Willems HJ, Faber GH, Wemer J and Faber DB. Comparison of equilibrium dialysis, ultrafiltration, and gel permeation chromatography for the determination of free fractions of phenobarbital and phenytoin. *Journal of Pharmaceutical Science* (1985) **74**: 692–694.

20 Bardy AH, Hiilesmaa VK, Teramo K and Neuvonen PJ. Protein binding of antiepileptic drugs during pregnancy, labor, and puerperium. *Therapeutic Drug Monitor* (1990) **12**: 40–46.

21 Kodama Y, Koike Y, Kimoto H, Yasunaga F, Takeyama M, Teraoka I and Fujii I. Binding parameters of valproic acid to serum protein in healthy adults at steady state. *Therapeutic Drug Monitor* (1992) **14**: 55–60.

8.6 Acute Spinal Epidural Abscess – A Neurosurgical Emergency

C. Veremakis and Subhash Todi

History

A 30-year-old white male, insulin-dependent diabetic, presented to the emergency room with low back pain of a few days duration. The pain was localized to the lower back, constant in nature, with no radiation. The patient denied any numbness or weakness in his legs. He gave a history of straining his back while picking up a heavy weight one week earlier, but had only mild discomfort in the back lasting one day. He had been feeling generally unwell for about a week with 'flu-like symptoms.

Physical examination revealed a low grade temperature and localized tenderness over the mid-lumbar spine. Spinal movements were restricted because of pain. Neurological examination of the legs was normal with intact, deep tendon reflexes and downgoing plantar responses.

Laboratory results showed a mild peripheral leukocytosis. Lumbar spine films were normal. A diagnosis of musculoskeletal pain was made, with a recommendation for bed rest and analgesics.

The patient returned to the emergency room the next morning with increasing pain that radiated into the upper right thigh. He also experienced some paraesthesia in the same region. Physical examination revealed persistent spinal tenderness, but no sensory loss or motor weakness in the legs. He was admitted to hospital with a diagnosis of acute neuritis/disc prolapse. A spinal CT scan was arranged for the next day. That night the patient complained that he was unable to move his right foot. Neurological examination showed marked weakness of the right leg with sluggish knee and ankle reflexes. The right plantar response was equivocal. He also had patchy sensory loss over his right thigh.

Further detailed examination revealed a small abscess over the lower abdomen at the site of the insulin injections. An urgent MRI revealed a posterior epidural mass of decreased signal intensity in T1 weighted images extending from L1 to L4 vertebrae. Corresponding T2 weighted images delineated a mass of high signal intensity, highly indicative of a spinal epidural abscess. At the end of the MRI the patient developed left lower extremity weakness and complained of an inability to urinate.

Traps

- The failure to consider acute spinal epidural abscess in a high-risk patient with acute vertebral pain, despite the absence of neurological deficit.

- The additional failure to recognize the rapidity with which acute epidural abscess can progress, leading to permanent neurological damage.

Tricks

An acute spinal epidural abscess is a medical emergency. However, because it is rare (an incidence of approximately one or two cases per 10 000 hospital admissions)[1–3] many physicians will never see a case during their career. However, it is readily diagnosed with current imaging techniques, and eminently treatable, whereas delay in diagnosis and treatment can leave the patient with permanent neurological disability.

The 'trick' in diagnosing an acute spinal epidural abscess is in recognizing high-risk patients and considering the diagnosis in any patient presenting with acute vertebral pain or tenderness, radicular radiation and some evidence, albeit minimal, of an inflammatory process including fever, leukocytosis, elevated ESR, etc. On presentation, neurological examination may be normal.

The signs and symptoms of an acute spinal epidural abscess progress through four phases: (1) spinal ache; (2) root pain; (3) weakness; and (4) paralysis.[1,4–6] In most series spinal pain was the most frequent presenting symptom, occurring in more than two-thirds of patients.[7] The pain was described by most patients as the worst they had ever experienced: on a scale of 1 to 10, the pain was rated 9.5, and was described as 'worse than having a baby' by four female patients.[3] This characteristic of the spinal pain should alert the clinician of an underlying acute inflammatory process, and may help to differentiate it from other causes of acute spinal pain. The location of the pain was variable but most commonly presented in the lumbar region. Other symptoms like radicular pain and weakness were less consistent and present in less than a third of patients.[1,2,7] Most importantly, paralysis was present in only a few patients on admission.[7]

The other key feature in diagnosing acute spinal epidural abscess is the presence of an underlying predisposing factor and/or a source of infection. In one series these were present in more than 80% of cases.[1] The predisposing factors may be local (such as recent spinal surgery, epidural anesthesia or lumbar tap) or systemic (such as diabetes, intravenous drug abuse, cirrhosis or alcoholism). In most series the source of infection was usually a skin or soft tissue infection, such as a furuncle, with hematogenous dissemination to the spinal epidural space.[7]

Mild peripheral leukocytosis, with left shift, was present in less than half of cases on presentation.[7] In some series an elevated ESR ($> 30 \, \mathrm{mm \, L^{-1}}$) was present in all cases on presentation; although very non-specific, it may help to differentiate from a non-inflammatory cause of back pain.[1,2] Blood cultures are positive in about 40% of cases, mainly for *Staphylococcus aureus*, and should always be taken before starting antibiotic therapy.[1,2,7]

Plain radiographic films of the spine, and bone scans, are neither sensitive nor specific, do not lead to appropriate management decisions and waste valuable time. Lumbar tap also has these disadvantages and may be harmful by predisposing to meningeal spread of infection and neurological deterioration.[1,2,7]

The crucial point to recognize in the critically ill patient is the potential for a precipitous progression to paralysis, within a few hours, in an otherwise stable patient presenting only with pain.[7–9] This deterioration can occur, despite the patient being on antibiotics. Mechanical compression alone is not an adequate explanation for such rapid progress, and many authors suggest a vascular mechanism.[1,10] At autopsy, Russel and colleagues saw no arterial compromise, but did find venous compression resulting in thrombosis, and thrombophlebitis involving the epidural space and the spinal cord, with venous infarction.[1,11] These findings may explain the rapidity and irreversibility of paralysis seen in some patients. Thus, the disastrous sequelae of this disease are a combination of compression and ischemia acting in synergy.

At the present time, spinal MRI with gadolinium enhancement is the diagnostic imaging technique of choice in suspected acute spinal epidural abscess.[1,7,12–18] It is as sensitive (92%) as a CT myelogram, and has the advantage of distinguishing other entities which can have similar presentations, such as disc herniation, spinal hematoma, transverse myelitis, infarction at the cord, syrinx and spinal tumor. Moreover, it obviates the need for a lumbar puncture required for myelography, avoids exposure to contrast, and often provides greater detail in demarcating the extent of the lesion. It also helps in differentiating abscess from the inflammatory edema of vertebral osteomyelitis, an important distinction if surgery is being contemplated.[7]

Surgical decompression combined with antibiotics remains the treatment of choice.[1] Since progression of disease is unpredictable and neurological abnormalities may be irreversible, many authorities believe that surgery should be performed on an urgent basis, no matter what the degree of neurological dysfunction.[3,7,19,20] Surgical treatment usually consists of decompressive laminectomy, and complete debridement of all the infected tissue. The antibiotic courage must include *Staphylococcus aureus*, as it is the commonest organism in most studies.[1,2,4,7] In patients after spinal surgery and in IV drug abusers, *Staphylococcus epidermidis* and Gram-negative organisms, such as Enterobacter, should be considered.[7] There are no controlled clinical trials that examine the ideal duration of antibiotic therapy in this condition. In most studies, the majority of patients responded to a 4–6 week course of IV antibiotics, with many physicians preferring to give several additional weeks of oral therapy, especially if vetebral osteomyelitis is present.

There is an overwhelming agreement in the literature[3,7,21] that the final neurological outcome is related to the severity of impairment before appropriate treatment is delivered. For example, patients who recovered after surgery were paralyzed for 0.2 days (95% CInt 0–0.4 days), as opposed to those who did not recover function or died where the paralysis was present an average of 0.5 days (95% CInt 0.3–0.8 days) and 1.9 days (95% CInt 0.5–3.3 days), respectively.[2,22,23] Nevertheless, delays in diagnosis still occur in a relatively high proportion of cases.[4] In one study the diagnosis of spinal epidural abscess was initially entertained in only a quarter of patients with the subsequent diagnosis.[7]

Screening all patients with back pain with MRI is prohibitively expensive. Patients with uncomplicated back pain, especially in the absence of radicular symptoms, or neurological deficit, and no evidence of an inflammatory process can be managed conservatively. But patients should be told to report immediately if the pain increases in severity, or if they develop root pain or weakness. On the other hand, high-risk patients with back pain which is severe, associated with root pain or some evidence of an inflammatory process should be intensively investigated for a source of infection and any underlying spinal or systemic disease; any suspicion warrants immediate MRI scan. Hopefully, this approach will decrease the unacceptably high morbidity and mortality associated with this potentially treatable entity.

Follow-up

After two blood cultures had been taken the patient was started on intravenous vancomycin, ceftazidime and gentamicin. He was taken to the operating room for a posterior decompressive laminectomy. Pus was found in the posterior epidural space, which eventually grew *Staphylococcus aureus*.

References

1 Halvin ML, Kaminski HJ, *et al*. Spinal epidural abscess: a ten year perspective. *Neurosurgery* (1990) **27**: 177–184.

2 Maslen DR, Jones SR, *et al*. Spinal epidural abscess: optimizing patient care. *Archives of Internal Medicine* (1993) **153**: 1713–1721.

3 Baker S and Ojemann RG. Spinal epidural abscess. *New England Journal of Medicine* (1975) **293**: 463–468.

4 McGee-Collett M and Johnston IJ. Spinal epidural abscess: presentation and treatment, a report of 21 cases. *Medical Journal of Australia* (1991) **155**: 14–17.

5 Rankin RM, Flothow PG, *et al*. Pyogenic infection of the spinal epidural space. *Western Journal of Surgery, Obstetrics and Gynaecology* (1946) **54**: 320–323.

6 Heusner AP. Non tuberculous spinal epidural infections. *New England Journal of Medicine* (1948) **239**: 845–853.

7 Darouiche RO, Hamill RJ, *et al*. Bacterial spinal epidural abscess: review of 43 cases and literature survey. *Medicine* (1992) **71**: 369–368.

8 Phillips GE and Jefferson A. Acute spinal epidural abscess: Observation from fourteen cases. *Postgraduate Medical Journal* (1979) **55**: 712–715.

9 Simpson RK, Azordegan PA, *et al*. Rapid onset of quadriplegia from a paraspinal epidural abscess. *Spine* (1991) **16**: 1002–1005.

10 Lasker BR and Harter DH. Cervical epidural abscess. *Neurology* (1987) **37**: 1747–1753.

11 Russell NA and Naughan R. Spinal epidural infection. *Canadian Journal of Neurological Science* (1979) **6**: 325–328.

12 Angtuaco E, McConell J, *et al*. MR imaging of spinal epidural abscess. *Radiology (abstr.)* (1987) **165**: 411.

13 Post MJD and Montaivo BM. Spinal infection: evaluation with MR imaging and intraoperative spinal US. *Radiology* (abstr.) (1987) **165**: 322.

14 Erntell M, Holtas S, *et al*. Magnetic resonance imaging in the diagnosis of spinal epidural abscess. *Scandinavian Journal of Infectious Diseases* (1988) **20**: 323–327.

15 Hanigan WC and Asner NG. Magnetic resonance imaging and the non operative treatment of spinal epidural abscess. *Surgical Neurology* (1990) **34**: 408–413.

16 Haughton VM. MR imaging of the spine. *Radiology* (1988) **166**: 297–301.

17 Post MJD and Quencer RMJ. Gadolinium enhanced MR in spinal infection. *Computer Assisted Tomography* (1990) **14**: 721–729.

18 Sharif HS. Role of MR imaging in the management of spinal infections. *American Journal of Roentgenology* (1992) **158**: 1333–1345.

19 Del Curling O and Gower DJ. Changing concepts in spinal epidural abscess: a report of 29 cases. *Neurosurgery* (1990) **27**: 185–192.

20 Hakin RN and Burt AA. Acute spinal epidural abscess. *Paraplegia* (1979) **17**: 330–336.

21 Danner RL and Hartman BJ. Update of spinal epidural abscess: 35 cases and review of the literature. *Review of Infectious Diseases* (1987) **9**: 265–274.

22 Siao P and Yagnik P. Spinal epidural abscess. *Journal of Emergency Medicine* (1988) **6**: 391–396.

23 Slade WR and Lonano F. Acute spinal epidural abscess. *Journal of the National Medical Association* (1990) **82**: 713–716.

9 Drug Interactions in Intensive Care

9.1 Substrate Competition between Drugs
S.E. Bakewell

History

A 70-year-old retired gentleman was referred to hospital by his general practitioner, complaining of increasing shortness of breath over the past few months. He was seen on two occasions. On the first he was discharged home and on the second he was admitted to a general medical ward.

He had a past medical history of pulmonary tuberculosis diagnosed almost 50 years before, for which he had been treated with streptomycin and para-amino salicylic acid for six months and bilateral artificial pneumothoraces. Seven years earlier he had been diagnosed as having late-onset asthma and atrial fibrillation, for which he had been started on digoxin. He was seen regularly in the chest clinic, and a CT scan of his chest four years before showed calcified pleura bilaterally and fibrotic changes, particularly in the upper lobes of both lungs. He led an independent lifestyle with a good quality of life, although this had deteriorated over the three to four months before admission.

Two recent chest infections had been treated by his general practitioner with oral steroids and antibiotics. He had made a good recovery from the first infection five months before, but had not recovered fully from the second illness three months later. Small amounts of white sputum were being expectorated which did not contain any blood. A peak expiratory flow rate (PEFR) of 300 L min^{-1} was measured (a normal value for him when well being 350–375 L min^{-1}). He was taking digoxin 0.125 mg and aspirin 150 mg once a day, and used a beclazone 250 inhaler twice a day, and a salbutamol [albuterol] inhaler as needed. Another three-week course of oral steroids prescribed by his general practitioner had just been finished. At the first assessment he was not found to be clinically septic or hypoxic, and was discharged home with an outpatients appointment for the chest clinic.

He was assessed again five days later and was admitted to an acute medical ward with severe shortness of breath, being only able to walk a few meters. On examination he looked comfortable at rest and was apyrexial; however, he had central cyanosis, with an oxygen saturation of 80% breathing air. This improved to 89% when the inspired oxygen concentration ($F_{I}O_2$) was increased to 0.24. He was in atrial fibrillation with an apical rate of 120/minute, and had a blood pressure of 170/85 mmHg. On auscultation of his chest he was found to have bronchial breathing at his right lung base. His PEFR was 360 L min^{-1}.

Initial investigations showed a hemoglobin of 13.5 g dL^{-1} and an increased white cell count of 14.5 x 10^9 L^{-1}, with a neutrophilia. He had a creatinine concentration of 114 µmol L^{-1} [1.5 mg dL^{-1}] and a urea concentration of 7.2 mmol L^{-1} [43.2 mg dL^{-1}]. The chest radiograph showed widespread scarring and calcification and probable consolidation of the right lower zone. The working diagnosis was underlying chronic lung disease with a community acquired pneumonia, although the possibility of a reactivation of the tuberculosis was considered.

The F_IO_2 was increased to 0.3, and regular nebulized salbutamol (2.5 mg 6 hourly) and antibiotic therapy with intravenous cefotaxime 1 g 8 hourly and oral clarithromycin 500 mg twice a day was started. Sputum and early morning urine specimens were sent for microscopy, including an auramine phenol stain to exclude acid-fast bacilli, and culture. Over the next four days his condition deteriorated further with increasing dyspnea at rest, a fever of 38.7°C and an increasing white cell count. Arterial blood gases performed on an F_IO_2 of 0.85 showed a P_aO_2 of 6.3 kPa [47 mmHg] and a P_aCO_2 of 5.0 kPa [37.5 mmHg]. He was therefore admitted to the intensive care unit.

On arrival at the ICU he was centrally cyanosed and had an apical heart rate of 140/minute. He was tachypneic with a respiratory rate of 60/minute, speaking with single words only and using his accessory muscles of respiration. There was bronchial breathing in his left mid and lower zones and right lower zone, and course crackles over both lower zones. The chest radiograph showed increased opacification of his right lung field.

His trachea was intubated and his lungs were ventilated on a pressure-limited, volume control mode. He was initially sedated with intravenous midazolam and morphine as required, although the morphine was changed to alfentanil two days later. No causative organism had yet been isolated so a fiber-optic bronchoscopy and bronchoalveolar lavage was performed. The antibiotic regimen was reviewed, and the oral clarithromycin changed to intravenous erythromycin 1 g 6 hourly in addition to the cefotaxime. Intravenous hydrocortisone 25 mg 6 hourly was started after a short synacthen test showed adrenal insufficiency. The atrial fibrillation was controlled with an intravenous amiodarone infusion. He was profoundly oliguric on admission to the ICU and despite aggressive resuscitation he developed acute renal failure, which was presumed to have been caused by dehydration. Ultrasound examination of his kidneys was unremarkable. Continuous veno-venous hemodiafiltration was started two days later, and was continued intermittently throughout the admission.

He remained on the ICU for 28 days. In addition to the renal failure the other main problems were his poor response to aggressive management of his pneumonia and difficulty with his weaning, which was compounded by inadvertent oversedation. Causative organisms for the initial pneumonia and an ICU-acquired pneumonia by day 18 were not isolated, and cultures for *Mycobacterium tuberculosis* were negative. He had a total of 13 days of intravenous cefotaxime and 10 days of intravenous erythromycin (the dose of erythromycin was reduced to 500 mg 6 hourly on day 4 in view of renal failure). On day 18 he started a five-day course of intravenous ciprofloxacin 200 mg twice daily and further intravenous erythromycin 500 mg 6 hourly. On day 26 *Citrobacter freundii* was cultured from a tracheal aspirate and a *Klebsiella* and *Citrobacter freundii* from the tracheostomy site, which were treated with intravenous ceftazidime 1 g 8 hourly.

His condition improved at first, but on day 8 he failed a trial of tracheal extubation, and a surgical tracheostomy was performed two days later to aid weaning from the ventilator. On day 21 the mode of ventilation was changed to high-frequency jet ventilation. He was mainly sedated with midazolam (both as an intravenous infusion and bolus intravenous injections as required), with this being supplemented by either alfentanil, fentanyl or morphine. Propofol was used at times of attempted weaning. On day 18 he was found to be unrousable, so all sedation was stopped. He slowly woke over the next ten days but remained drowsy and unresponsive. His concious level did, however, improve dramatically after flumazenil 200 μg intravenously on three separate occasions, showing that his coma was caused by benzodiazepine toxicity.

Trap

There was an interaction between the midazolam being used for sedation and erythromycin, resulting in oversedation and a prolonged requirement for intermittent positive-pressure ventilation.

Tricks

There are several factors which probably contributed to a reduced clearance of midazolam in this patient, such as renal impairment, advancing age and the use of enzyme inhibitors (erythromycin and amiodarone). Careful titration of the dose of midazolam against the response, especially when using an infusion, and anticipation of the interaction with erythromycin may have helped to avert this problem.

Midazolam is a short-acting, water-soluble 1,4-benzodiazepine with anxiolytic and hypnotic properties, which is widely used for premedication, induction of anesthesia and sedation for ventilation on the ICU.[1–3] The brief duration of action is a result of the extensive metabolism by a cytochrome P450,[4] which normally results in an elimination half-life of 1.5–2.5 hours, although this has been shown to be prolonged in some postoperative patients.[2] In the UK it is used by either the intravenous or the intramuscular route (via which it has 90% bioavailability) because it is not available as an oral preparation. When taken orally, there is extensive first-pass metabolism with an oral bioavailability of less than 50%.[1]

Erythromycin is a macrolide antibiotic and is the drug of choice in *Mycoplasma pneumoniae* pneumonia, legionnaires' disease, *Campylobacter fetus* and *jejuni* enteritis and infantile *Chlamydia trachomatis* pneumonia. It may also be used to treat streptococcal infections and syphilis, and for prophylaxis against rheumatic fever and endocarditis. Erythromycin has been shown to inhibit the metabolism of some drugs in the liver and also drug metabolism by microorganisms in the gut, either through its antibiotic effect or as a result of complex formation and inactivation of drug-oxidizing enzymes.[5]

Midazolam is extensively metabolized, with less than 0.03% being excreted unchanged in the urine.[6] The metabolism of midazolam and triazolam to their 1'-hydroxy and 4-hydroxy metabolites was studied in microsomes of 15 human livers by Kronbach and colleagues, who found that it was predominantly mediated by cytochrome P450-3A4 (CYP3A4).[4] Midazolam 1'-hydroxylation can also be catalyzed by CYP3A5, an enzyme which is only detectable in the liver of 20–30% of adults.[6]

Cytochromes P450 are a group of hemoprotein isoenzymes which are responsible for the oxidative metabolism of a large number of endogenous and exogenous compounds. The expression and function of these isoenzymes is regulated by many factors, such as hormones, genetic factors and exogenous and endogenous inducers and inhibitors, resulting in large differences between individuals. Kronbach and colleagues found that this interindividual variation in catalytic activity correlated with variable amounts of protein recognized by polyclonal and monoclonal antibody against human CYP3A4. They concluded that the clinically important variability in midazolam and triazolam metabolism was most likely to be caused by variable levels of CYP3A4 and closely related proteins.[4]

1'-Hydroxy midazolam is the major metabolite of midazolam, and accounts for 98% of the metabolites found in urine.[2,6] It had been thought that the 1'-hydroxy and 4-hydroxy metabolites did not contribute significantly to the pharmacological effect of midazolam, as they are conjugated rapidly and excreted through the kidney.[2,3] However, recent work by Bauer and colleagues has suggested that the conjugated metabolites may in fact have a sedative effect.[7] Caution is advised in renal failure.

The metabolism of midazolam has been shown to be inhibited by many drugs, including erythromycin,[2,6] cyclosporin [cyclosporine],[2,6] lignocaine [lidocaine],[2,6] dihydropyridine calcium channel antagonists,[2,6] phenothiazine-type neuroleptics,[2] H_2 receptor antagonists (cimetidine having a more pronounced effect than ranitidine),[2,8] amiodarone,[1,2] ketoconazole,[2] verapamil[2] and theophylline.[2] Immunoinhibition studies have shown that nifedipine,[2] diltiazem,[9] cyclosporine[2] and lignocaine[2] are oxidized by an identical or closely related isoenzyme of the CYP3A subfamily. The major CYP3A enzyme present in human liver is CYP3A4.[6]

The erythromycin breath test measures the ability of the patient to demethylate erythromycin by measuring exhaled $^{14}CO_2$ production after intravenous ^{14}C-N-methyl-erythromycin administration. CYP3A4 catalyzes this reaction and consequently the test reflects CYP3A4 activity.[6,10] This has been used as a guide for cyclosporin dosing, as CYP3A4 activity largely accounts for the relationship between dose of cyclosporine and blood levels for each individual patient.[10] The erythromycin breath test shows a broad unimodal distribution of enzyme activity in the population. This is different to the bimodal distribution of debrisoquin [debrisoquine] metabolism which is impaired in 8–10% of the caucasian population.[10,11] Debrisoquine is specifically metabolized by CYP 450IID6, a form of P450 distinct from P4503A.[9]

There is at least a ten-fold variability in the liver content and catalytic activity of CYP3A4 between individuals. Lown and colleagues[6] tested the hypothesis that this may in part account for the known interpatient differences in midazolam kinetics. Using intravenous midazolam and the erythromycin breath test to assess CYP3A4 activity, they found a significant correlation between the breath test results and hence CYP3A4 activity and weight-adjusted clearance of both total and unbound midazolam. Transient sedation and memory impairment were experienced by some patients, but this did not correlate with either total or free plasma midazolam levels seen at that time. This was felt to be consistent with the view that factors other than blood levels, such as the density of γ-aminobutyric acid receptors in the brain, are more important in determining the psychometric aspects of the response to midazolam. Individuals with low CYP3A4 activity may be at increased risk of prolonged hypnotic, sedative and amnesic effects after treatment with midazolam, and this could be predicted by the erythromycin breath test.[6]

No consistent effect of ageing on liver CYP3A activity has been shown,[10] but the elimination half-life of benzodiazepines is increased in the elderly.[12] In addition, elderly patients with impaired cardiovascular function and poor psychomotor ability are more at risk of increased pharmacodynamic effects from midazolam.[13] A reduction in liver perfusion has not been strongly implicated as a cause for reduced metabolism of midazolam, although it is thought to contribute in some situations.[3]

During infusions of midazolam it has been shown that extensive redistribution of the drug occurs. At first the plasma concentration of the metabolite may be low, but a gradual increase to maximum is seen, with the plasma concentration of metabolite being maintained for some hours after the infusion is stopped.[14] To avoid accumulation, careful titration of the dose is needed.

Erythromycin has been shown to be a specific inhibitor of CYP3A. It is metabolized to a nitroso derivative (presumably by CYP3A) which binds irreversibly to the heme iron and deactivates the cytochrome.[9] This affects the oxidative metabolism of several drugs that are metabolized mainly by CYP3A, such as midazolam,[1,2,11,15] theophylline,[5,11,13,16] alfentanil,[11,17] methylpredniso-lone,[5,13] carbamazepine,[5,13] and warfarin.[5] This inhibition may result in an increased plasma concentration, prolonged elimination half-life and enhanced effects of these drugs.

Olkkola and colleagues[1] investigated the interaction between oral erythro-mycin given regularly for one week and a single dose of midazolam given by either the oral or the intravenous route in two double-blind, randomized, cross-over studies. They showed that after oral midazolam the area under the midazolam concentration–time curve was increased by more than four times and the maximum plasma concentration by more than two times, compared with the placebo phase. The elimination half-life of midazolam was also prolonged from 2.4 to 5.7 hours. The higher plasma concentrations during treatment with erythromycin were associated with profound sedative effects and a significant deterioration in all psychomotor tests. This confirmed that erythromycin significantly affects the pharmacokinetics of oral midazolam and increases its pharmacodynamic effects.

After intravenous midazolam, erythromycin reduced the plasma clearance of midazolam by 54% and increased the elimination half-life from 3.5 to 6.2 hours. However, only a weak interaction was shown between erythromycin and intravenous midazolam on psychomotor tests. It is the interaction between oral midazolam and erythromycin which is most marked, and it is felt to reflect an increase in oral bioavailability and a decrease in the plasma clearance of midazolam. When midazolam was given intravenously, it bypassed the altered presystemic metabolism and there were only minor changes in pharmacodynamic parameters.[1]

Other studies and case reports have confirmed this pharmacokinetic–pharmacodynamic interaction between midazolam and erythromycin.[3,15,18] It has been shown that even a single dose of erythromycin in combination with midazolam 10 mg orally impairs psychomotor performance more than giving midazolam 15 mg alone.[13]

The ability of erythromycin and other macrolides to inhibit hepatic oxidative metabolism of susceptible drugs by the formation of complexes with CYP3A mainly depends on the affinity of the macrolide concerned for the CYP enzyme system. The macrolide antibiotics can be divided into three groups according to their affinity for CYP.[19] The first group (e.g. erythromycin, troleandomycin [triacetyloleandomycin]) forms an inactive CYP complex leading to inhibition of metabolism of other drugs. The second group (e.g. josamycin, roxithromycin) has lower affinity for CYP and forms inactive complexes to a lesser extent. Clinically, this is supported by the findings that although roxithromycin does enhance the effects of midazolam, it was less marked than the effect of erythromycin.[13,20] The third group (e.g. azithromycin, spiramycin) does not affect the enzymes and is believed to be unable to modify the pharmacokinetics of drugs. This was confirmed by Mattila and colleagues,[19] who found that azithromycin did not enhance the effects of midazolam on performance or on subjective sedation compared with erythromycin.

The metabolism of midazolam can be affected by many factors, and this leads to clinically important effects. In our patient, the contributing factors were likely to be inhibition of CYP3A4 activity by erythromycin and amiodarone and reduced renal clearance of midazolam, exacerbated by the use of a midazolam infusion. Although only minor changes in pharmacodynamic parameters have been observed after the combination of intravenous midazolam and erythromycin, it is prudent to carefully and regularly adjust the dose of midazolam in response to its effect on the patient. The use of one of the newer macrolide antibiotics might have avoided the prolonged sedation and requirement for intermittent positive-pressure ventilation.

Follow-up

The patient's poor response to intensive therapy resulted in the decision to withdraw active treatment, and the patient died on day 28. A hospital postmortem was performed which confirmed the cause of death as severe bilateral confluent pneumonia and ischemic heart disease. The pleural cavities showed extensive fibrosis and egg-shell calcification of both visceral and parietal pleura, with a focus of old TB in the right apical region. Both kidneys looked normal.

References

1 Olkkola KT, Aranko K, Luurila H, Hiller A, Saarnivaara L, Himberg JJ and Neuvonen PJ. A potentially hazardous interaction between erythromycin and midazolam. *Clinical Pharmacology and Therapeutics* (1993) **53**: 298–305.
2 Gascon MP and Dayer P. *In vitro* forecasting of drugs which may interfere with the biotransformation of midazolam. *European Journal of Clinical Pharmacology* (1991) **41**: 573–578.
3 Byatt CM, Lewis LD, Dawling S and Cochrane GM. Accumulation of midazolam after repeated dosage in patients receiving mechanical ventilation in an intensive care unit. *British Medical Journal* (1984) **289**: 799–800.
4 Kronbach T, Mathys D, Umeno M, Gonzalez FJ and Meyer UA. Oxidation of midazolam and triazolam by human liver cytochrome P450111A4. *Molecular Pharmacology* (1989) **36**: 89–96.
5 Ludden TM. Pharmacokinetic interactions of the macrolide antibiotics. *Clinical Pharmacokinetics* (1985) **10**: 63–79.
6 Lown KS, Thummel KE, Benedict PE, Shen DD, Turgeon DK, Berent S and Watkins PB. The erythromycin breath test predicts the clearance of midazolam. *Clinical Pharmacology and Therapeutics* (1995) **57**: 16–24.
7 Bauer TM, Ritz R, Haberthür C, Ha HR, Hunkeler W, Sleight AJ, Scollo-Lavizzari G and Haefeli WE. Prolonged sedation due to accumulation of conjugated metabolites of midazolam. *Lancet* (1995) **346**: 145–147.
8 Fee JPH, Collier PS, Howard PJ and Dundee JW. Cimetidine and ranitidine increase midazolam bioavailability. *Clinical Pharmacology and Therapeutics* (1987) **41**: 80–84.
9 Pichard L, Fabre I, Fabre G, Domergue J, Saint Aubert B, Mourad G and Maurel P. Cyclosporin A drug interactions: screening for inducers and inhibitors of cytochrome P450 (cyclosporin A oxidase) in primary cultures of human hepatocytes and in liver microsomes. *Drug Metabolism and Disposition* (1990) **18**: 595–606.
10 Watkins PB, Hamilton TA, Annesley TM, Ellis CN, Kolars JC and Voorhees JJ. The erythromycin breath test as a predictor of cyclosporine blood levels. *Clinical Pharmacology and Therapeutics* (1990) **48**: 120–129.
11 Wood M. Midazolam and erythromycin [letter]. *British Journal of Anaesthesia* (1991) **67**: 131.
12 Moon CAL. [Letter]. *British Medical Journal* (1984) **289**: 1309.
13 Mattila MJ, Idänpään-Heikkilä JJ, Tömwall M and Vanakoski J. Oral single doses of erythromycin and roxithromycin may increase the effects of midazolam on human performance. *Pharmacology and Toxicology* (1993) **73**: 180–185.
14 Byrne AJ, Yeoman PM and Mace P. Accumulation of midazolam in patients receiving mechanical ventilation [letter]. *British Medical Journal* (1984) **289**: 1309.
15 Hiller A, Olkkola KT, Isohanni P and Saarnivaara L. Unconciousness associated with midazolam and erythromycin. *British Journal of Anaesthesia* (1990) **65**: 826–828.
16 Prince RA, Wing DS, Weinberger MM, Hendeles LS and Riegelman S. Effects of erythromycin on theophylline kinetics. *Journal of Allergy and Clinical Immunology* (1981) **68**: 427–431.
17 Bartkowski RR, Goldberg ME, Larijani GE and Boerner T. Inhibition of alfentanil metabolism by erythromycin. *Clinical Pharmacology and Therapeutics* (1989) **46**: 99–102.
18 Aranko K, Olkkola KT, Hiller A and Saarnivaara L. Clinically important interaction

between erythromycin and midazolam. *British Journal of Clinical Pharmacology* (1992) **33**: 217–218.

19 Mattila MJ, Vanakoski J and Idänpään-Heikkilä JJ. Azithromycin does not alter the effects of oral midazolam on human performance. *European Journal of Clinical Pharmacology* (1994) **47**: 49–52.

20 Backman JT, Aranko K, Himberg JJ and Olkkola KT. A pharmacokinetic interaction between roxithromycin and midazolam. *European Journal of Clinical Pharmacology* (1994) **46**: 551–555.

9.2 Drug Interaction Mimicking Sepsis
P. Diesel and G.R. Park

History

A 30-year-old man needed a liver transplant for polyarteritis nodosa. Before operation he was wasted, with a body weight approximately 70% of that expected. Surgery was complicated by profuse bleeding after operation, that tamponaded his abdomen and caused renal failure. He needed ventilatory support for almost two weeks before he could be weaned from his ventilator and return to the ward.

He developed a chest infection 20 days later and needed readmission to the intensive care unit for this. At this time he was having continuous jerking movements and was hallucinating (seeing snakes all the time). He was also hypotensive.

On admission to the intensive care unit a pulmonary artery and arterial catheter was inserted. The hemodynamic variables shown in Table 9.2.1 were obtained.

Although infection was thought to be likely, he was afebrile (36.9°C [98.4°F]), had a normal white cell count ($8.6 \times 10^9 \, L^{-1}$) and did not have the systemic upset (an obtunded concious level, tachypnea, etc.) associated with sepsis. Therefore other causes for his hypotension and hallucinations were sought.

A review of this patients' drug chart showed that he was getting cyclosporine [cyclosporin] (immunosuppression), erythromycin (chest infection), diazepam (hallucinations), nifedipine (hypertension), prochlorperazine (nausea), amitryptilline (depression), codeine (diarrhea) and metoclopramide (nausea).

Trap

Drugs are well recognized as a cause of hallucinations. They can also cause jerky limb movements. Hemodynamic disturbances can also be caused by drugs. During anesthesia, hypotension caused by intravenous and volatile anesthetic agents is well recognized. This is often not recognized outside of the operating

Table 9.2.1. Hemodynamic variables in this patient at the time of admission

Mean arterial blood pressure	60 mmHg
Heart rate	120/minute
Cardiac index	$4.5 \, L \, min^{-1}$
Pulmonary artery occlusion pressure	12 mmHg
Right atrial pressure	12 mmHg
Systemic vascular resistance index	852 dyn-sec cm^{-5}
DO$_{21}$	$800 \, mL \, min^{-1} \, m^{-2}$

theater when similar and other drugs are given. Even drugs that normally only have a limited effect on the cardiovascular system can cause a profound hemodynamic disturbance when they accumulate. We therefore felt that this patient had a drug-induced syndrome mimicking the sepsis syndrome.

Tricks

The patient with liver disease has several problems with drugs. There may be a reduction in their elimination caused by both impaired hepatic function and, because of this, a reduction in renal function.[1-3] In addition, there is a change in the receptors in the central nervous system causing increased sensitivity to these drugs.[4] The impaired hepatic function may be caused by a reduction in liver blood flow (reducing delivery of the drug to the liver) or because of a change in the enzymes that metabolize these drugs.

Drugs are metabolized from lipophilic active compounds by enzymes to make them more water soluble. This enables them to be excreted in the urine and bile. Furthermore, the increased polarity means that they cannot cross membranes and are therefore inactive.

Two types of enzymes are typically used in this process. The first are the cytochromes P450. These are hemoproteins that add oxygen to drugs in oxidation, hydroxylation and similar reactions. There are about 28 of these so far described in man, and between them they metabolize about 250 000 compounds.[5-8] The second group of enzymes are involved in conjugation reactions, such as glucuronidation and sulfation;[9] like the cytochromes P450, each enzyme metabolizes many compounds. Some drugs are only metabolized by one type of enzyme. However, many are metabolized first by the cytochrome P450 system and then by the conjugation enzymes. For these and the drugs only metabolized by cytochromes P450 abnormalities of this enzyme will delay metabolism.

Cytochromes P450 are affected by many different factors including hypoxia, inflammatory mediators, hormones (including exogenous corticosteroids), other drugs and interferon.[2,10-12] Most of these factors will decrease the amount of enzyme present or reduce its activity, but some will induce it. All these factors are likely to be present in this patient. In addition, some enzymes are missing in some patients because of a pharmacogenetic abnormality.

Two cytochromes P450 were important in this patient: cytochromes P4503A4 and 2D6. These two metabolize many of the drugs given to this patient (Table 9.2.2).

Many drugs given to this patient compete for the same enzyme. This will lead to a reduction in the metabolism of the drug and a potential increase in its toxicity. In addition, in a patient after liver transplantation the amount of enzyme present is likely to be reduced, causing a further reduction in metabolism and exacerbating the problem of drug accumulation.

Cytochromes P450 have evolved over many millions of years and some are now of no evolutionary benefit.[13] For these enzymes pharmacogenetic

Table 9.2.2. Some drugs metabolized by cytochromes P4503A4 and 2D6. Some of these pathways may be minor pathways of elimination

Drugs metabolized by cytochrome P4503A4	Drugs metabolized by cyctochrome P4502D6
Cyclosporine	Prochlorperazine
Erythromycin	Amitryptilline
Diazepam	Codeine
Nifedipine	Beta blockers
Alfentanil	Debrisoquin
Midazolam	

abnormalities can develop without any overt signs. Cytochrome P4502D6 is subject to an abnormality of its gene.[14] It metabolizes the antihypertensive drug debrisoquine. When this was first given to humans one of the volunteers became hypotensive and remained so for a long time. No metabolites were found in that volunteer's urine. Although debrisoquin is not used in the critically ill patient many other drugs metabolized by it are. It is possible that the transplanted liver in this patient had a pharmacogenetic abnormality, since it occurs with a frequency of 10% in our population. The chance of this is increased since he needed a further admission later for the same problem. This cytochrome P450 is also important for the metabolism of inactive to active drugs. In this patient the codeine he was given first has to be metabolized to morphine to be active.[6] This is done by cytochrome 2D6 and thus in 10% of patients this drug will be ineffective as an analgesic.

Although many drugs and other xenobiotics are metabolized by cytochromes P450 there is as yet no easy bedside measure of their activities. There are tests of single cytochrome P450 activity: one example is the MEGX test. For this, lidocaine [lignocaine] 1 mg kg is given and 15 minutes later a single blood sample is taken. The main metabolite of lidocaine – monoethylglycinexylidide – is measured in this way. Its rate of production has been used as an indicator of liver function. Unfortunately, it only measures the activity of cytochrome P4503A.

There is not a large amount of knowledge about which drugs are safe to give to patients with acute liver disease. In addition, the need for many drugs in these seriously ill patients will give rise to other difficulties with drug interactions. Further difficulties will be caused by pharmacogenetic abnormalities in the enzymes. The potential for drug-induced disease is thus enormous.

Follow-up

Broad-spectrum antibiotic treatment with ciprofloxacillin and metronidazole was started in this patient, in case he should be infected. In addition, he was volume resuscitated with a gelatin solution so that his pulmonary artery occlusion pressure increased to 15 mmHg. The major treatment was to stop all of the other drugs that he was being given, except cyclosporine. It was not possible to stop his cyclosporine, since to do so would have caused him to reject his transplanted liver.

Over the next three days he improved. There was no source of infection ever identified and he showed no clinical or laboratory evidence of infection. Unfortunately, when the patient returned to the ward some of these drugs were restarted. Three weeks later he needed readmission for a further episode of hypotension, hallucinations and jerky limb movements caused by drugs!

References

1 Bodenham A, Shelly MP and Park GR. The altered pharmacokinetics and pharmacodynamics of drugs commonly used in critically ill patients. *Clinical Pharmacokinetics* (1988) **14**: 347–373.

2 Park GR and Elston A. What controls drug metabolism in the critically ill patient? *Care of the Critically Ill* (1991) **7**: 212.

3 Penfold NW and Park GR. The effects of organ failure on drug metabolism. *Current Opinion in Anaesthetics* (1991) **3**: 235–240.

4 Park GR. Pharmacokinetics and pharmacodynamics in the critically ill patient. *Xenobiotica* (1993) **23**: 1195–1230.

5 Coon MJ, Ding X, Pernecky SJ and Vaz ADN. Cytochrome P450: progress and predictions. *FASEB Journal* (1992) **6**: 669–673.

6 Cholerton S, Daly AK and Idle JR. The role of individual human cytochromes P450 in drug metabolism and clinical response. *TIPs* (1992) **13**: 434–439.

7 Guengerich FP. Characterisation of human cytochrome P450 enzymes. *FASEB Journal* (1992) **6**: 745–748.

8 George J and Farrel GC. Role of human hepatic cytochromes P450 in drug metabolism and toxicity. *Australian and New Zealand Journal of Medicine* (1991) **21**: 356–362.

9 Gibson GG and Skett P. Techniques and experiments illustrating drug metabolism. In: *Introduction to Drug Metabolism*. London: Chapman and Hall, pp 239–284, 1986.

10 Park GR, Pichard L, Tinel M, Larroque C, Elston A, Domerque J, Dexionne B and Maurel P. What changes drug metabolism in critically ill patients? Two preliminary studies in isolated hepatocytes. *Anaesthesia* (1994) **49**: 188–191.

11 Park GR, Laroche C, Elston A, Domergue J and Maurel P. Serum from critically ill humans changes the metabolism of progesterone in cultured human hepatocytes. *Journal of Basic Clinical Physiological Pharmacology* (1992) **3**: P132.

12 Gallenkamp H, Epping J, Fuchshofen-Rockel M, Heusler H and Richter E. Zytochrom P450-Gehalt und Arzneimittelmetabolismus der Leber im Schock. *Deutsche Gesellschaft in Medizin* (1982) **88**: 1093–1096.

13 Meyer UA. Genotype or phenotype: the definition of a pharmacogenetic polymorphism. *Pharmacogenetics* (1991) **1**: 66–67.

14 Gonzalez FJ, Skoda RC, Kimura S, Umeno M, Zanger UM, Nebert DW, Gelboin HV, Hardwick JP and Meyer US. Characterization of the common genetic defect in humans deficient in debrisoquine metabolism. *Nature* (1988) **331**: 442–446.

9.3 Seizures caused by Interaction between Theophylline and Quinolone Antibiotics

N.D. Murphy and J.G. Cunniffe

History

A 37-year-old woman with a 13-year history of asthma was admitted to the hospital with a severe acute attack. Before her admission she had had a three-day history of increasing shortness of breath and an unproductive cough. Her general practitioner had started her on prednisolone 30 mg a day. Apart from a few hospital admissions early in the course of her disease, her asthma had been well controlled and she had not needed a course of oral steroids for the past five years. She had undergone allergy analysis, which had shown a sensitivity to aspirin.

On examination she was apyrexial, dyspneic, but able to talk in sentences. She had a tachycardia of 120 beats/minute and was using her accessory muscles to breathe. Her chest was hyperexpanded and on auscultation there was a prolonged bilateral expiratory wheeze. Her peak expiratory flow was $60 \, mL \, s^{-1}$. The initial laboratory investigations were normal and her chest radiograph did not show any signs of infection.

Treatment was started with nebulized salbutamol [albuterol] (5 mg 2 hourly), ipratropium bromide (500 µg 4 hourly), hydrocortisone (250 mg 6 hourly), salbutamol (by infusion: 5 µg per minute), aminophylline (250 mg bolus followed by an infusion of 350 mg per hour). Erythromycin (500 mg 8 hourly) and cefotaxime (1 g 8 hourly) were started to cover the possibility of a community acquired pneumonia. These were latter stopped.

When the patient failed to respond to this treatment she was admitted to the intensive care unit for closer observation. Daily investigations included: full blood count, urea and electrolyte estimations, aminophylline concentrations, four-hourly arterial blood gas (ABG) measurements and a chest radiograph.

After 24 hours both her clinical state and the ABGs had deteriorated. Her trachea was intubated and ventilatory support started. The bronchospasm remained severe despite maximum conventional therapy and isoflurane was added to the inspired gas five days later, both to sedate her and in an attempt to improve the bronchospasm. The next day she developed a fever and blood cultures were taken. Chest radiograph appearances suggested a hospital-acquired pneumonia and ciprofloxacin 200 mg twice daily was started. The next day *Escherichia coli* was grown from her blood. By this time her bronchspasm had resolved and the isoflurane was stopped. She awoke rapidly and was weaned from the ventilator over a short period. The patient was noted to be weak and there was marked muscle wasting but her ABGs remained satisfactory and she was observed.

Twelve hours later the patient had a *grand mal* epileptic fit. The seizure was stopped after 90 seconds with 5 mg of intravenous diazepam. Investigations after the seizure, including a lumbar puncture, were normal. Neurological examination showed profound weakness but did not reveal any focal abnormality.

Trap

There was a failure to note the increase in the patient's plasma concentration of aminophylline, measured daily, before the seizure and after the introduction of ciprofloxacin (Figure 9.3.1), and to make the necessary adjustments in the dose.

Trick

Aminophylline can cause seizures even within the normal therapeutic range, especially when it interacts with other drugs.

Aminophylline is a mixture of the therapeutically active theophylline and ethylene-diamine that increases water solubility. Measurement of plasma concentration is essential, especially if the patient has previously been taking oral theophylline.

Fluoroquinolones are a class of antibiotic structurally related to nalidixic acid. They exhibit bactericidal activity principally by inhibiting bacterial DNA gyrase. Compared to naladixic acid these newer compounds exhibit high potency, a lower incidence of resistance, high oral bioavailability, extensive tissue penetration, low protein binding and long elimination half-lives. Their excellent activity against Gram-negative pathogens, including Enterobacteriaceae and *Pseudomonas aeruginosa*, make them useful agents in the critically ill, particularly in the treatment of ventilator-associated pneumonia.

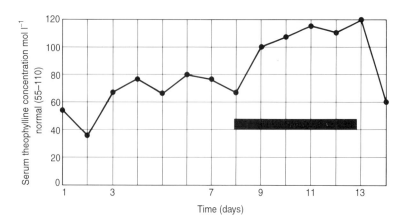

Figure 9.3.1. The increase in plasma theophylline concentration after the introduction of ciprofloxacin (black bar).

Quinolones are generally well tolerated but may give rise to side-effects including seizures, usually in patients with a predisposing factor such as a brain tumor, epilepsy, metabolic imbalance, anoxia or severe cerebral arteriosclerosis. Their effect on the CNS is caused by antagonism of gamma-aminobutyric acid (GABA) at both pre- and postsynaptic receptors.[1] Quinolones should be used with caution in patients with a history of CNS disorders,[2] and high dose regimens should probably be avoided.

Theophylline (and its soluble derivative aminophylline) remains a useful agent in the management of reversible obstructive lung disease. However, it has a narrow therapeutic range $(10\text{–}20\,\text{mg L}^{-1}$ $[55\text{–}110\,\mu\text{mol L}^{-1}])$ and side-effects such as tachycardia, restlessness, vomiting, headache and seizures are frequently seen. In ventilated, sedated patients the first indications of toxicity may be the onset of convulsions, which may occur within the therapeutic range.[3] As with quinolones, theophylline appears to act on the CNS by inhibition of GABA receptor binding.[3]

Both quinolones and theophylline are commonly used in the ICU. As both compounds cause convulsions through the same mechanism, additional CNS toxicity may be seen when they are used in combination. A further problem is that certain quinolones may decrease the clearance of theophylline, leading to elevated and potentially toxic serum concentrations. Many drugs have been found to influence theophylline metabolism because of an interaction with one or more variants of the cytochrome P450 enzyme system. This was first noted with a quinolone in 1984, when there were reports of toxicity associated with enoxacin and theophylline combinations.[4,5] The mechanism of interaction appears to be competition between the 4-oxo metabolite of the quinolone group and theophylline during demethylation at cytochrome P450. Enoxacin appears to be the most potent inhibitor in the quinolone group, consistently decreasing theophylline clearance by more than 50%.[6,7] Ciprofloxacin and pefloxacin reduce the clearance of theophylline by approximately 20–30%,[6] although in some subjects, particularly the elderly, the clearance may be reduced even more.[8,9] Convulsions caused by the interaction between ciprofloxacin and theophylline are extensively documented in the literature.[10] It has been suggested that a 30% reduction in theophylline dosage should be considered if ciprofloxacin is coadministered.[11] Certainly, plasma theophylline levels should be monitored and signs and symptoms of toxicity acted upon. Decreased theophylline clearance may persist for as long as five days after stopping ciprofloxacin therapy.[11]

Many additional quinolones have been investigated for interaction with theophylline. Norfloxacin[12,13] and ofloxacin,[14,15] do not have a significant effect on theophylline clearance. Of the newer agents sparfloxacin,[16,17] lomefloxacin,[18,19] fleroxacin[20,21] and levofloxacin[22] do not require theophylline dosage adjustment.

Only 10% of theophylline is excreted unchanged in the urine, the rest being metabolized in the liver to inactive xanthine derivatives.[23] Theophylline shows capacity-limited or restrictive hepatic elimination. This means that it has a low intrinsic clearance by the liver and its metabolism is unaffected by liver blood flow. However, it is profoundly influenced by changes in hepatic enzyme activity. In addition to fluoroquinolones, other drugs that decrease theophylline clearance include erythromycin, cimetidine and oral contraceptives. The effects of these agents appear to be additive.[24] Increased clearance of theophylline is seen with barbiturates, phenytoin and activated charcoal.

The interaction between ciprofloxacin and theophylline is now well recognized in the medical literature, and is noted in the data sheets for these compounds. Despite this, life-threatening interactions continue to occur, and there has been at least one death attributed to the use of these agents in combination.[25] The convulsions in our patient were almost certainly caused by the interaction between ciprofloxacin and aminophylline, even though the serum theophylline level was only just outside the recommended range. In retrospect, the dosage of aminophylline should have been reduced when the ciprofloxacin was started, or when the gradual increase in the serum theophylline level was noted. An alternative would have been to have used a different fluoroquinolone, such as ofloxacin, that does not alter theophylline metabolism significantly.[14,15] Unfortunately, ofloxacin is not as active as ciprofloxacin against important ICU pathogens such as *Pseudomonas aeruginosa*[26]. Future compounds such as sparfloxacin may hold the key to optimal antimicrobial activity without influencing theophylline excretion.[16]

Critically ill patients are given many drugs and interactions will inevitably occur. Sedation and ventilation of patients can result in the early indications of toxicity being missed. It is vital for staff to avoid combinations of drugs that may interact and, if such combinations need to be administered, to monitor patients carefully.

Follow-up

No more fits were seen after the diazepam was given. The aminophylline was stopped and plasma concentrations decreased (Figure 9.3.1). It was reintroduced at a lower dose 24 h later. The patient was discharged to the ward after a further 24 h and made an uneventful recovery.

References

1 Christ W. Central nervous system toxicity of quinolones; human and animal findings. *Journal of Antimicrobial Chemotherapy* (1990) **26** (Suppl B): 219–225.

2 Shimada J and Hori S. Adverse effects of fluoroquinolones. *Progress in Drug Research* (1992) **38**: 133–143.

3 Semel JD and Allen N. Seizures in patients simultaneously receiving theophylline and imipenem or ciprofloxacin or metronidazole. *Southern Medical Journal* (1991) **84**: 465–468.

4 Wijnands WJ, Van Herwaarden CL and Vree TB. Enoxacin raises plasma theophylline concentrations. *Lancet* (1984) **2**: 108–109.

5 Maesen FP, Teengs JP, Baur C and Davies BI. Quinolones and raised plasma concentrations of theophylline. *Lancet* (1984) **2**: 530.

6 Edwards DJ, Bowles SK, Svensson CK and Rybak MJ. Inhibition of drug metabolism by quinolone antibiotics. *Clinical Pharmacokinetics* (1988) **15**: 194–204.

7 Davey PG. Overview of drug interactions with the quinolones. *Journal of Antimicrobial Chemotherapy* (1988) **22** (Suppl C): 97–107.

8 Rybak MJ, Bowles SK and Chandrasekar PH. Increased theophylline concentrations secondary to ciprofloxacin. *Drug Intelligence and Clinical Pharmacy* (1987) **21**: 879–881.

9 Raoof S, Wollschlager C and Khan FA. Ciprofloxacin increases serum levels of theophylline. *American Journal of Medicine* (1987) **82**: 115–118.

10 Grasela TH and Dreis MW. An evaluation of the quinolone–theophylline interaction using the Food and Drug Administration spontaneous reporting system. *Archives of Internal Medicine* (1992) **152**: 617–621.

11 Hulisz D and Miller K. Update on quinolone drug interactions. *American Pharmacy* (1990) **9**: 34–36.

12 Bowles SK, Popovski Z, Rybak MJ, Beckman HB and Edwards DJ. Effect of norfloxacin on theophylline pharmacokinetics at steady state. *Antimicrobial Agents and Chemotherapy* (1988) **32**: 510–512.

13 Janknegt R. Drug interactions with quinolones. *Journal of Antimicrobial Chemotherapy* (1990) **26** (Suppl D): 7–29.

14 Tack KJ and Smith JA. The safety profile of ofloxacin. *American Journal of Medicine* (1989) **87**: 78S–81S.

15 Lamp KC, Bailey EM and Rybak MJ. Ofloxacin clinical pharmacokinetics. *Clinical Pharmacokinetics* (1992) **22**: 32–46.

16 Shimada J, Nogita T and Ishibashi Y. Clinical pharmacokinetics of sparfloxacin. *Clinical Pharmacokinetics* (1993) **25**: 358–369.

17 Takagi K, Yamaki K, Nadai M, Kuzuya T and Hasegawa T. Effects of a new quinolone sparfloxacin, on the pharmacokinetics of theophylline in asthmatic patients. *Antimicrobial Agents and Chemotherapy* (1991) **35**: 1137–1141.

18 Wadworth AN and Goa KL. Lomefloxacin. A review of its antibacterial activity, pharmacokinetic properties and therapeutic use. *Drugs* (1991) **42**: 1018–1060.

19 Rizk E. The US clinical experience with lomefloxacin. *American Journal of Medicine* (1992) **92**: 130S–135S.

20 Nightingale CH. Overview of the pharmacokinetics of fleroxacin. *American Journal of Medicine* (1993) **94**: 38S–43S.

21 Stuck AE, Kim DK and Frey FJ. Fleroxacin clinical pharmacokinetics. *Clinical Pharmacokinetics* (1992) **22**: 116–131.

22 Davis R and Bryson HM. Levofloxacin. A review of its antibacterial activity, pharmacokinetics and therapeutic efficacy. *Drugs* (1994) **47**: 677–700.

23 Davis RL, Quenzer RW, Kelly HW and Powell JR. Effects of the addition of ciprofloxacin on theophylline pharmacokinetics in subjects inhibited by cimetidine. *Annals of Pharmacotherapy* (1992) **26**: 11–13.

24 Upton RA. Pharmacokinetic interactions between theophylline and other medication (part 1). *Clinical Pharmacokinetics* (1991) **20**: 66–80.

25 Holden R. Probable fatal interaction between ciprofloxacin and theophylline. *British Medical Journal* (1988) **297**: 1339.

26 Wolfson JS and Hooper DC. Comparative pharmacokinetics of ofloxacin and ciprofloxacin. *American Journal of Medicine* (1989) **87**: 31S–36S.

9.4 Residual Neuromuscular Blockade
P.H. Carroll and B.F. Matta

History

A 71-year-old man was admitted to the intensive care unit after an emergency repair of a leaking abdominal aortic aneurysm. The patient had been waiting for elective repair of his aneurysm when he developed acute lower back pain two days before his emergency admission. He had a long-standing history of angina, hypertension and peripheral vascular disease, and had suffered a myocardial infarction in 1992. Despite ureteric stent insertion for the treatment of renal outflow obstruction in 1994, he had suffered from chronic renal failure necessitating regular hemodialysis. Previous general anesthesia had been uneventful.

Daily medications included simvastin 10 mg, amlodipine besylate 5 mg, aspirin 75 mg and temazepam 10 mg. Sublingual glycerol trinitrate was used as required. Shortly before his emergency admission, the patient had undergone hemodialysis and his urea and electrolytes were satisfactory.

After instituting routine monitoring (ECG, invasive blood pressure, central venous pressure), and having estimated the patient's weight at 70 kg, a rapid sequence induction was performed using fentanyl 500 µg, thiopentone [thiopental] 50 mg and suxamethonium [succinylcholine] 100 mg. Once the trachea was intubated and the tube secured, pancuronium 8 mg was administered after evidence of return of neuromuscular function. Flucloxacillin 1 g and gentamicin 80 mg were administered for antibiotic prophylaxis. Two hours after the start of surgery, pancuronium 4 mg was given after the patient coughed. The remainder of the surgery and anesthesia were uneventful with 1300 mL blood loss. The patient received midazolam 5 mg before transfer to the ICU for stabilization and overnight ventilation.

On arrival to the ICU (02:45 h), the patient was hemodynamically stable with normal blood pressure and good gas exchange: pH 7.40 [H^+ 40 nmol L^{-1}], P_aO_2 of 17.2 kPa [129 mmHg] and P_aCO_2 of 4.7 kPa [35 mmHg] on an F_IO_2 of 0.5 and minute volume of 10 L min^{-1}. The patient's hematocrit was 30%, potassium of 4.4 mmol L^{-1}, urea (BUN) of 19.7 mmol L^{-1} [118 mg dL^{-1}] and creatinine of 964 µmol L^{-1} [12.5 mg dL^{-1}]. Coagulation and liver function tests were within normal limits. Core temperature was 36.2°C [97.1°F]. Sedation and analgesia were started immediately with a propofol bolus of 0.5 mg kg^{-1} followed by an infusion of 1 mg kg^{-1} h^{-1} and an alfentanil infusion of 10–30 µg kg^{-1}. Boluses of midazolam 0.05 mg kg^{-1} were used for 'top-up' sedation when necessary. Throughout his operation and his stay in intensive care, the patient remained oliguric and no further gentamicin was given.

As the patient remained hemodynamically stable with good gas exchange and pinpoint pupils, propofol was stopped in preparation for tracheal extubation.

One hour later, the patient became hypertensive, tachycardic, sweaty and his pupils dilated. No associated movement or respiratory efforts were visible. Propofol sedation was restarted and the provisional diagnosis of residual neuromuscular blockade was confirmed by a nerve stimulator. Neostigmine 2.5 mg and glycopyrrolate [glycopyrronium] 500 µg were given with almost immediate eye opening and good respiratory effort. Efforts to wean the patient off the ventilator started but unfortunately, 45 minutes after the administration of neostigmine and glycopyrrolate, neuromuscular blockade had returned. Sedation was then restarted with regular assessment of neuromuscular activity. The patient's trachea was eventually extubated at 14:00 h (8 hours after admission to the ICU) after full neuromuscular activity had returned.

Traps

There are four main traps associated with this case:

- Prolonged neuromuscular blockade in patient with compromised renal function.
- The potentiation of neuromuscular blockade by the aminoglycoside antibiotics.
- The potential failure to recognize residual paralysis in a patient on the ICU with a poor respiratory effort and lack of response, with potential awareness.
- Recurarization after giving the relatively short acting antagonist, neostigmine.

Tricks

Pupillary dilatation associated with hypertension and a tachycardia alerted the clinicians to the possibility of residual neuromuscular blockade. The earlier use of a nerve stimulator would have prevented the risk of this patient being aware. It would also have assisted with the subsequent monitoring of the neuromuscular function. Fortunately, the amnesic effects of the propofol and midazolam ensured the patient had no recall of events.

Poor renal function is a well-recognized cause of prolonged neuromuscular blockade. Other factors that may prolong the duration of non-depolarizing muscle relaxants include pre-existing liver disease, inhalational anesthetic agents, hypokalemia, hypocalcemia, acidosis, hypothermia and the administration of aminoglycoside antibiotics. Muscle relaxants that are totally dependent on renal excretion are obviously more affected than those that undergo some hepatic or plasma metabolism.

Although pancuronium undergoes hepatic metabolism to its 3-hydroxy, 17-hydroxy and 3,17-hydroxy derivatives,[1,2] there is some evidence to suggest that up to 50% of the injected dose appears unchanged in the urine.[3] The neuromuscular blockade produced by pancuronium may be prolonged by up to

40 minutes in patients undergoing renal transplantation,[4] and paralysis of up to 4 hours has been reported in anephric patients.[5] The prolonged neuromuscular blockade produced by pancuronium has been linked to reduced renal excretion of its active metabolites (which are half as potent as pancuronium), altered protein binding and bioavailability found in patients with renal impairment. This, coupled with the availability of muscle relaxants independent of renal function (mainly atracurium), has prompted some authors to recommend avoiding the use of pancuronium in patients with renal impairment.[6]

In this patient, the prolonged action of pancuronium by renal impairment and the use of gentamicin was not considered to be a problem, as a period of postoperative mechanical ventilation in the intensive care unit was planned. Admittedly, the duration of neuromuscular blockade was longer than anticipated. Awareness, prevented by adequate sedation, could have been a problem had the possibility of residual paralysis in this patient not been recognized. The change in pupil size on stopping sedation was the only pointer to residual muscle paralysis as the hypertension and tachycardia seen would also have been present in the absence of residual muscle paralysis. The change in pupil size served as a good indicator of depth of sedation in this case.

The patient did receive both midazolam and propofol and remembered nothing afterwards on direct questioning. Both propofol and midazolam produce amnesia, but by different mechanisms. The amnesia produced by propofol is related to the depth of sedation, while midazolam has a specific amnesic effect.[7]

Postoperative respiratory dysfunction and/or the lack of cerebral response in patients receiving intensive care is commonly attributed to oversedation with benzodiazepines, opioids or anesthetic agents, especially in those patients who are critically ill with altered drug pharmacokinetic and pharmacodynamic properties. This relatively common trap may allow the unsuspecting to forget residual paralysis as a cause of slow awakening after stopping of sedation.

The problem of being paralyzed and aware is further exaggerated by the much smaller doses of sedative drugs used in the critically ill when compared to those required to produce anesthesia. The smaller doses are often dictated by unstable hemodynamics and the fear of drug accumulation. As long as the possibility of residual muscle blockade is entertained early on as a possible cause of slow awakening, this 'trap' can be successfully avoided.

Another 'trap' was recurarization after the action of neostigmine had worn off. Although the duration of neostigmine may be prolonged by renal impairment, recurarization is a potential problem when very long-acting muscle relaxants are used. A possible scenario would have been tracheal extubation followed by recurarization and the need for reintubation of the trachea. Careful observation of respiratory and neuromuscular function prevented this happening in this case.

Once the diagnosis of prolonged muscle relaxation is made, it is best to leave the patient sedated and the lungs ventilated until neuromuscular blockade has worn off completely, thus obviating the need for reversal.

In summary, the possibility of residual muscle blockade must always be ruled out in patients receiving intensive therapy before sedation is stopped. This is particularly important in patients with renal and/or hepatic impairment, in whom long-acting muscle relaxants dependent on renal or hepatic excretion are used. Careful observation of hemodynamic changes and pupil size, coupled with neuromuscular function tests, will inevitably reduce the risk of awareness while paralyzed.

Follow-up

After a period of stable hemodynamics and good gas exchange, the patient was transferred to the high dependency unit where he remained for a 24-hour period before transfer to the general surgical ward. The patient had no evidence of recall.

References

1 Calvey TN and Williams NE. Drugs that act on the neuromuscular junction. In *Principles and Practice of Pharmacology for Anaesthetists*. Oxford, Blackwell, 1987, Chapter 8, pp 159–186.
2 Atkinson RS, Rushman GB and Alfred Lee J (eds). The muscle relaxants. In *Synopsis of Anaesthesia*. Bristol, Wright, 1987, Chapter 14, p 270–271.
3 McLeod K, Watson MJ and Rawlins MD. Pharmacokinetics of pancuronium in patients with impaired renal function. *British Journal of Anaesthesia* (1976) **48**: 341–345.
4 Millar RD, Stevens WC and Way WL. The effect of renal failure and hyperkalaemia on the duration of pancuronium bromide in man. *Anaesthesia and Analgesia* (1973) **52**: 661–666.
5 Somogyi AA, Shanks CA and Triggs EJ. The effect of renal failure on the disposition and neuromuscular blocking action of pancuronium bromide. *European Journal of Clinical Pharmacology* (1977) **12**: 23–29.
6 Aitkenhead AR and Smith G (eds). Neuromuscular blockade. In *Textbook of Anaesthesia*. Edinburgh, Churchill Livingstone, 1990, Chapter 12, pp 211–224.
7 Polster MR, Gray PA, O'Sullivan G, McCarthy R and Park GR. Comparison of the sedative and amnesic effects of midazolam and propofol. *British Journal of Anaesthesia* (1993) **70**: 612–616.

10 Nutritional Failure

10.1 Acute Recent Upper Gastrointestinal Bleeding in a Patient with Known Esophageal Varices

G. Dobb and N. Watkins

History

A 23-year-old woman was referred to the intensive care unit with hemorrhagic shock and acute upper gastrointestinal bleeding. Her background history was of autoimmune chronic active hepatitis since the age of 14, complicated by biopsy-proven cirrhosis and progressive liver dysfunction. There was no history of blood transfusion, excessive ethanol intake or serological evidence of viral hepatitis. The portal hypertension was complicated by splenomegaly, hypersplenism and esophageal varices documented at endoscopy. She had been admitted 12 months before this episode with upper gastrointestinal bleeding and had undergone a successful course of endoscopic sclerotherapy for bleeding varices. There had been no episodes of hepatic encephalopathy. At the time of the current admission, she was under consideration for liver transplantation. There was no other significant medical history.

She had presented on this occasion with collapse and hematemesis. Having been well since her last clinic visit, she developed sudden onset of nausea followed by a large hematemesis of bright red blood. She then became drowsy and was unable to stand. In the ambulance she was noted to be tachycardic, shocked, peripherally cyanosed and responded only to pain. On arrival at the emergency department she was resuscitated with intravenous colloid and crystalloid fluids, supplemental oxygen and airway management. With fluid resuscitation, her systolic blood pressure increased from 50 to 90 mmHg but her pulse rate remained at 150/minute. A Minnesota tube was inserted in the emergency department, blood was sent for cross-matching and she was then referred to the intensive care unit for further management.

Resuscitation continued after admission to the ICU where examination revealed a 23-year-old woman of normal build who was mildly jaundiced. She was obtunded but maintaining a patent airway despite the presence of the Minnesota tube. Her peripheries were cold and vasoconstricted. She had a pulse of 150/minute, a blood pressure of 90 mmHg systolic, a temperature of 35.5°C and an S_aO_2 of 97% while receiving oxygen by face mask. The respiratory rate was 28/minute and of a normal pattern. Bright red blood was present around the mouth and was easily aspirated from the orogastric tube. There were spider nevi over the chest and back. Cardiovascular and respiratory examinations were otherwise normal. The abdomen was soft without tenderness or peritonism. A liver edge was palpable 4 cm below the costal margin, and a spleen was tippable. There was no evidence of ascites. Rectal examination demonstrated hemorrhoids and melena. Neurological examination demonstrated purposeful responses to pain in all four limbs, but not to voice. Pupils were 3 mm and reactive to light. The optic fundi could not be seen. Tone in the limbs was normal with brisk reflexes bilaterally. The plantar responses were downgoing. The investigations at this time are shown in Table 10.1.1.

Rapid fluid resuscitation through two 14-gauge cannulae was given in the form of 5% albumin, packed red cells and crystalloid and coagulation corrected with fresh frozen plasma and platelets. In order to secure the airway, elective tracheal intubation was performed assisted by midazolam and suxamethonium, followed by controlled ventilation and sedation with intravenous propofol. Intravenous ranitidine and somatostatin were given by infusion. After fluid resuscitation and intubation, an urgent esophagogastroduodeoscopy was performed by a gastroenterologist in the ICU. This showed two small esophageal varices which were not bleeding. Gastroscopy revealed large fundal varices and extensive portal gastropathy. There was evidence of recent hemorrhage but no active bleeding was seen. The fundal varices were not amenable to injection sclerotherapy, and it was not possible to determine the site of recent hemorrhage. The Minnesota tube was replaced and the gastric lumen re-inflated.

Further episodes of cardiovascular instability suggestive of bleeding despite near-normal coagulation indices followed the endoscopy. After consultation with a transplant hepatologist and surgeon, the patient was referred for an emergency transjugular intrahepatic portosystemic stent shunt which was performed successfully. The bleeding stopped, with some resolution of the portal gastropathy seen on endoscopy. Lactulose was given through a nasogastric tube. Doppler ultrasound demonstrated flow across the shunt seven days after the procedure. Sustained increases in aspartate aminotransferase and bilirubin were seen, but coagulation returned to normal without continuing replacement of clotting factors. Although the bleeding stopped, the patient's stay in the ICU was complicated by severe respiratory failure associated with bilateral lung infiltrates and sepsis syndrome. No systemic bacterial infection was identified, and acute lung injury associated with shock, massive transfusion and possible pulmonary aspiration of stomach contents was the working diagnosis.

Table 10.1.1. Investigations on admission to the intensive care unit

Arterial blood gases: F_IO_2 0.5, H^+ 51 nmol L^{-1} [pH 7.29], $P_{a}O_2$ 4.4 kPa [33 mmHg], $P_{a}O_2$ 20.5 kPa [154 mmHg], base excess -7 mmol L^{-1}, $S_{a}O_2$ 98%

Plasma lactate: 5 mmol L^{-1}

Hematology: hemoglobin 12 g dL^{-1}, white blood cell count 15 × $10^9 L^{-1}$ platelets 80 × $10^9 L^{-1}$, INR 2.5, prothrombin time 16 s, APTT 45 s, fibrinogen 1.5 g L^{-1}, FDPs negative.

Plasma biochemistry: sodium 135 mmol L^{-1}, potassium 3.4 mmol L^{-1}, bicarbonate 19 mmol L^{-1}, urea 9 mmol L^{-1} [BUN 54 mg dL^{-1}], creatinine 1.63 mg dL^{-1} [125 μmol L^{-1}], glucose 144 mg dL^{-1} [8 mmol L^{-1}], albumin 29 g L^{-1}, calcium 2.0 mmol L^{-1} [8 mg dL^{-1}], AST 158 U L^{-1}, alkaline phosphatase 190 U L^{-1}, bilirubin 64 μmol L^{-1} [3.8 mg dL^{-1}], ammonia 45 μmol L^{-1}.

Traps

1. This patient had signs of compensated shock on admission to the ICU.
2. The Minnesota tube failed to stop the bleeding from her gastrointestinal tract.
3. Pulmonary aspiration of gastric contents occurred despite early tracheal intubation.

Tricks

1. The two likely causes of compensated shock are inadequate resuscitation or continuing bleeding. The conclusion that continuing fluid replacement is needed is supported by the lactic acidosis but this investigation does not replace careful clinical assessment.
2. Using a Minnesota tube[1] may produce a false sense of security when bleeding is caused by lesions other than esophageal varices. It is of doubtful value in the management of gastric varices, and of no value in the treatment of portal gastropathy.
3. A significant gastrointestinal bleed can precipitate hepatic encephalopathy and an acute deterioration in liver function. Protection of the airway is essential to avoid complications such as aspiration pneumonitis. This is particularly important when endoscopy or angiography are undertaken because the intravenous sedation used during these procedures may further compromise the airway. Similarly, the airway compromise associated with a Minnesota or similar tube in obtunded patients should lead to prompt endotracheal intubation.

This patient demonstrates the difficulties of managing severe upper gastrointestinal hemorrhage in the setting of known portal hypertension. Bleeding can be torrential with hypovolemic shock a major threat to life in the first minutes following presentation. In addition, the bleeding may not be immediately amenable to surgical management, making coordination between critical care physicians, endoscopists, hepatologists and surgeons essential.

Essential points when managing gastrointestinal hemorrhage in patients with portal hypertension are:

- Attention to resuscitation, including airway management, fluid replacement and treatment of coagulopathy.
- Diagnosis of the source of bleeding.
- Local management of the hemorrhage by surgical or endoscopic means, if possible.
- Reduction in portal pressure by medical, surgical or radiological techniques.
- Management of complications including hepatic encephalopathy and liver failure.

An endoscopy is an essential component of the management in all cases. Portal hypertension can produce bleeding in almost any part of the gastrointestinal tract,[2] and it is therefore essential to localize the bleeding site in order to give appropriate therapy. In addition, patients with chronic liver disease are no less at risk from developing bleeding from peptic ulcer disease. Never assume that gastrointestinal bleeding in a patient with portal hypertension is caused by esophageal varices. In a series of 222 patients with upper gastrointestinal bleeding and esophageal varices, the varices were the cause of bleeding in 65%, gastroduodenal erosions in 15% and gastric or duodenal ulcers 10%. A variety of other lesions were the cause in the remaining 10%.[3]

Bleeding esophageal varices can be managed endoscopically by skilled interventional endoscopists.[4] This must occur as soon as possible to prevent ongoing bleeding and coagulopathy. Endoscopic sclerotherapy and endoscopic ligation are alternative techniques, with ligation appearing to give better results in skilled hands while sclerotherapy is technically less demanding.[5]

Bleeding from gastric varices or portal gastropathy can be very difficult to stop endoscopically. Portal gastropathy should always be considered in the differential diagnosis of gastrointestinal bleeding in patients with known portal hypertension.

Medical treatment of portal hypertension in association with acute gastrointestinal bleeding should not replace or delay definitive management by either endoscopic techniques or surgery. Pharmacological treatment of portal hypertension has been used as an adjunctive therapy, predominantly for variceal bleeding. Intravenous vasopressin decreases portal pressure in animal models, but its efficacy is not established by clinical trials, and its use can be associated with cardiovascular side-effects. Propranalol may reduce the incidence of re-bleeding in the long term, but its use in bleeding of unstable patients is associated with hemodynamic instability. Somatostatin analogs lower splanchnic blood flow in animals and man, and they are free or adverse cardiovascular effects. Their efficacy in the management of acute variceal hemorrhage is not conclusively established.[6] Octreotide infusion, when combined with sclerotherapy, reduced the risk of re-bleeding from varices but did not improve 15-day survival.[7]

Transjugular intrahepatic portosystemic stent shunts (TIPSS) are gaining increasing acceptance in the management of portal hypertension.[8] The procedure requires specialized radiological expertise and it is therefore not available outside tertiary referral institutions. Early studies have suggested that it may be effective in reducing both portal pressure and the incidence of re-bleeding. Re-bleeding after TIPSS occurs in 10–20% of patients and is usually associated with shunt narrowing or thrombosis.[9] At present, indications include bleeding from gastric varices, the onset of active variceal bleeding not controlled by sclerotherapy and hemorrhage from portal hypertensive gastropathy refractory to propranolol. Avoiding a laparotomy and vascular anastamoses makes subsequent liver transplantation technically easier. Complications include intra-abdominal hemorrhage, haemobilia, hepatic encephalopathy short migration and hemolysis. Surgical options in the management of variceal hemorrhage depend in part on the expertise and preference of the surgeon. They include:

- Esophageal transection and re-anastamosis.

- Surgical portosystemic shunt.
- Emergency liver transplantation.

Follow-up

After 11 days of mechanical ventilation, the patient was weaned from the ventilator and her trachea extubated. She then awaited elective liver transplantation.

References

1 Garden OJ and Carter DC. Balloon tamponade and vasoactive drugs in the control of acute variceal haemorrhage. *Ballière's Clinical Gastroenterology* (1992) **6**: 451–463.
2 Collini FJ and Brener B. Portal hypertension. *Surgical Gynecology and Obstetrics* (1990) **170**: 177–192.
3 Sutton FM. Upper gastrointestinal bleeding in patients with esophageal varices: What is the most common source? *American Journal of Medicine* (1987) **83**: 273–275.
4 Heaton ND and Howard ER. Complications and limitations of injection sclerotherapy in portal hypertension. *Gut* (1993) **34**: 7–10.
5 Stiegmann GV, Goff JS, Michaletz-Onody PA, Korula J, Lieberman D, Saeed ZA, Reveille RM, Sun JH and Lowenstein SR. Endoscopic sclerotherapy as compared with endoscopic ligation for bleeding esophageal varices. *New England Journal of Medicine* (1992) **326**: 1527–1532.
6 Burroughs AK and Panagou E. Pharmacological therapy for portal hypertension: rationale and results. *Seminars in Gastrointestinal Disease* (1995) **6**: 148–164.
7 Besson I, Ingrand P, Person B, *et al.* Sclerotherapy with or without octreotide for acute varical bleeding. *New England Journal of Medicine* (1995) **333**: 555–560.
8 McCormick PA, Dick R, Chin J, Irving JD, McIntyre N, Hobbs KEF and Burroughs AK. Transjugular intrahepatic portosystemic stent-shunt. *British Journal of Hospital Medicine* (1993) **19**: 791–797.
9 Hayes PC, Redhead PN and Finlayson NDC. Transjugular intrahepatic portosystemic stent shunts. *Gut* (1994) **35**: 445–446.

10.2 Acute Recurrent Gastrointestinal Bleed in an Intubated Patient

G. Dobb

History

A 58-year-old accounts clerk presented with a 3-day history of fever, cough and increasing breathlessness. She had a long history of asthma and had also been a heavy cigarette smoker (20–30 per day for 28 years). Recent treatment included slow release theophylline, beclomethasone by inhaler, salbutamol [albutenol] as required by inhaler, prednisolone 10 mg per day, and warfarin and digoxin for atrial fibrillation. Despite this treatment her normal exercise tolerance was limited to about 100 m slow walking on the level, but she was able to drive to work and do her own shopping with her husband's assistance. When seen by her usual respiratory physician 6 weeks previously, respiratory function tests showed an FEV_1 of 0.65 L and FVC of 1.4 L.

On admission to a medical ward she was noted to have a somewhat Cushingoid appearance and atrophic skin with telangiectasia and ecchymoses. Her temperature was 38.7°C [101.7°F], pulse 115/minute irregular, arterial pressure 135/85 mmHg, JVP slightly elevated, normal heart sounds and some slight ankle edema. Examination of the chest was consistent with the chest radiograph, which showed consolidation in the right lower lobe and early consolidation in the left perihilar region with hyperlucent lung fields elsewhere and evidence of bullae in both upper zones. She was given oxygen by face mask and started on cefotaxime 1 g 8 hourly and erythromycin 500 mg 8 hourly.

After admission to the ward she appeared to become less distressed and was noted by the nursing staff to be sleeping peacefully, but when the evening meal was delivered she was unrousable. Urgent review by the medical registrar found her to have a pulse of 130/minute irregular, arterial pressure 160/100 mmHg, and to have very shallow respiration. Arterial blood gases were P_aO_2 8.5 kPa [64 mmHg], P_aCO_2 13.9 kPa [104 mmHg]. She was intubated, ventilated and transferred to the intensive care unit for ongoing management.

Over the next four days antibiotic treatment was continued with cefotaxime after identification of a pneumococcus from early sputum cultures. There appeared to be a clinical response with her temperature decreasing to 37.5–38°C [99.5–100.4°F] and a decreasing white blood cell count. However, she remained ventilator-dependent and tolerated the tracheal tube poorly, and therefore needed moderately heavy sedation. Attempts to establish enteral feeding through a nasogastric tube were frustrated by intermittent large aspirates resulting in absorption of less than half the target volume. Other treatment included parenteral steroids, increased to 60 mg prednisolone per day, intravenous aminophylline, nebulized salbutamol 4 hourly, warfarin and digoxin.

On the fourth day small amounts of 'coffee grounds' were noted in the nasogastric aspirate. On day five she suddenly regurgitated fresh blood and over 500 ml was aspirated through the nasogastric tube. This was accompanied by a decrease in arterial pressure to 95/60 mmHg. The nasogastric tube was connected to a drainage bag after aspiration of a further 200 ml of fresh blood. A steady flow of 100–150 mL of fresh blood every 15 minutes continued to drain into the drainage bag. Her investigations at this time are shown in Table 10.2.1.

There was a short delay in gaining adequate intravenous access. Ideally, two large-bore cannulae should have been inserted but with her atrophic skin it had been noted that she had 'fragile' veins and after a few days of peripheral intravenous access and antibiotics using an 18-gauge cannula no suitable veins for anything larger were found. An 8FG pulmonary artery catheter introducer was therefore inserted into the right internal jugular vein, together with a triple lumen central venous catheter. During this time arterial pressure decreased to 70/40 mmHg and the initial CVP measurement was zero. Rapid fluid resuscitation with 500 mL Hemaccel® and 4 units of fresh frozen plasma ordered to correct the prolonged prothrombin time brought the arterial pressure to 120/65 mmHg and CVP to 9 mmHg. Omeprazole 40 mg was given intravenously.

Urgent endoscopy was arranged. This showed numerous superficial gastric erosions with some minor oozing of blood from the surface of the larger ones. A considerable amount of blood and blood clot in the stomach made the examination technically difficult but, because there did not appear to be sufficient cause for the volume of hemorrhage in the stomach and because the esophagus was normal, the endoscope was passed into the duodenum. Considerable distortion was evident from chronic duodenal ulceration, but there was also a deep acute ulcer with some minor continuing ooze from a vessel in the ulcer base.

A lesion with this appearance has an 85% chance of re-bleeding[1] if there is no active intervention. The oozing vessel was treated by laser photocoagulation, and after this she was transfused with 3 units of packed cells for a hemoglobin of 62 g L^{-1}.

Controlled studies have failed to show an effect of acid secretion inhibitors on the recurrence or continuation of upper gastrointestinal bleeding (UGIB). Nevertheless, most gastroenterologists continue to advise their use, arguing that if an ulcer is present, treatment may as well start at the earliest opportunity. There is good evidence that inhibition of acid and pepsin secretion should promote clot formation. Below a pH of 5.4 both coagulation and platelet aggregation are severely inhibited.[2]

Table 10.2.1. Investigations

Hemoglobin 94 g L^{-1}, white blood cell count 13.4 × 10^9 L^{-1}, platelets 97 × 10^9 L^{-1}

Sodium 134 mmol L^{-1}, potassium 4.2 mmol L^{-1}, chloride 99 mmol L^{-1}, urea 9.4 mmol L^{-1}, creatinine 87 µmol L^{-1}

Calcium 2.14 mmol L^{-1}, phosphate 0.7 mmol L^{-1}, albumin 31 g L^{-1}

Bilirubin 28 µmol L^{-1}, alkaline phosphatase 314 IU L^{-1}, AST 54 IU L^{-1}

Both the gastroenterologists and general surgical team were asked to review the patient. Over the next hour the rate of blood loss decreased as evidenced by loss from the nasogastric tube. This was accompanied by relative hemodynamic stability, although a further 2 units of fresh frozen plasma were given to correct a repeated INR of 2.4.

Fifteen hours after endoscopy and laser photocoagulation, further fresh blood appeared in the nasogastric tube. This was quickly followed by increasing tachycardia, hypotension and peripheral vasoconstriction. Despite the rapid infusion of fluid the systolic arterial pressure remained 90–100 mmHg. Investigations at this time were:

Hemoglobin 91 g dL^{-1}, white blood cell count 12.3 × 10^9 L^{-1},
    platelets 84 × 10^9 L^{-1}
INR 1.4, APTT 43 s (control 35 s), fibrinogen 1.8 g L^{-1}

A further 6 units of blood were cross-matched. After an urgent surgical review with discussion of the available options, including repeat endoscopy with endoscopic intervention to try and control the bleeding again, she was transferred to the operating room where the ulcer was undersewn then a vagotomy and pyloroplasty performed. Once the bleeding was controlled further infusion of blood and colloid resulted in the heart rate decreasing to 95/minute with an arterial pressure of 130/75 mmHg and a CVP of 10 mmHg.

Trap 1

Even though the frequency of UGIB in critically ill patients appears to have decreased, patients with prolonged respiratory failure and coagulopathy are a high-risk population. The need for UGIB prophylaxis should be considered until nasogastric feeding is fully established in 'at risk' patients.

Trap 2

It should never be assumed that stress ulceration is the cause of UGIB in a critically ill patient. Endoscopic studies have shown a very high frequency of gastric erosions in critically ill patients. However, Peura and Johnson[3] found erosions in 74% of medical intensive care patients, so the finding of these lesions should not curtail a search for other causes of significant bleeding that exist in the remaining 26% of patients. In this patient, gastric erosions were present as well as another cause for her significant UGIB.

Tricks

The patient had a number of 'risk factors' for UGIB. Many factors have been associated with UGIB in critically ill patients (Table 10.2.2). Scoring systems

Table 10.2.2. Risk factors for upper gastrointestinal hemorrhage from stress ulceration (modified from Tryba[4])

History of ulcer	Gastroenterological disease
Acute renal insufficiency	Respiratory failure
Burn >25%	Transplantation
Head injury (alone) with neurological deficit	Coagulopathy
Severe infection	Intracranial bleeding
Severe multiple trauma	Transfusion (>4 units of blood)
Cardiogenic shock	Anticoagulation with heparin
Pancreatitis	Hemoglobin <10 for >24 hours
Kidney disease	More than one episode with arterial pressure <100 mmHg for >1 hour

based on the number and severity of risk factors present have been suggested as a means of providing an overall estimate of the risk.[4] However, these have been somewhat discredited in recent times. The proposed risk factors were identified by a retrospective review of the records of cohorts of patients with UGIB without comparison to a control group, or from prospective series and clinical trials in which the odds ratio and confidence limits for the risk of bleeding associated with 'risk factors' are not reported. In a more recent study examining the risk factors for UGIB, only prolonged mechanical ventilation and coagulopathy were found to be predictive of UGIB.[5]

This patient had both respiratory failure and a coagulopathy. A case might therefore have been made for UGIB prophylaxis. The choice of prophylaxis is between H_2-antagonists, sucralfate and antacids. Other drugs have been used (M1-receptor antagonists, proton pump inhibitors) but these, like the H_2-antagonists, act to reduce gastric acid secretion. Such drugs, together with the antacids which neutralize gastric acid, have the effect of increasing the pH of gastric contents. In most clinical trials the use of these drugs reduces the frequency of UGIB to about 2%. Sucralfate appears equally effective in preventing UGIB but does not increase gastric pH significantly. This, together with mild antibacterial activity, may account for a lower frequency of bacterial overgrowth in the stomach using sucralfate than the pH increasing agents. This, in turn, may account for an apparent decrease in the frequency of nosocomial pneumonia in patients receiving UGIB prophylaxis with sucralfate when compared to, for example, H_2-receptor antagonists.[6] However, the cause of nosocomial pneumonia is complex and factors other than bacterial colonization of gastric contents almost certainly play a role, e.g. volume of gastric contents, history of gastro-esophageal reflux, presence of a large-bore nasogastric tube.

Studies in the 1980s reported overt UGIB in approximately 15% of critically ill patients not given prophylaxis against UGIB;[7] this reduced to 2–3% using H_2-antagonists or antacid prophylaxis. More recent studies have found a much lower frequency of UGIB in critically ill patients.[8] UGIB is unusual in patients who have been established on enteral feeds[9] but it should be noted that this patient was largely intolerant of nasogastric feeding.

Electrocoagulation, heat coagulation and injection of absolute alcohol are alternatives to laser photocoagulation. No difference between these methods has been shown in clinical trials.[1,10] The choice of treatment therefore tends to depend on the endoscopist's preferences, experience and the equipment available. A meta-analysis of trials of laser photocoagulation found re-bleeding, progression to surgery and mortality were all significantly less with photocoagulation than in controls.[11]

Continued or recurrent bleeding after endoscopic intervention is an indication for urgent surgery. Although the mortality after surgery is high, the limited physiological reserves suggest that early surgery, before the onset of significant multiple organ dysfunction, is likely to give better results than saving surgery for a last resort after multiple transfusions and in the presence of dilutional coagulopathy or activated thrombolysis.

Approximately half the critically ill patients who have significant UGIB will die. Their tolerance of significant bleeding is reduced by diminished physiological reserves. UGIB in critically ill patients must be treated as an emergency with vigorous resuscitation, investigation and urgent definitive treatment when appropriate. A pause in the bleeding is not a reason to delay investigation.

Acute UGIB induces a hypercoagulable state[12] which will enhance the chances of spontaneous clotting at a bleeding point. Transfused blood, particularly if it has been stored for some time, contains activated fibrinolytics. There is evidence that early blood transfusion results in more prolonged and greater bleeding from upper gastrointestinal lesions. A policy of delaying blood transfusion and only using other fluids until the hemoglobin concentration is less than $8\,\mathrm{g\,dL^{-1}}$ appears to provide the best outcome.[13]

Rapid correction of a high INR when there is acute hemorrhage is best achieved by infusion of clotting factors. Vitamin K is the antidote to warfarin, but it takes too long to be effective when there is significant bleeding. If vitamin K is given to a patient who will need ongoing anticoagulation, only 1 or 2 mg should be given. If larger doses (e.g. 10 mg) are given, difficulties may occur with subsequent anticoagulation.

Follow-up

A percutaneous tracheostomy was performed one day after the UGIB because it was apparent that weaning from mechanical ventilation was likely to be prolonged. After the tracheostomy sedation was no longer needed. Weaning from ventilation proceeded through decreasing synchronized intermittent mandatory ventilation and decreasing pressure support. There was gradual resolution of the pulmonary consolidation, and 15 days after the UGIB the tracheostomy was removed, followed by discharge from the intensive care unit one day later. Repeat endoscopy before the patient's discharge home from the hospital showed healing of the duodenal ulcer.

References

1 Gupta PK and Fleischer DE. Nonvariceal upper gastrointestinal bleeding. *Medical Clinics of North America* (1993) **77**: 973–992.

2 Kaplan MM and May JR. The influence of pH control on the prevention and management of gastrointestinal bleeding. *Journal of Intensive Care Medicine* (1990) **5**: S28–S33.

3 Peura DA and Johnson LF. Cimetidine for prevention and treatment of gastroduodenal mucosal lesions in patients in an intensive care unit. *Annals of Internal Medicine* (1985) **103**: 173–177.

4 Tryba M. Risk of acute stress bleeding and nosocomial pneumonia in ventilated intensive care patients. *American Journal of Medicine* (1987) **83** (Suppl. 3B): 117–124.

5 Marshell JC, Leasa D, Hall R, Winton TL, Rutledge F, Todd TJ, Roy P, Cook DJ, Fuller HD, Guyatt GH. Risk factors for gastrointestinal bleeding in critically ill patients. Canadian Critical Care Trials Group. *New England Journal of Medicine* (1994) **330**: 377–381.

6 Manning M, Burke RA, Garvin GM, Kunches LM, Farber HW, Wedel SA, McCabe WR, Driks MR, Craven DE, Celli BR Nosocomial pneumonia in intubated patients given sucralfate as compared with antacids or histamine type 2 blockers. *New England Journal of Medicine* (1987) **317**: 1376–1382.

7 Shuman RB, Schuster DP and Zuckerman GR. Prophylactic therapy for stress ulcer bleeding: a reappraisal. *Annals of Internal Medicine* (1987) **106**: 562–567.

8 Zandstra DF and Stoutenbeek CP. The virtual absence of stress ulceration related bleeding in intensive care unit patients receiving prolonged mechanical ventilation without any prophylaxis. A prospective cohort study. *Intensive Care Medicine* (1994) **20**: 335–340.

9 Pingleton SK and Hadzima SK. Enteral alimentation and gastrointestinal bleeding in mechanically ventilated patients. *Critical Care Medicine* (1983) **11**: 13–16.

10 Palmer KR and Choudari CP. Endoscopic intervention in bleeding peptic ulcer. *Gut* (1995) **37**: 161–164.

11 Henry DA and White I. Endoscopic coagulation for gastrointestinal bleeding. *New England Journal of Medicine* (1988) **318**: 186–187.

12 Henricksson AE, Nilsson TK and Svensson JO. Time course of clotting and fibrinolytic markers in acute upper gastrointestinal bleeding: relation to diagnosis and blood transfusion treatment. *Blood Coagulation and Fibrinolysis* (1993) **4**: 877–880.

13 Henricksson AE and Svensson JO. Upper gastrointestinal bleeding. With special reference to blood transfusion. *European Journal of Surgery* (1991) **157**: 193–196.

10.3 Acute Pancreatitis Presenting as Hypotension and Pyrexia
G. Dobb

History

A 52-year-old school teacher was first seen by intensive care medical staff on the surgical ward at the request of the surgeon. Five days previously she had undergone laparoscopic cholecystectomy for recurrent right upper quadrant abdominal pain associated with multiple small gall bladder calculi demonstrated on abdominal ultrasound. The procedure was uncomplicated apart from transient hypotension to a systolic arterial pressure of 70 mmHg during abdominal insufflation which had responded slowly to infusion of 1 liter of 0.9% saline. She was discharged home the day after surgery but returned on the third postoperative day with abdominal pain, nausea and fever (38.7°C [101.7°F]). Abdominal tenderness was greatest in the right upper quadrant and a presumptive diagnosis of cholangitis was made. Management included fasting, intravenous fluids and antibiotic treatment with cefotaxime 1 g 8 hourly and metronidazole 500 mg 12 hourly intravenously. Over the 24 hours before being seen she had developed oliguria unresponsive to successive fluid challenges, resulting in a total of a 5 L positive fluid balance since admission. In the previous 12 hours there had been a progressive increase in respiratory rate to 40/minute on oxygen via a Hudson mask at 12L min^{-1} and a decrease in arterial pressure which had remained in the range of 85–90 mmHg systolic despite the fluid challenges. The abdominal pain and tenderness were now more widespread, though still greatest in the upper abdomen and fever had increased to 40.5°C [104.9°F].

Her past history included hypertension (usual treatment captopril 25 mg 8 hourly), ankle swelling (frusemide [furosemide] 40 mg daily) and non-insulin dependent diabetes ('diet controlled'), together with appendicectomy, hysterectomy and tonsillectomy carried out more than 10 years previously. Her investigations at this time are shown in Table 10.3.1.

Abdominal ultrasound (from earlier the same day) was of limited use because of extensive bowel gas. No calculi were seen in the common bile duct though this was somewhat dilated, being at the upper limit of normal. There was no evidence of renal obstruction. Blood cultures showed no growth after three days.

A primary diagnosis of pancreatitis was made.

Arrangements were made for the patient to be transferred to the intensive care unit (ICU). While this was being organized, a long central line was inserted through her only remaining visible vein which was in the right cubital fossa. An initial CVP reading was 2 cmH$_2$O. A dopamine infusion was started through the central catheter, rapidly increasing to 10 µg kg^{-1} min^{-1} with systolic arterial pressure increasing to 100–105 mmHg. During transfer from bed to trolley in the ward the other intravenous cannula used for infusion of fluids was inadvertently removed.

Table 10.3.1. Investigations

Hemoglobin 96 g dL^{-1}, white blood cell count 15.2 × 10^{9}L^{-1}, 92% neutrophils with left shift, platelets 127 × 10^{9}L^{-1}.

INR 1.4, APTT 44 s (control 35 s), fibrinogen 44 g L^{-1}.

Sodium 133 mmol L^{-1}, potassium 5.2 mmol L^{-1}, bicarbonate 13 mmol L^{-1}, urea 20.1 mmol L^{-1}, BUN 120.6 mg dL^{-1}, creatinine 304 μmol L^{-1} [4.0 mg dL^{-1}].

pH 7.28 [H$^+$ 53 nmol L^{-1}], P_aCO$_2$ 28 mmHg [3.7 kPa], P_aO$_2$ 54 mmHg [7.2 kPa], base excess −12 mmol L^{-1}, bicarbonate 12 mmol L^{-1}.

Blood sugar 18.4 mmol L^{-1} [calcium 1.82 mmol L^{-1}], phosphate 0.5 mmol L^{-1}, albumin 30 g L^{-1}, bilirubin 44 μmol L^{-1} [2.6 mg dL^{-1}], alkaline phosphatase 428 U L^{-1}, AST 98 U L^{-1} amylase 2416 U L^{-1}.

On arrival in the ICU the patient was very distressed, tachypneic and somewhat confused. A nasogastric tube was inserted as a prelude to a trial of CPAP. Through the nasogastric tube was aspirated a large quantity of gas and 1–1.5 L of light brown fluid. There was an immediate slowing in the respiratory rate to 34/minute and further slowing after application of mask CPAP 5 cmH$_2$O ($F_{IO_{2.5}}$ 50%) to 28/minute.

At this time she could tolerate lying flat for a short time to have a triple lumen central venous catheter and a 9FG catheter introducer inserted through the left subclavian vein. The CVP was 1–3 mmHg, though it was difficult to read because of marked inspiratory swings. Infusion of 1.6 L of colloid over the next hour in 200 mL boluses resulted in the CVP increasing to 14 mmHg but she remained tachycardic, increasing amounts of dopamine were required to support the arterial pressure (increasing to 16 μg kg^{-1} min^{-1}), urine output was 8 mL for the hour and respiratory rate increased to 40/minute.

Urgent investigations showed:

pH 7.07 [H$^+$ 85 nmol L^{-1}], P_aCO$_2$ 6 kPa [45 mmHg], P_aO$_2$ 8.1 kPa [61 mmHg], base excess −20 mmol L^{-1}, sodium 130 mmol L^{-1}, potassium 6.4 mmol L^{-1}, blood glucose 18.4 mmol L^{-1} [331 mg dL^{-1}].

A trial of 10 cmH$_2$O CPAP failed to halt the increasing tachypnea. It was decided to start mechanical ventilation.

Concurrently, 50% dextrose 20 mL, soluble insulin 10 units and calcium chloride 5 mmol were given because of the hyperkalemia. After tracheal intubation, satisfactory arterial blood gases were obtained with an F_IO_2 of 0.6, 10 cmH$_2$O of PEEP on pressure control ventilation. Continuous venovenous hemodiafiltration was started for continuing hyperkalemia and oliguria, and total parenteral nutrition (TPN) started (10% amino acids 750 mL, 50% dextrose 750 mL plus electrolytes, multivitamins and trace elements over 24 hours). Further hypotension stabilized with a systolic arterial pressure of 115 mmHg and mean pressure of 70 mmHg after starting first adrenaline [epinephrine], increasing to 10 μg min^{-1} and then noradrenaline [norepinephrine] to $12 \, \mu g \, min^{-1}$. A pulmonary artery catheter was inserted showing a PAOP of 12 mmHg and a cardiac index of $5.7 \, L \, min^{-1} \, m^{-2}$.

Over the next three days, hemodiafiltration continued because she became anuric, ventilation was unchanged and there was some stabilization of hemodynamic function with epinephrine being weaned off and norepinephrine being decreased to $4 \, \mu g \, min^{-1}$ with the cardiac index remaining high ($4.9 \, L \, min^{-1} \, m^{-2}$). Hyperglycemia remained a problem (18–26 mmol L^{-1}) [324–468 mg dL^{-1}] despite an insulin infusion increasing from 2 to 6 units per hour. The TPN was modified to provide 50% dextrose 500 mL and 10% of amino acids 1000 mL over 24 hours. On this, blood glucose concentrations were 10–12 mmol L^{-1} [180–216 mg dL^{-1}] on insulin 2–3 units per hour. There was increasing jaundice with the total bilirubin increasing to 167 µmol L^{-1} [9.8 mg dL^{-1}].

A repeat ultrasound was technically unsatisfactory. An abdominal CT scan was arranged. Moderate pleural effusions were seen on the upper scans, there was marked dilatation of the common bile duct and the suggestion of a calculus at the lower end. Dilated loops of bowel, extensive pancreatitis and retroperitoneal edema were seen. Endoscopic retrograde cholangiopancreatography (ERCP) demonstrated an obstructing calculus which was removed endoscopically after sphincterotomy of the ampulla.

Over the next 48 hours the plasma bilirubin decreased to 82 µmol L^{-1} [4.8 mg dL^{-1}], but there was otherwise little overall change. Inotropic drug infusions, mechanical ventilation, hemodiafiltration and TPN continued. At the end of this period there was sudden onset of pyrexia to 39.7°C [103.5°F] accompanied by increasing inotropic drug requirements to maintain arterial pressure. The CVP was 8 mmHg and on re-inserting a pulmonary artery flotation catheter the PAOP was 14 mmHg after 500 mL of colloid with a cardiac index of $5.2 \, L \, min^{-1} \, m^{-2}$. All other intravascular catheters were changed and the tips sent for culture (no subsequent growth). A chest radiograph showed changes consistent with ARDS/acute lung injury but no focal abnormalities, and sputum sample microscopy revealed many leukocytes but no bacteria were seen. No bacteria were seen in the 12 mL of urine obtained from in–out bladder catheterization. Blood cultures subsequently grew *Escherichia coli*.

After taking the samples for culture, imipenem 500 mg 6 hourly was started and a repeat abdominal CT scan was performed. The CT scan showed a greatly enlarged pancreas, peri-pancreatic fat necrosis, extensive retroperitoneal edema and small amounts of fluid in the paracolic gutters. Fine needle aspirates from the pancreas subsequently grew *E. coli* and *Klebsiella* spp. The patient was taken to the operating room for debridement of her pancreas.

On return to the ICU the patient's condition was very unstable with a temperature of 40.2°C, arterial pressure being supported by adrenaline $40 \, \mu g \, min^{-1}$ and noradrenaline $25 \, \mu g \, min^{-1}$. The PAOP was 12 mmHg despite 4.2 L of blood and colloid being given during surgery (hemoglobin 12.4 g dL^{-1}, estimated intra-operative blood loss 540 mL). Worsening arterial oxygenation had resulted in the F_IO_2 being increased to 100% with 10 cmH$_2$O PEEP (pH 7.18 [H$^+$ 64 nmol L^{-1}], P_aCO_2 48 mmHg [6.4 kPa], P_aO_2 63 mmHg [8.4 kPa], lactate 6.2 mmol L^{-1}). A chest radiograph showed extensive bilateral pulmonary infiltrates with interstitial and alveolar edema. Continuous hemodiafiltration was restarted with a negative balance of $100 \, \text{mL} \, \text{h}^{-1}$. This was well tolerated and over the next 12 hours there was a gradual improvement in oxygenation (F_1O_2 reduced to 0.6) and a decrease in the rates of catecholamine infusion to adrenaline $15 \, \mu\text{g} \, \text{min}^{-1}$, noradrenaline $5 \, \mu\text{g} \, \text{min}^{-1}$ (cardiac index $4.6 \, \text{L} \, \text{min}^{-1} \, \text{m}^{-2}$, mean arterial pressure $76 \, \text{mmHg}$, PAOP $11 \, \text{mmHg}$, lactate $3.7 \, \text{mmol} \, \text{L}^{-1}$). Over the next 36 hours there was little change with her remaining febrile. A repeat laparotomy and surgical debridement were performed at this time and again after a further two days. Each was followed by a brief period of instability, but after the last laparotomy core temperature decreased to 37–$38°\text{C}$ [98.6–$100.4°\text{F}$] and the catecholamine infusions could gradually be weaned off.

Traps

Most surgeons do not insert a nasogastric tube in patients with mild or moderate pancreatitis and there is evidence that a nasogastric tube is unnecessary. Severe pancreatitis, especially when it is associated with renal failure, may cause acute gastric dilatation. In this patient, diabetic autonomic neuropathy could have been a contributory cause. Acute gastric dilatation exacerbates respiratory distress.

Patients with anything other than a normal mental state undergoing mask CPAP should have a nasogastric tube inserted to reduce the risks of vomiting or regurgitation with a close-fitting mask in place. Some centers routinely place a nasogastric tube when mask CPAP is used.

Edema and swelling of the head of the pancreas during severe pancreatitis often cause some obstruction to the bile duct. This, together with elements of ischemic or septic hepatitis and absorption of hematoma associated with hemorrhagic pancreatitis almost invariably causes an increased plasma bilirubin concentration sufficient to cause mild jaundice. More severe jaundice should provoke a search for a specific cause. While post-cholecystectomy pancreatitis is well recognized, there should be particular concern in a patient with this history and laboratory findings that biliary obstruction by a missed gallstone underlies both the pancreatitis and increasing jaundice.

Tricks

It is common for ultrasound to be unsatisfactory during the early phase of pancreatitis. At this time, for instance, only two-thirds of the gall bladder calculi present will be visualized and the pancreas cannot be seen in up to 40% of patients because of overlying bowel gas.

Indications for ERCP in pancreatitis include:

1. Suspicion of gallstone induced pancreatitis, not improving by 24 hours after admission.
2. Traumatic pancreatitis, to evaluate pancreatic duct disruption.

Infection of necrotic pancreas is a relatively early (as early as the first week) complication, whereas pancreatic abscesses and pseudocysts are later complications. Fine needle aspiration of necrotic pancreatic tissue is not an established technique but has proved useful on occasion for confirming infection of the necrotic pancreatic mass and identifying the organisms involved.

Antibiotics vary in their penetration of pancreatic tissue. A study of pancreatic samples taken at the time of surgery[1] found the lowest tissue concentrations for aminoglycosides and the highest concentrations for imipenem and quinolones. Intermediate concentrations of broad-spectrum penicillins and third-generation cephalosporins were found. The most common bacterial isolates were *E. coli* (26%), *Pseudomonas* spp. (16%), anaerobic organisms (16%), *Staphylococcus aureus* (15%), *Klebsiella* spp. (10%) and *Proteus* spp. (10%).

The place of prophylactic antibiotics in severe pancreatitis has been uncertain. Clinical trials in the 1970s showed no benefit but this may have been because of the antibiotic used (ampicillin). A more recent clinical trial[2] using imipenem, has shown a decreased frequency of infection in necrotic pancreatitis and it is possible that this patient might have benefitted from earlier prophylactic use of imipenem.

Experimental studies suggest that both bacterial translocation from the gut and hematogenous seeding have a role in the infection of necrotic pancreas.[3] A clinical trial of selective decontamination of the digestive tract by oral norfloxacin, colistin and amphotericin shows a significant reduction in Gram-negative bacterial pancreatic infection in patients given selective decontamination.[4] After adjustment for illness severity, selective decontamination was associated with an improved outcome in treated patients. This treatment has still to achieve widespread acceptance.

When Gram-negative organisms were seen in the fine needle aspirate, extensive discussions were held with the surgical team and the patient's family. Because of the extensive nature of the infection it was thought unlikely that percutaneous catheter drainage would be of any benefit. On the other hand, extensive surgery in the presence of multiple organ failure and hemodynamic instability would clearly carry a high risk. The decision was made to proceed to surgical debridement of necrotic tissue.

The place of surgery in severe pancreatitis is somewhat controversial[5] but there appears to be a consensus that survival is improved by surgical debridement when the necrotic pancreas becomes infected. Interpretation of published results from surgical intervention in acute severe pancreatitis is complicated by the variety of underlying causes and variation in the proportions of, for example, obstructive gallstone-associated pancreatitis and alcohol-associated pancreatitis from different countries and different centers.[6,7] Patients with alcohol-associated pancreatitis, in particular, tend to have more concurrent disease and a poorer initial nutritional status than those with pancreatitis of other etiologies. It is an impression that patients with alcohol-associated pancreatitis cope badly with the protracted course and repeated surgery that often follow surgical intervention in necrotic hemorrhagic pancreatitis.

A feeding jejunostomy should be created at the time of laparotomy to

permit subsequent enteral nutrition. Low-fat formulae such as Precision HN®
(Sandoz Nutrition), Criticare HN® (Mead Johnson) or Vivonex HN® (Norwich
Eaton) are recommended.[8] Enteral feeding must be started slowly and with
careful observation. Even low-fat feeds cause pancreatic exocrine stimulation.

As with other surgical approaches to severe pancreatitis, the place of repeat
laparotomy and debridement has not been established.[9] However, on basic
surgical principles it seems sound practice to ensure that all necrotic and infected
material has been removed to the fullest possible extent if a surgical approach is
used.

Semi-elective tracheal intubation of a patient with severe respiratory distress
and metabolic acidosis should only be undertaken by appropriately skilled and
experienced staff. It is a procedure which carries a significant risk of cardiac
arrhythmia or severe hypoxemia if there is any delay in inserting the tracheal
tube. Sedative drugs given to facilitate tracheal intubation may cause a reduction
in sympathetic tone and hypotension.

Hyperkalemia provided an additional threat in this patient. Any worsening of
metabolic or respiratory acidosis would further increase the plasma potassium
concentration. A $0.4\,\mathrm{mmol\,L^{-1}}$ increase in plasma potassium concentration for
every 0.1 decrease in pH is commonly quoted. Although the place of sodium
bicarbonate treatment of metabolic acidosis is controversial, many would give, say,
100 mmol of sodium bicarbonate before attempting tracheal intubation to decrease
the metabolic acidosis and potassium concentration.

Suxamethonium should not be used in hyperkalemic patients. It will further
increase the plasma potassium concentration, increasing the risk of cardiac
arrhythmias. Alternative approaches to tracheal intubation are sedation and
muscle paralysis using a neuromuscular blocking agent such as atacurium 50 mg
or vecuronium 10–12 mg intravenously to achieve optimum conditions for
tracheal intubation, or awake tracheal intubation using local anesthesia. Attempts
at awake intubation are often tolerated very poorly by patients with severe
respiratory distress unless they are mentally obtunded. The choice of method for
tracheal intubation under these circumstances is best left to the preference and
experience of the doctor concerned.

Follow-up

There was a slow improvement in respiratory function and, from 12 days after the
final laparotomy, a steady increase in urine output. Hemodiafiltration was stopped
at this time and extubation occurred 24 hours later. The patient was discharged to
the surgical ward 2 weeks after the final laparotomy with enteral feeding re-
established, but still needing regular subcutaneous insulin to control blood
glucose.

References

1 Isenmann R, Vanek E, Grimm H, Schlegel P, Friess T, Beger HG, Buchler M, Malfertheiner P, Friess H. Human pancreatitic tissue concentration of bactericidal antibiotics. *Gastroenterology* (1992) **103**:1902–1908.
2 Perderzoli P, Bassi C, Vesentini S and Campedelli A. A randomized multicenter clinical trial of antibiotic prophylaxis of septic complications in acute necrotizing pancreatitis with imipenem. *Surgery in Gynecology and Obstetrics* (1993) **176**: 480–483.
3 Foitzik T, Fernandez-del-Castillo C, Ferraro MJ, Mithofer K, Rattner DW and Warshaw AL. Pathogenesis and prevention of early pancreatic infection in experimental acute necrotizing pancreatitis. *Annals of Surgery* (1995) **222**: 179–185.
4 Luiten EJT, Hop WCJ, Lange JF and Bruining HA. Controlled clinical trial of selective decontamination for the treatment of severe acute pancreatitis. *Annals of Surgery* (1995) **222**: 57–65.
5 Steinberg W and Tenner S. Acute pancreatitis. *New England Journal of Medicine* (1994) **330**: 1198–1210.
6 Miller BJ, Henderson A, Strong RW, Fielding GA, Di Marco AM and O'Loughlin BS. Necrotizing pancreatitis: operating for life. *Journal of Surgery* (1994) **18**: 906–910.
7 Sarr MG, Nagorney DM, Mucha P, Farnell MB and Johnson CD. Acute necrotizing pancreatitis: management by planned, staged pancreatic necrosectomy/debridement and delayed primary wound closure over drains. *British Journal of Surgery* (1994) **78**: 576–581.
8 Pisters PW and Ranson JH. Nutritional support for acute pancreatitis. *Surgery, Gynecology and Obstetrics* (1992) **175**: 275–284.
9 D'Egidio A and Schein M. Surgical strategies in the treatment of pancreatic necrosis and infection. *British Journal of Surgery* (1991) **78**: 133–137.

10.4 Ileus Complicating Septic Shock
G. Dobb

History

A 63-year-old fork-lift truck driver had presented with a three-day history of feeling unwell with fever, anorexia and increasing left lower quadrant abdominal pain. On examination his temperature was 38.4°C [101.1°F], pulse 115/minute, arterial pressure 125/60 mmHg, the chest was clear and the abdomen tender in the left iliac fossa without overt peritonism. He was admitted for observation, permitted to eat and drink and started on amoxycillin 1 g 8 hourly and metronidazole 500 mg 12 hourly for a presumed diagnosis of diverticulitis.

Over the next 24 hours the patient remained febrile, tachycardic and anorexic. He complained of increasing abdominal pain, worst in the left lower quadrant. When seen by a duty resident in the evening he was prescribed pethidine 50–100 mg intramuscularly as required, and a differential diagnosis of diverticulitis or renal colic was recorded. When eventually seen by his admitting surgical team after the morning operating list, he had a temperature of 39.7°C [103.5°F], pulse 136/minute, blood pressure 85/4 mmHg, JVP was not visible at 45°, the peripheries were somewhat constricted and the chest remained clear. Abdominal examination revealed tenderness, guarding and peritonism maximal in the left lower quadrant. His investigations are shown in Table 10.4.1.

Further hemodynamic deterioration led to admission to the intensive care unit for resuscitation before surgery. Empiric antibiotic treatment of ticarcillin-clavulanic acid 3.1 g 8 hourly and gentamicin 240 mg daily was started. At laparotomy a diverticular abscess involving the sigmoid colon was found and it was commented that there was a moderate amount of turbid peritoneal fluid. Sigmoid colectomy with primary anastomosis and a defunctioning transverse colostomy was carried out. Despite further fluid resuscitation to a CVP of 12 mmHg and dopamine to 10 μg kg^{-1} min^{-1} the arterial pressure remained 100–105/50–55 mmHg and he returned to the ICU intubated and ventilated.

Over the next five days there was gradual hemodynamic improvement with weaning from inotropic support and extubation was possible, though arterial oxygenation remained marginal on high-flow oxygen (P_aO_2 62 mmHg [6.2 KPa],

Table 10.4.1. Investigations

Hemoglobin 16.2 g dL^{-1}, white blood cell count 30.2 × 10^9 L^{-1}.

Sodium 144 mmol L^{-1}, potassium 4.8 mmol L^{-1}, urea 9.4 mmol L^{-1} [BUN 56.4 mg L^{-1}], creatinine 94 μmol L^{-1} [1.2 mg dL^{-1}].

CSU: protein ++, 2 WBCs per high power field, no bacteria seen

Blood cultures subsequently grew *Escherichia coli* and *Enterococcus faecalis*

P_aCO_2 46 mmHg [6.1 kPa]). A chest radiograph demonstrated bilateral lower zone atelectasis. Attempts to establish nasogastric feeding between 24 and 72 hours after admission were unsuccessful. Nasogastric aspirates remained high and bowel sounds scant. Over days 5 and 6 the patient complained of increasing nausea and abdominal discomfort. He developed a fever varying between 37.6°C [99.7°F] and 38.9°C [102.2°F] accompanied by tachycardia and a decrease in arterial pressure from 150/90 to 110/70 mmHg. When reviewed by his surgical team he was noted to be mildly jaundiced, to have moderate dependent edema and abdominal distension. The colostomy was edematous, but pink. The surgical incision was noted to be red with a small amount of fluid oozing from the bottom end. There was generalized abdominal tenderness with mild rebound and bowel sounds were noted to be absent.

The investigations ordered are shown in Table 10.4.2.

When reviewed by the general surgeons there was considerable debate regarding the merits of proceeding to an immediate laparotomy. In general it was thought that the abdominal findings were consistent with an ileus, but it was difficult to exclude an intra-abdominal or pelvic collection as a cause for the fever and hemodynamic deterioration. There was also concern about the abdominal wound. It was finally decided that the staples would be removed from 5 cm of the abdominal wound, antibiotics would be continued, the biochemical abnormalities would be corrected and further regular surgical review would occur. The central venous catheter was replaced with a new triple-lumen catheter and the tip of the old catheter sent for culture.

Over the next six hours sodium chloride 300 mmol was given by the addition of 20% sodium chloride to 0.9% saline 500 mL. To this was also added potassium dihydrogen phosphate 60 mmol. Repeat investigations after this were:

Table 10.4.2. Investigations on day 6

Hemoglobin 98 g dL^{-1}, white blood cell count 28.2 × 10^9 L^{-1}, 97% neutrophils with pronounced left shift, platelets 57 × 10^9 L^{-1}.

Sodium 127 mmol L^{-1}, potassium 2.8 mmol L^{-1}, chloride 87 mmol L^{-1}, urea 4.2 mmol L^{-1} [BUN 25.2 mg dL^{-1}], creatinine 116 µmol L^{-1} [1.5 mg dL^{-1}].

Calcium 1.98 mmol L^{-1}, phosphate 0.4 mmol L^{-1}, albumin 23 g L^{-1}, bilirubin 48 µmol L^{-1} [2.8 mg dL^{-1}], alkaline phosphatase 148 U L^{-1}, AST 45 U L^{-1}.

Blood cultures: growth of *Pseudomonas aeruginosa* and coagulase-negative staphylococci at 48 hours

Wound swab: growth of *Pseudomonas aeruginosa* and large number of yeasts seen on direct microscopy

Urine culture: moderate proteinuria, but no growth

Abdominal radiographs: no free gas. Loss of psoas outline consistent with free intraperitoneal fluid. Moderately distended loops of bowel with multiple fluid levels

Abdominal CT scan: confirmed free intraperitoneal fluid. A possible small pelvic abscess was seen. Swelling around the surgical wound site was noted but artefact from skin staples prevented clear images

Sodium 134 mmol L^{-1}, potassium 3.4 mmol L^{-1}, chloride 94 mmol L^{-1}, urea 4.3 mmol L^{-1} [25.8 mg dL^{-1}], creatinine 110 μmol L^{-1} [1.43 mg dL^{-1}], calcium 2.01 mmol L^{-1}, phosphate 0.8 mmol L^{-1}, albumin 24 g L^{-1}

Turbid fluid continued to be lost from the abdominal wound. To simplify nursing care and prevent fluid running down the abdominal wall, a small corrugated drain was pushed into the wound and a plastic collection bag positioned over this. The patient remained febrile and his abdomen remained distended, silent and generally tender with rebound. Total parenteral nutrition was started because of the period of fasting and ongoing abdominal problems.

After further surgical review a repeat laparotomy was arranged. Within the abdominal wound were a number of loculi of turbid fluid. Microbiological cultures of these subsequently grew *Pseudomonas aeruginosa*. No localized collections were found in the abdomen, but the bowel was noted to be generally flaccid and distended with large amounts of intraluminal fluid and gas. A moderate amount of turbid peritoneal fluid was present (cultures: *Pseudomonas aeruginosa* and *Candida albicans* isolated). This was sucked out, the abdomen washed out with 5 L of 0.9% saline and drainage tubes placed in both subphrenic spaces and the pelvis. A careful search for leaks failed to reveal any bowel perforation and the anastomosis was intact. During surgery he remained reasonably hemodynamically stable, although there were periods of arterial pressure decreasing to 95–100 mmHg systolic initially, responding to infusion of colloid to a CVP of 15 mmHg and then to dopamine increasing to 12 μg kg^{-1} min^{-1}. At the end of surgery the patient returned to the ICU intubated and ventilated and on a dopamine infusion still at 12 μg kg^{-1} min^{-1}. His investigations showed:

Sodium 135 mmol L^{-1}, potassium 3.3 mmol L^{-1}, chloride 94 mmol L^{-1}, urea 5.6 mmol L^{-1} [BUN 33.6 mg dL^{-1}], creatinine 108 μmol L^{-1} [1.4 mg dL^{-1}], P_aO_2 84 mmHg [11.2 kPa] (F_IO_2 0.5), P_aCO_2 38 mmHg [5.1 kPa], base excess –6 mmol L^{-1}, lactate 4.2 mmol L^{-1}.

A plasma magnesium concentration subsequently measured on the sample was 0.41 mmol L^{-1}.

The subsequent management of the patient included the addition of intravenous amphotericin B to the other antimicrobials, total parenteral nutrition and magnesium supplements which restored the plasma magnesium concentration to 0.8 mmol L^{-1} 36 hours later. After 24 hours it was possible to gradually reduce the rate of dopamine infusion and his body temperature decreased to 37–37.5°C [98.6–99.5°F]. The abdomen remained somewhat distended and silent with large nasogastric aspirates. Three days after the last laparotomy a nasoenteric feeding tube was inserted under fluoroscopic control. There was some difficulty in getting the tube to pass through the pylorus.

Trap 1

Ileus is unlikely to improve until the biochemical abnormalities are corrected. Hyponatremia, hypokalemia, hypocalcemia and hypomagnesemia can all produce paralytic ileus.

Trap 2

Hypomagnesemia is a well-recognized cause of paralytic ileus. It is also associated with persistent hypokalemia which is difficult to correct until the hypomagnesemia is corrected. This is because of the role played by magnesium in Na^+/K^+ exchange.

Trap 3

Bowel sounds are a poor indicator of bowel activity in mechanically ventilated patients. It is also usual for small bowel activity to return before colonic with gastroparesis being the last to recover.

Tricks

This patient had a number of potential causes of ileus. This is common in postoperative patients. Causes of ileus are summarized in Table 10.4.3. The ileus that normally follows laparotomy and bowel surgery or handling usually resolves spontaneously within 2–3 days. The duration of surgery and the amount of bowel handling do not affect the duration of ileus.[1] Division of the abdominal muscles inhibits the bowel migratory motor complexes and these are totally abolished when the peritoneum is opened. High plasma catecholamine concentrations may play a part in causing ileus. A combination of α-adrenergic blockade and parasympathetic stimulation appears to stimulate resumption of colonic motor function. After cardiac surgery, splanchnic hypoperfusion with visceral ischemia has been implicated as the cause of ileus and other abdominal complications.[2] Splanchnic hypoperfusion may well be implicated as the cause of ileus in other settings. Drugs associated with ileus include opiates, phenothiazines and calcium

Table 10.4.3. Causes of ileus

Laparotomy with bowel surgery or handling	Drugs
Electrolyte abnormalities	Trauma
Peritonitis	Spinal cord damage
Intestinal ischemia	Retroperitoneal hemorrhage
General or spinal anesthesia	Hypothyroidism

antagonists. The opiates and phenothiazines are commonly used as analgesics and antiemetics in postoperative patients.

Prolonged ileus with stasis of bowel contents, absence of enteral nutrition, and use of antibiotics favors the overgrowth of potentially pathogenic bacteria in the bowel.[3] These same factors also favor bacterial translocation. The evidence for the process of bacterial translocation from the lumen of the bowel to the mesenteric lymph nodes and other sites is best established in experimental models, but there is also evidence that this process occurs in man, for example, during bowel obstruction[4] or after major abdominal trauma.[5] It is tempting to suggest that the site of origin of the *Pseudomonas aeruginosa* isolated from a variety of sites and the *Candida albicans* isolated from peritoneal fluid was the lumen of the bowel.

A prophylactic antimicrobial combination applied to the mouth and stomach, 'selective decontamination of the digestive tract' (SDD) – commonly using amphotericin, tobramycin and polymyxin in a paste applied to the mouth and as a mixture for injection through a nasogastric tube[6] – is designed to prevent proliferation of Gram-negative organisms and *Candida* spp. in the digestive tract while preserving the normal flora. In a large number of clinical trials this prophylactic antibiotic regimen has reduced the frequency of pneumonia and purulent tracheobronchitis in intensive care unit patients. Such a regimen would be expected to reduce the number of potentially pathogenic microorganisms that might translocate under suitable circumstances and so reduce the frequency of systemic sepsis, multiple organ failure and death. However, effects on these end-points have still to be conclusively shown in clinical trials. Meta-analyses of published clinical trials suggest there may be a 10–20% reduction in mortality in patients given SDD, but this has not reached conventional statistical significance.

Insertion of a nasoenteric feeding tube frequently permits enteral feeding when gastric aspirates remain large. It can be difficult to pass and erythromycin 200 mg given intravenously over 10 minutes may allow an enteric feeding tube to be passed through the gastric antrum, its tip eventually passing to the proximal jejunum. Erythromycin has potent prokinetic effects and can be of great assistance in the placing of enteric feeding tubes.[7]

Follow-up

Enteral feeding was established, followed within 24 hours by passage of flatus. Parenteral feeding was stopped, and after a short period of reducing SIMV and pressure support it was possible to extubate the patient. Recovery was complicated by a continuing gastroparesis and a period of diarrhea. No cause was found for the diarrhea – *Clostridium difficile* was not isolated and no toxin was detected—and the gastroparesis eventually (8 days after the final laparotomy) recovered a day after starting cisapride 10 mg 6 hourly through the nasogastric tube. He was discharged back to the surgical ward at this time and subsequently made an uneventful recovery.

References

1 Condon RE, Cowles VE, Schulte WJ, Frantzides CT, Mahoney JL and Sarna SK. Resolution of postoperative ileus in humans. *Annals of Surgery* (1986) **203**: 574–581.
2 Christenson JT, Schmuziger M, Maurice J, Simonet F and Velebit V. Postoperative visceral hypotension: the common cause of gastrointestinal complications after cardiac surgery. *Thoracic and Cardiovascular Surgery* (1994) **42**: 152–157.
3 Marshall JC, Christou NV and Meakins JL. The gastrointestinal tract. The 'undrained abscess' of multiple organ failure. *Annals of Surgery* (1993) **218**: 111–119.
4 Deitch EA, Bridges WM, Ma JW, Ma L, Berg RD and Specian RD. Obstructed intestine as a reservoir for systemic infection. *American Journal of Surgery* (1990) **159**: 394–401.
5 Reed LL, Martin M, Manglano R, Newson B, Kocka F and Barrett J. Bacterial translocation following abdominal trauma in humans. *Circulation and Shock* (1994) **42**: 1–6.
6 Donnelly JP. Selective decontamination of the digestive tract and its role in antimicrobial prophylaxis. *Journal of Antimicrobical Chemotherapy* (1993) **31**: 813–829.
7 Stern MA and Wolf DC. Erythromycin as a prokinetic agent: a prospective randomised, controlled study of efficacy in nasoenteric tube placement. *American Journal of Gastroenterology* (1994) **89**: 2011–2013.

10.5 Hollow Viscus Perforation and Multiple Abdominal Abscesses
G. Dobb and N. Watkins

History

A 69-year-old man was referred to the intensive care unit after a laparotomy for an acute abdomen. Other medical problems were type II diabetes, hypertension and cigarette-induced lung disease with some degree of chronic airflow limitation. For one week before admission he had complained of intermittent colicky lower abdominal pain and fever. There had been no rectal bleeding, but he had had intermittent constipation for one month. On the day before admission, his family physician had noted left lower quadrant tenderness without peritonism, and a temperature of 37.9°C [100.2°F]. He suspected acute diverticulitis and prescribed an oral cephalosporin.

That night the patient deteriorated markedly with sudden onset of abdominal pain associated with distension and rigidity. He was taken by ambulance to the emergency department where he was noted to be pale, sweaty and was complaining of severe abdominal pain. His pulse rate was 150/minute, systolic pressure 85 mmHg, respiration rate 46/minute and temperature 35.8°C [96.4°F]. Abdominal examination revealed a distended tense abdomen with diffuse guarding and rigidity, particularly prominent in the lower abdomen. Rectal examination demonstrated diffuse tenderness. An urgent surgical opinion confirmed the diagnosis of peritonitis. At laparotomy an acute peritonitis, extensive diverticular disease, a perforated descending colon and excessive fecal contamination of the peritoneum was found. Despite fluid resuscitation, which included 1 liter colloid, 1 liter crystalloid and 2 units of packed red cells, he was hemodynamically unstable during surgery, and an adrenaline [epinephrine] infusion was started.

After resection of the perforated large bowel, peritoneal lavage and fashioning of a defunctioning colostomy, the abdomen was closed and he was transferred to the ICU. Intravenous ticarcillin/clavulanate 3.1 g 8 hourly and tobramycin 320 mg daily were given.

Assessment in the ICU revealed a ventilated man with cold peripheries, pulse 140/minute, arterial pressure 100/50 mmHg, temperature of 34.9°C [94.8°F] and an S_aO_2 of 96% on an F_IO_2 of 0.75. The central venous pressure was 8 mmHg. Intravenous adrenaline was being infused at $15 \, \mu g \, min^{-1}$. Cardiovascular and respiratory examinations were otherwise non-contributory. The abdomen was distended and tense with absent bowel sounds. When a urinary catheter was inserted there was only 40 mL of urine. A pulmonary artery catheter was inserted, and the initial findings are summarized in Table 10.5.1 and the investigations in Table 10.5.2.

At the initial assessment the pulmonary artery wedge pressure and cardiac

Table 10.5.1. Initial findings

Pulse 150/minute	Cardiac index $2.5\,\mathrm{L\,min^{-1}\,m^{-2}}$
Central venous pressure $8\,\mathrm{mmHg}$	
PA $19\,\mathrm{mmHg}$	RVSWI $3\,\mathrm{g\,m^{-1}\,m^{-2}}$
PAOP $7\,\mathrm{mmHg}$	LVSWI $14\,\mathrm{g\,m^{-1}\,m^{-2}}$
Blood pressure $67\,\mathrm{mmHg}$	PVRI $391\,\mathrm{dyn\text{-}sec\,cm^{-5}\,m^{-2}}$
Cardiac output $5.0\,\mathrm{L/minute}$	SVRI $1924\,\mathrm{dyn\text{-}sec\,cm^{-5}\,m^{-2}}$

Table 10.5.2. Investigations immediately after surgery

pH 7.11 [H^+ $82\,\mathrm{nmol\,L^{-1}}$], P_aCO_2 $35\,\mathrm{mmHg}$ [$4.7\,\mathrm{kPa}$], P_aO_2 $78\,\mathrm{mmHg}$ [$10.4\,\mathrm{kPa}$] (F_IO_2 0.75), base excess $-9\,\mathrm{mmol\,L^{-1}}$, S_aO_2 95%

Plasma lactate $7\,\mathrm{mmol\,L^{-1}}$

Hemoglobin $8\,\mathrm{g\,dL^{-1}}$, white blood cell count $1.2\times10^9\,\mathrm{L^{-1}}$, platelets $98\times10^9\,\mathrm{L^{-1}}$

INR 1.9, PT 15s, APTT 31s, fibrinogen $2.1\,\mathrm{g\,L^{-1}}$, FDPs negative

Sodium $145\,\mathrm{mmol\,L^{-1}}$, potassium $5.1\,\mathrm{mmol\,L^{-1}}$, bicarbonate $15\,\mathrm{mmol\,L^{-1}}$, urea $13\,\mathrm{mmol\,L^{-1}}$ [BUN $78\,\mathrm{mg\,dL^{-1}}$], creatinine $254\,\mathrm{\mu mol\,L^{-1}}$ [$3.3\,\mathrm{mg\,dL^{-1}}$]

Glucose $8\,\mathrm{mmol\,L^{-1}}$ [$144\,\mathrm{mg\,dL^{-1}}$]

Albumin $31\,\mathrm{g\,L^{-1}}$, calcium $2.2\,\mathrm{mmol\,L^{-1}}$, AST $68\,\mathrm{U\,L^{-1}}$, alkaline phosphatase $85\,\mathrm{U\,L^{-1}}$, bilirubin $18\,\mathrm{\mu mol\,L^{-1}}$ [$1.1\,\mathrm{mg\,dL^{-1}}$]

Chest radiograph: intubated trachea, CVC and PA catheters in place. Diffuse interstitial infiltrate

Blood cultures: negative

index were low indicating inadequate volume replacement in a patient with sepsis, an inappropriately low cardiac index given the degree of sepsis and a degree of acute lung injury and respiratory failure. Further fluid resuscitation in the form of colloid, packed red cells and fresh frozen plasma was given, increasing central filling pressures and cardiac index. However, he remained dependent on inotropic drugs and, despite fluid resuscitation, epinephrine in increasing doses was required to maintain systemic blood pressure. The severity of the respiratory failure remained static, with some progression of the bilateral infiltrates on chest radiography, and F_IO_2 requirements between 0.6 and 0.8 with the addition of $10\,\mathrm{cmH_2O}$ of PEEP.

Persistent clinical and laboratory markers of sepsis syndrome were evident by the third day after laparotomy. By this time, epinephrine requirements had increased markedly, and norepinephrine [noradrenaline] was added to the inotropic therapy in order to maintain systolic blood pressure. On the fourth day after the first laparotomy, he returned to the operating room where a repeat laparotomy showed diffuse inflammatory change within the peritoneal cavity and small bowel serosa with an early abscess in the splenic bed which was drained.

Intravenous antibiotics were changed to imipenem 500 mg 8 hourly and tobramycin.

Renal failure developed in the five days after admission, and continuous venovenous hemodiafiltration was started to facilitate fluid management and the administration of intravenous nutrition. Repeat laparotomy and a laparostomy were performed. No localized collection was identified this time, but operative swabs submitted for culture demonstrated a growth of *Pseudomonas aeruginosa, Enterobacter cloacae, Enterococcus faecium* and *Candida albicans.* Intravenous amphotericin was added to the antibiotic treatment. Some improvement in cardiovascular function followed, but further deterioration occurred on day 8.

At day 12, sepsis syndrome and inotrope dependence persisted, and no extra-abdominal source of infection could be identified. An abdominal CT scan was performed, demonstrating several small pelvic abscesses and a subcutaneous collection adjacent to the colostomy. The collections were drained surgically, and operative specimens demonstrated a persistent growth of *Enterococcus faecium* and *Candida albicans,* which was also recovered from blood cultures the following day.

Traps

1. When the patient returned from the operating theater he showed all the signs of hypovolemic shock. To maintain his blood pressure he had been started on adrenaline.
2. In the first 72 h after operation he developed signs of sepsis that did not respond to treatment.
3. After his laparotomy on day 4 his antibiotic regimen was changed to imipenem.
4. Beware of fungal infection. In patients with severe bacterial peritonitis, superinfection with *Candida albicans* is a potential problem.
5. Persistent sepsis needs aggressive investigation.

Tricks

1. Hypovolemia is a common feature of such patients on admission to the ICU after laparotomy. This may present as an inappropriately low cardiac output and systemic oxygen delivery with reduced cardiac filling pressures. If oxygenation can be adequately maintained with ventilatory support, aggressive fluid resuscitation is indicated with full hemodynamic monitoring in an effort to improve organ perfusion and systemic oxygenation.
2. In the first 72 h after a laparotomy for fecal soiling of the peritoneum, sepsis syndrome and septic shock are more likely to be due to the initial infectious episode than to recurrent, localized abdominal sepsis. During this period, attention should be given to adequate fluid resuscitation, optimum cardiovascular support, appropriate antibiotic treatment and early intravenous nutrition. However, clinical deterioration should precipitate repeat laparotomy.

3. The antibiotic treatment should cover enterococci. The second- and third-generation cephalosporins are not effective against these organisms. Enterococci with multiple antibiotic resistance are an emerging problem. *Enterococcus faecium* is resistant to imipenem. It tends to emerge as a pathogen under circumstances such as those described here. Other imipenem-resistant organisms include *Xanthomonas* spp. and coagulase-negative staphylococci. These organisms and fungi should be specifically targeted when signs of sepsis occur or persist in patients treated with imipenem.

4. If *Candida albicans* infection is suspected, early and prompt antifungal therapy is indicated. Isolation of *Candida* spp. from operative swabs as a minimum highlights the need for repeated microbiological surveillance of the abdominal cavity (swabs from the laparotomy or abdominal drains) and a high index of suspicion for systemic infection rather than colonization.

5. Persistent sepsis syndrome requires a systematic approach. A prompt and thorough search for extra-abdominal sources of infection should be undertaken, with regular blood cultures to detect any blood-borne infection. If the conclusion is that intra-abdominal sepsis is present, the differential diagnosis should include:

   (a)   localized bacterial infection or abscess;
   (b)   infection with a resistant organism, such as *Candida*;
   (c)   an intra-abdominal vascular event such as infarction of the small bowel; and
   (d)   a surgical complication, e.g. an anastomotic leak.

This patient demonstrated many of the difficulties in the management of severe abdominal sepsis.[1] Delays in presentation with severe peritonitis are associated with an increased incidence of multiple organ failure and death, as well as operative complications. Prompt, adequate resuscitation followed by definitive surgical management are essential if outcome is to be improved. Fecal peritonitis carries a high mortality despite aggressive surgical and medical therapy. In cases such as this, multiple abdominal abscesses and ongoing sepsis syndrome with multiple organ dysfunction are common sequelae.

The place of planned relaparotomy in the management of intraperitoneal infection (a 'second look') remains controversial. In a recent non-randomized comparison of relaparotomy with laparotomy on demand,[2] complications were more frequent in those patients managed with planned relaparotomy but the trend to increased mortality – 21% as against 13% – did not reach statistical significance. Ideally, randomized prospective studies are needed but until then this study appears to provide the best available evidence.

Important points in the management of severe bacterial peritonitis with multiple abdominal abscesses are:

1. Attention to resuscitation, including airway management, adequate oxygenation, optimum fluid replacement and appropriate inotropic support.
2. Prompt, definitive surgical intervention.

3. Appropriate antibiotic therapy.
4. Re-exploration of the abdomen when indicated by clinical findings and the results of abdominal imaging procedures.

Appropriate antibiotics are a key component of the management of severe peritonitis.[3,4] Proximal viscus perforations characteristically produce a sterile peritonitis, although patients taking long-term H_2-receptor antagonists may have Gram-negative or fungal colonization of the stomach. In contrast, massive bacterial contamination occurs in distal perforations. Distal small bowel or colonic contents contain 10^{12} organisms per gram, with an anaerobe to aerobe ratio of $100:1$. It is therefore essential that the initial empirical treatment provides broad cover against aerobic Gram-negative bacteria and activity against anaerobes. In contrast to the cultures obtained from bowel contents, peritoneal cultures from patients with peritonitis associated with a perforated hollow viscus demonstrate a predominance of facultative anaerobes including *Escherichia coli*, non-enterococcal streptococci, *Enterobacter* spp. and *Candida albicans*.

Common antibiotic regimens include an aminoglycoside with an anti-anaerobic agent (e.g. metronidazole, clindamycin), a second- or third-generation cephalosporin with an anti-anaerobic agent, carbapenems, or β-lactam/β-lactamase inhibitor combinations.[3] In recent clinical trials ciprofloxacin/metronidazole achieved similar results to imipenem/cilastatin in achieving a 'clinical cure'.[5,6] This later study was randomized, but open. Given the effect of other factors such as nutritional status and appropriate surgery on clinical outcome, this finding should be treated with caution.

Imaging of the abdomen has an important role in the postoperative management of peritonitis associated with a perforated viscus.[7] As a general principle, it should be remembered that imaging modalities are usually unable to distinguish between sterile fluid collections and infected collections. This is particularly true of CT scanning within the first seven days after laparotomy. In addition, the risks of transporting critically ill patients to the radiology department for imaging procedures should be weighed against the potential diagnostic benefits. Portable abdominal ultrasound performed by an experienced radiologist may be a practical alternative.

The choice of imaging procedure is determined by the question being asked, the fitness of the patient to be moved to the radiology department, and available expertise. Although useful in diagnosing pseudo-obstruction, ileus and occasionally ischemic bowel, plain abdominal radiography is unlikely to be helpful in the diagnosis of intra-abdominal abscesses following hollow viscus perforation. Ultrasound has the advantage of being rapid, inexpensive and portable. Major technical limitations occur in patients who have developed a postoperative ileus, in the obese, and in those with multiple stomas or an open abdomen. In most cases, optimal views can be obtained in the subphrenic and pelvic spaces. In general, ultrasonography has a high sensitivity when adequate images are obtained for abdominal abscesses, but lower specificity.[8,9]

Faster CT scanners have increased its popularity in the diagnosis of intra-abdominal abscesses. CT scanning is more effective in displaying and localizing abnormalities and better at guiding percutaneous drainage than ultrasound.[10] However, false negative and positive rates are in the order of at least 10% in postoperative patients. In one review, CT scans did not demonstrate abscesses before the eighth postoperative day, only 55% of examinations added to the pre-operative diagnosis and more than 70% were of no benefit to the patient.[10] Clinical judgement should be taken into account when interpreting an equivocal or negative CT scan. Areas of the abdomen which are well demonstrated with CT scanning include the subphrenic and subhepatic spaces, the paracolic gutters and the pelvis.

With both ultrasonography and CT scanning the most difficult abscesses to localize are the multiple small abscesses that may complicate widespread intra-abdominal fecal contamination. Commonly, these occur between loops of bowel and in intermesenteric folds. Adhesions can make repeat laparotomy technically demanding. Laparostomy with daily or second daily re-exploration and lavage has been advocated as a means of minimizing early adhesions and reducing abscess formation,[11] but there is no conclusive evidence that this results in better outcomes than a more conventional approach. The reported survival has been 33–93%, with most case series being in the range of 60–75%.

When the abscesses localized by ultrasonograph CT scan are single or few, percutaneous drainage provides an alternative to repeat laparotomy. While Schecter and colleagues[12] found that CT scan-guided percutaneous drainage was sufficient in 80% of patients with intra-abdominal abscesses and ultrasound-guided drainage has been successful in nearly 90%,[13] not all have achieved such good results. For example, McLean and others[14] found that only 33% of a small series of postoperative intra-abdominal abscesses could be managed with percutaneous drainage alone. They also concluded that operative management was preferable if there was any possibility of anastomotic dehiscence. In critically ill patients needing intensive care considerable clinical judgement is needed to balance the benefits of a less invasive approach against the hazards of delayed definitive treatment in patients with diminished physiological reserves. This is usually best achieved by close consultation between the intensivists, surgeons and radiologists involved.

Follow-up

Despite maximum supportive therapy, the patient died of intractable septic shock and cardiovascular failure on day 13.

References

1 Nathens AB and Rotstein OD. Therapeutic options in peritonitis. *Surgical Clinics of North America* (1994) **74**: 677–692.

2 Hau T, Ohmann C, Wolmershauser A, Wacha H and Yang Q for the Peritonitis Study Group of the Surgical Infection Society – Europe. Planned relaparotomy vs

relaparotomy on demand in the treatment of intra-abdominal infection. *Archives of Surgery* (1995) **130**: 1193–1197.

3 Bohnen JMA, Solomkin JS and Dellinger EP. Guidelines for clinical care: anti-infective agents for intra-abdominal infection. A Surgical Infection Society policy statement. *Archives of Surgery* (1992) **127**: 83–94.

4 Mosdell DM, Morris DM, Voltura A, *et al.* Antibiotic treatment for surgical peritonitis. *Annals of Surgery* (1991) **214**: 543–556.

5 Eklund AE and Nord CE. A randomized multicenter trial of piperacillin/tazobactam versus imipenem/cilastatin in the treatment of severe intra-abdominal infections. Swedish Study Group. *Journal of Antimicrobial Chemotherapy* (1993) **31** (Suppl A): 79–85.

6 Solomkin JS, Reinhart HH, Dellinger EP, *et al.* and the Intra-abdominal Infection Study Group. Results of a randomized trial comparing sequential intravenous/oral treatment with ciprofloxacin plus metronidazole to imipenem/cilastatin for intra-abdominal infections. *Annals of Surgery* (1996) **223**: 303–315.

7 Fry DE. Noninvasive imaging tests in the diagnosis and treatment of intra-abdominal abscesses in the post-operative patient. *Surgical Clinics of North America* (1994) **74**: 693–709.

8 Dewbury KC and Joseph AE. The role of ultrasound scanning. *Scandinavian Journal of Gastroenterology* (1994) **203** (Suppl): 5–10.

9 Gazelle GS and Mueller PR. Abdominal abscesses. Imaging and intervention. *Radiology Clinics of North America* (1994) **32**: 913–932.

10 Zingas AP. Computed tomography of the abdomen in the critically ill. *Critical Care Clinics* (1994) **10**: 321–339.

11 Schein M, Saadia R and Decker GGA. The open management of the septic abdomen. *Surgery Gynecology and Obstetrics* (1986) **1634**: 587–592.

12 Schecter S, Eisenstat TE, Oliver GC, Rubin RJ and Salvati EP. Computerized tomographic scan-guided drainage of intra-abdominal abscesses. Preoperative and postoperative modalities in colon and rectal surgery. *Colon Rectum* (1994) **37**: 984–988.

13 Goletti O, Lippolia PV, ChiaGhiselli G, *et al.* Percutaneous ultrasound guided drainage of intra-abdominal abscesses. *British Journal of Surgery* (1993) **80**: 336–339.

14 McLean TR, Simmons K and Svensson LG. Management of post-operative intra-abdominal abcesses by routine percutaneous drainage. *Surgery Gynecology and Obstetrics* (1993) **176**: 167–171.

11 Obstetric Critical Care

11.1 Pre-Eclampsia
D.G. Greig and Maire P. Shelly

History

A 26-year-old woman developed ankle edema during the 21st week of her first pregnancy. Within 5 weeks, her diastolic blood pressure was 100 mmHg and she had mild proteinuria. At 26 weeks' gestation she was admitted to another hospital with increasing peripheral edema and hypertension. Her diastolic blood pressure increased to 110 mmHg and was treated with labetolol. During her hospitalization, she received steroids to hasten fetal maturity. However, at 30 weeks' gestation she suddenly felt anxious, restless and unwell. On examination, she was hyperreflexic and her blood pressure varied between 150/105 and 180/110 mmHg. A good urine output was maintained but her respiratory rate increased to 31 minute and her oxygen saturation decreased to 90%. Intravenous hydrallazine controlled her blood pressure and phenytoin was given prophylactically in view of the hyperreflexia.

Fetal distress necessitated an urgent Cesarean section under general anesthesia. Perioperatively, her oxygen saturation varied between 93% and 95% with an F_IO_2 of 1.0. She was oliguric and received 2 L cystalloid. A 2.8 kg baby boy was delivered and taken to the special care baby unit. At the end of the procedure, she was allowed to wake and her trachea was extubated. Her blood pressure was 180/110 mmHg with an oxygen saturation of 90% on an F_IO_2 of 1.0, and she was restless. Because of this, her trachea was reintubated, mechanical ventilation was restarted and she was transferred to the intensive care unit.

On admission to the ICU, she was restless and poorly sedated. She responded purposefully to pain but not to voice; her pupils were equal in size and reactive to light. She was sedated with propofol and alfentanil to ensure comfort, to reduce the risk of hypertension and to allow effective ventilation. Once sedated, her heart rate was 89/minute, mean arterial blood pressure was 95 mmHg and temperature 36.3°C [97.3°F]. Examination revealed fine basal crackles on both sides of the chest. A chest radiograph (Figure 11.1.1) demonstrated pulmonary edema.

A pulmonary artery catheter was inserted and results obtained as shown in Table 11.1.1. Initial blood gases with F_IO_2 of 1.0 showed H^+ 38 nmol L^{-1} [pH 7.42], P_aO_2 26.0 kPa [195 mmHg], P_aCO_2 4.9 kPa [36.8 mmHg], base excess of 0.1 mmol L^{-1}. Biochemistry results and coagulation screen were within normal limits; her hemoglobin concentration (Hb) was 10.7 g dL^{-1} and her white blood cell count was 21.5 × $10^9 L^{-1}$.

Her pulmonary edema was treated with controlled ventilation with 7.5 cmH$_2$O of PEEP. A bolus of frusemide [furosemide] 20 mg was given intravenously and a continuous infusion of dopamine started at a rate of 2.5 µg kg^{-1}

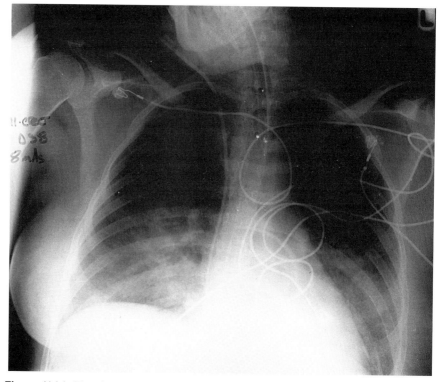

Figure 11.1.1. The chest radiograph of the patient with pre-eclampsia after admission to ICU. There are electrocardiograph wires, a pulmonary artery catheter, an endotracheal tube and a nasogastric tube. Patchy shadowing in both lung fields suggests pulmonary edema.

Table 11.1.1. Hemodynamic variables in the patient at admission

Heart rate	91/minute
Mean arterial blood pressure	97 mmHg
Pulmonary artery occlusion pressure	18 mmHg
MPAP	27 mmHg
Cardiac index	$4.4\,L\,min^{-1}\,m^{-2}$
Systemic vascular resistance index	$795\,dyn\text{-}sec\,cm^{-5}$
Blood lactate	$0.8\,mmol\,L^{-1}$

min^{-1}. This gave a 7-hour diuresis of 2400 mL. Over this period, her MAP increased to 110 mmHg with a heart rate of 115/minute, PAOP 16 mmHg, MPAP 28 mmHg, cardiac index $6.8\,L\,min^{-1}\,m^{-2}$, SVR 547 $dyn\text{-}sec\,cm^{-5}$. Over the same period her $F_{I}O_2$ was reduced to 0.4 and PEEP to $2.5\,cmH_2O$ with good arterial oxygenation.

The next day, the dopamine infusion and her sedation were stopped. Her trachea was extubated uneventfully. The only problem at this stage was hypertension, with an arterial pressure of 170/105 mmHg. This was treated first with intravenous bolus doses of esmolol 20 mg and hydrallazine 10 mg and subsequently with continuous intravenous infusions of both agents. This regimen controlled her arterial pressure at about 160/85 mmHg.

Trap 1

This patient had an early presentation of her pre-eclampsia which then progressed over 9 weeks. An early presentation carries a poor fetal prognosis so she was closely monitored. The use of steroids to hasten fetal lung maturity has been shown to reduce fetal mortality and morbidity without maternal complications.

The progression of pre-eclampsia can only be halted by delivery of the placenta but the timing of delivery has to be a decision based on individual maternal and fetal risk factors. Control of this patient's blood pressure was important to reduce the risk of cerebral hemorrhage and to extend the pregnancy. However, when she developed evidence of worsening hypertension, cerebral irritation and hyperreflexia and impaired gas exchange, her delivery was precipitated. In view of her preoperative evidence of pre-eclampsia and intraoperative hypoxemia, postoperative tracheal extubation was risky. The risks included regurgitation and aspiration of gastric contents because of altered conscious level, persistent hypoxemia and recurrent hypertension.

Trick 1

A longer period of gradual awakening would have allowed the patient's blood pressure and oxygen saturation to be monitored as she woke. Her trachea could have been safely extubated if these parameters had remained within acceptable limits and she regained a normal conscious level. In fact she became irritable, hypertensive and her hypoxemia worsened. Under these circumstances it would have been safer to resedate her without tracheal extubation and the risks of regurgitation and aspiration.

Trap 2

Pulmonary edema may occur in pre-eclampsia due to fluid overload into the non-compliant circulation, reabsorption of edema fluid into the circulation, or renal failure. This patient's renal function was normal. Therefore, there was a choice: to remove fluid from the circulation, or to expand the circulation which should be regaining compliance after placental delivery.

Trick 2

In fact both courses of action were followed. Fluid was removed by diuretic treatment. The relatively small dose of frusemide needed to produce a significant diuresis is an indication of the increased extracellular water in this patient. It also points to a degree of spontaneous recovery after removal of the placenta. The sedative used to maintain comfort during ventilation was propofol. This has vasodilator properties and decreases afterload, as shown by the decrease in SVR. A potential problem with this approach is the risk of hypovolemia and hypoperfusion. Monitoring the circulation with a pulmonary artery catheter allowed additional fluid to be given if necessary to maintain perfusion.

Pre-eclampsia is a common problem and a major cause of maternal mortality. The diagnosis may be difficult since the classic combination of hypertension, proteinuria and peripheral edema is frequently absent. Pre-eclampsia should be suspected in any woman with any of those signs but differs from simple pregnancy-induced hypertension in terms of treatment and outcome. The rate of progression of pre-eclampsia is variable but it may lead to: eclampsia, cerebral hemorrhage, pulmonary edema, renal failure, fetal death, HELLP syndrome (hemolysis, elevated liver enzymes and low platelets) and disseminated intravascular coagulopathy (DIC).

The pathology of pre-eclampsia is complex and poorly understood. One proposed sequence is that implantation of the placenta is abnormal in some way, probably caused by immunological factors. This results in reduced placental perfusion and release of blood-borne substances into the maternal systemic circulation. These substances are thought to act on the vascular endothelium, increasing sensitivity to normally circulating vasopressors and causing profound vasospasm and reduced organ perfusion. In addition, altered endothelial permeability leads to edema and the loss of endothelial anticoagulant activity activates the coagulation cascade with the formation of microthrombi. These changes may reduce placental perfusion further and lead to a spiraling progression of disease.

Preoperatively, the patient was anxious and hyperreflexic; postoperatively she remained restless. Phenytoin was started preoperatively as prophylaxis against convulsions. This was continued postoperatively. Propofol was used as a sedative agent during ventilation and this also controlled her irritability. Propofol is relatively contraindicated in patients at risk of convulsions since it is associated with fits. There is evidence that propofol reduces central inhibitory output and allows unopposed excitatory impulses. However, this may be a peripheral phenomenon, since electroencephalograph recordings demonstrate no abnormal patterns during these fits. We used propofol for these reasons and for its hemodynamic advantages.

An alternative agent in the management of cerebral irritability is magnesium sulfate. This is widely used in the USA but only rarely in the UK. Since magnesium is not an anticonvulsant, the rationale for its use has been unclear. The pathology of cerebral irritability is presumed to be ischemia. If this is the case, magnesium sulfate is a logical treatment since it reverses cerebral vasospasm. The effect of magnesium can be difficult to monitor since it does not correlate with plasma levels.

While the patient was sedated and ventilated, her hypertension was controlled by propofol infusion. When she was woken and extubated, an alternative was necesssary. The choice was between a beta-adrenergic blocking agent, hydrallazine and nifedipine. We used esmolol, a beta blocker with a half-life of 20 minutes in combination with hydrallazine. Vasodilator hypotensive agents can produce a reflex tachycardia, particularly in the young, which may preserve the hypertension. The combination of vasodilator and beta blocker reduces this problem. Both agents can be given by continuous intravenous infusion and titrated separately to control blood pressure. Both agents were withdrawn gradually as her hypertension resolved. The duration of pre-eclamptic hypertension following delivery is variable and short-acting agents may be useful in case it resolves rapidly.

Follow-up

Over the next 12 hours the patient required an increasing amount of hydrallazine to control her arterial pressure. The esmolol maintained her heart rate at around 90/minute. After this her arterial pressure stabilized and the esmolol and subsequently the hydrallazine were withdrawn over 48 hours. Four days after admission, she was discharged to the ward with an arterial pressure of 145/85 mmHg on no treatment. Her son required a week of special care and was eventually discharged home at three weeks of age.

Bibliography

1 Roberts JM and Redman CWG. Pre-eclampsia: more than pregnancy-induced hypertension. *Lancet* (1993) **341**: 1147–1451.
2 Redman CWG and Roberts JM. Management of pre-eclampsia. *Lancet* (1993) **341**: 1451–1454.
3 Sibai BM. Hypertension in pregnancy. *Obstetric and Gynecology Clinics of North America* (1992) **19**: 615–632.

11.2   Amniotic Fluid Embolus

D.G. Greig and Maire P. Shelly

History

A 29-year-old woman was admitted to hospital at 32 weeks' gestation with a small vaginal bleed. Ultrasound scan demonstrated a placenta praevia impinging on, but not covering, the cervical canal. Three weeks later she had a significant vaginal bleed and underwent emergency Cesarian section under general anesthesia. During opening of the uterus, the arterial pressure decreased to 78/56 mmHg with a tachycardia of 140 beats/minute and her oxygen saturation decreased to 88%. She was given gelofusine 1.5 L which increased her systolic blood pressure to 85–90 mmHg; her heart rate was 125/minute. An arterial blood sample taken on an F_IO_2 of 1.0 showed a H^+ 64 nmol L^{-1} [pH of 7.2], $P_{a}O_2$ 14.3 kPa [107 mmHg], $P_{a}CO_2$ 7.1 kPa [53 mmHg], base excess -4.2 mmol L^{-1}. A healthy baby girl was delivered, hemostasis was achieved with some difficulty and surgery was completed. At the end of the procedure the patient was transferred to the intensive care unit (ICU).

On admission to the ICU, the patient was sedated and ventilated with an F_IO_2 of 1.0. Her peak airway pressure was 42 cmH$_2$O on synchronized intermittent mandatory ventilation. Arterial blood gas analysis was unchanged. Examination of the chest showed a mild expiratory wheeze and a chest radiograph demonstrated increased perihilar shadowing. The patient's heart rate was 115/minute and her arterial pressure was 92/51 mmHg. Her uterus was well contracted and the urine output for the first hour was 15 mL. Biochemical analysis of her blood was normal, her hemoglobin was 10.2 g dL^{-1}, white blood cell count 18.3 $\times$ 10^9 L^{-1}, platelet count 52 $\times$ 10^9 L^{-1}, prothrombin time (PT) 28 s, activated partial thromboplastin time (APTT) 48 s, fibrinogen 0.9 g L^{-1} and D-dimer screen for fibrinogen degradation products 6 mg L^{-1}. Her electrocardiogram was normal and the only abnormality on echocardiography was basal hypokinesia.

Because of her coagulopathy, 4 units of fresh frozen plasma and 6 units of platelets were given before insertion of monitoring lines. She also received 10 mg of vitamin K, and calcium to maintain an ionized calcium above the lower limit of normal. Her hemodynamic measurements were: HR 122/minute, MAP 63 mmHg, MPAP 32 mmHg, PAOP 24 mmHg, CI 3.6 L min^{-1} m^{-2}, SVR 1150 dyn-sec cm^{-5} and PVR 222 dyn-sec cm^{-5}; her lactate was at the upper end of the normal range. Pulmonary arterial blood was also sampled for cytological examination but analysis later showed no fetal material.

A dopamine infusion was started at 2 μg kg^{-1} min^{-1} and a dobutamine infusion at 4 μg kg^{-1} min^{-1}. These improved her MAP to 78 mmHg and her CI to 4.1 L min^{-1} m^{-2}. Her PAOP decreased to 20 mmHg, her MPAP to 27 mmHg and her lactate remained normal. She received 20 mg of frusemide [furosemide] and her urine output increased to 40 mL h^{-1}. Her ventilatory support was changed to pressure-controlled ventilation with a pressure of 32 cmH$_2$O, 5 cmH$_2$O PEEP, an F_IO$_2$ of 1.0 and an inspiratory : expiratory (I : E) ratio of 2 : 1. On this support, her respiratory status stabilized with a pH of 51nmol L^{-1} [7.29], P_aO$_2$ 13.4 kPa [101 mm Hg], P_aCO$_2$ 6.5 kPa [49 mm Hg] and base excess −3.3 mmol L^{-1}.

The next morning she was hemodynamically stable on dopamine and dobutamine with MAP 85 mmHg, MPAP 25 mmHg, PAOP 18 mmHg, CI 5.6 L min^{-1}, SVR 706 dyn-sec cm^{-5}, PVR 180 dyn-sec cm^{-5} and normal lactate. Her urine output was maintained at approximately 50 mL h^{-1}. Her coagulopathy remained a problem. Blood was oozing from the sites of line insertion and there was some vaginal bleeding. Her Hb had decreased to 8.8 g dL^{-1}, platelets were 44 × 10^9 L^{-1}, PT and APTT still increased at 25 and 45 s, fibrinogen 0.6 g L^{-1} and D-dimer 8 mg L^{-1}. She received 6 units of FFP and 4 units of platelets as well as 10 mg of vitamin K intravenously. Vaginal examination revealed no abnormality and no intrauterine collection was seen on ultrasound scan. Her respiratory condition and ventilatory support remained unchanged.

Over the next 24 hours the patient remained hemodynamically stable. Dobutamine was reduced to 2 µg kg^{-1} h^{-1} which maintained her CI at around 5 L min^{-1} m^{-2}, MAP between 85 and 90 mmHg and urine output 50–100 mL h^{-1}. Four units of FFP were given on two occasions to control vaginal bleeding. She received 2 units of blood and her Hb increased to 10.3 g dL^{-1}. Her respiratory function remained unchanged as did her ventilatory support.

Trap

This patient had disseminated intravascular coagulopathy, characterized by three features: thrombocytopenia, prolonged PT and APTT, and increased fibrinogen degradation products measured by D-dimer estimation with a decrease in fibrinogen concentration.

Trick

This patient had all three features of disseminated intravascular coagulation. Replacement of clotting factors and platelets is the mainstay of treatment. There is insufficient evidence to advocate routine treatment with agents such as heparin or ε-aminocaproic acid. Vitamin K is given to enable synthesis of clotting factors.

Calcium is an important cofactor in the clotting cascade and is chelated by citrate in transfused blood products. While transfused blood may no longer contain citrate as an anticoagulant, clotting factors do. Repeated administration of clotting factors requires monitoring of the ionized calcium concentration and replacement if the ionized calcium falls below 0.8 mmol L^{-1}. This patient required a total of 29 mmol of calcium to maintain her ionized calcium at an acceptable level.

Replacement of clotting factors is not usually necessary if the platelet count is greater than 50 × 10^9 L^{-1} and if the PT is less than 20 s. Correction of a coagulopathy should be guided clinically. Correction of even gross coagulation abnormalities may not be necessary unless the patient is bleeding or at risk of doing so, for instance, because of the need for line insertion.

Amniotic fluid embolus is a rare but catastrophic obstetric emergency. It usually presents with the sudden onset of hypotension, hypoxia and coagulopathy and has a mortality of 80%. The syndrome is started by the entrance of amniotic fluid or fetal debris into the maternal circulation. The response to this may depend more on an abnormal substance within the amniotic fluid than on the volume of fluid. It is thought that mediators such as leucotrienes and arachidonic acid metabolites are released and result in the clinical features. Initially, there is pulmonary vasospasm which causes pulmonary hypertension and hypoxia. This is followed by myocardial depression leading to evidence of left ventricular failure. The characteristic DIC develops rapidly. Trophoblastic tissue has thromboplastin-like effects and is thought to have a role in the development of DIC.

Amniotic fluid embolus can be rapidly fatal and diagnosis is often made at post-mortem. The differential diagnosis is between septic shock, pulmonary aspiration of gastric contents, myocardial infarction, pulmonary embolus and placental abruption. Amniotic fluid embolus is often a clinical diagnosis based on the clinical presentation and progress. This patient presented with sudden hypotension and hypoxemia. A coagulopathy was indicated by the difficulty with hemostasis but not investigated. Fetal material may be found in the maternal pulmonary circulation. This indicates amniotic fluid embolus but, since fetal material has been found in the lungs of patients with no clinical features of amniotic fluid embolism, it cannot be diagnostic.

Fortunately, the clinical course of this patient was not fulminant and she responded to initial fluid resuscitation and oxygen. Intraoperative fluid balance is critical. Excessive fluid may compromise myocardial function further and result in pulmonary edema. However, fluid administration is essential to avoid under-resuscitation if the patient's collapse is due to another cause. The response to fluid administration should be carefully monitored and, if the patient remains hypotensive, inotropic agents may be required. Further problems may arise from the rapidly developing coagulopathy. This may contraindicate the insertion of monitoring lines and complicate appropriate resuscitation. In this situation, an indication of myocardial performance can be obtained with a less invasive technique such as trans-esophageal echocardiography or esophageal doppler monitoring. The coagulopathy may also complicate delivery or surgery with excessive bleeding and difficult hemostasis. Although this woman responded to resuscitation measures, she was still hypotensive and hypoxic on admission to the ICU.

This patient was hypotensive as a result of her myocardial depression. She had an increased pulmonary artery occlusion pressure, a decreased cardiac index and a relatively high systemic vascular resistance. This responded to frusemide to reduce preload, dobutamine to increase myocardial contractility and sedation with propofol to control afterload. Her increased blood lactate and decreased urine output were evidence of organ hypoperfusion but these responded to resuscitation.

The early institution of monitoring in this case enabled early appropriate treatment of her hypotension. During insertion of a pulmonary artery catheter, it is important to remember to take a sample of pulmonary venous blood for cytological investigation. This may assist the diagnosis by finding fetal tissue in the maternal circulation.

The initial cause of this patient's hypoxia was pulmonary vasoconstriction as evidenced by her increased MPAP and PVR. This caused a ventilation–perfusion mismatch and hypoxia. The situation was exacerbated by her pulmonary edema secondary to myocardial depression. As the alveolar pulmonary edema responded to diuretic treatment and her pulmonary hypertension settled spontaneously, her oxygenation did not improve. This appeared to be because of the development of acute respiratory distress syndrome (ARDS). In the acute phase of amniotic fluid embolus, there is an increase in lung water out of proportion to the increase in PAOP. This suggests the early development of interstitial pulmonary edema which is part of the pathology of ARDS. The severity of her ARDS was indicated by her requirement for considerable ventilatory support to maintain adequate oxygenation.

Follow-up

The dopamine and dobutamine infusions were withdrawn gradually over the next two days and she remained hemodynamically stable and with a urine output of $50–100\,mL\,h^{-1}$. Her coagulopathy also improved slightly. She required no further blood transfusion and over 48 hours had 6 units of FFP and 4 units of platelets to control bleeding. Her clotting function had improved to a platelet count of $77 \times 10^9\,L^{-1}$, PT 21 s, APTT 41 s, fibrinogen $1.4\,g\,L^{-1}$ and D-dimer $4\,mg\,L^{-1}$; her Hb was $10.2\,g\,dL^{-1}$.

Her lungs did not improve until day 5. Throughout this time she remained on pressure controlled ventilation with a pressure of $32\,cmH_2O$, F_IO_2 1.0, PEEP $5\,cmH_2O$ and I : E ratio 2 : 1. Her chest radiograph showed diffuse patchy shadowing with the appearances of ARDS. On day 5 her F_IO_2 was reduced to 0.7 and her pressure control to $30\,cmH_2O$. On this support her arterial blood gas analysis was: H^+ $42\,nmol\,L^{-1}$ [pH 7.38], P_aO_2 $12.6\,kPa$ [95 mmHg], P_aCO_2 $6.35\,kPa$ [48 mmHg], and base excess $-1.8\,mmol\,L^{-1}$. Over the next 5 days the patient was weaned gradually from her ventilatory support. Her trachea was extubated on day 11 with a respiratory rate of 32/minute and a P_aO_2 of $14.7\,kPa$ [110 mmHg] on an F_IO_2 of 0.4. The next day, she was discharged to the ward where she required treatment for depression, but was later discharged home well.

Bibliography

1 Chatelain SM and Quirk JG. Amniotic and thromboembolism. *Clinical Obstetrics and Gynaecology* (1990) **33**: 473–481.
2 Masson RG. Amniotic fluid embolus. *Clinical Chest Medicine* (1992) **13**: 657–665.

11.3 Major Hemorrhage
D.G. Greig and Maire P. Shelly

History

A 32-year-old woman was admitted for an elective Cesarean section at 38 weeks' gestation. She had had four previous uneventful Cesarean sections and in this pregnancy, after a small bleed at 25 weeks' gestation, had an ultrasonographically confirmed placenta praevia almost completely covering the cervical os. At Cesarian section, a healthy baby girl was delivered but a placenta accreta was found. The placenta could not be removed entirely and the uterus failed to contract with massage and syntocinon. At this stage bleeding was excessive. A hysterectomy was performed to control uterine bleeding and hemostatic sutures controlled bleeding from the right side of the vaginal vault. Hemostasis was satisfactory at the end of the procedure.

Surgery lasted a total of 3 hours and the estimated intraoperative blood loss was 20 L. During this time, the patient had received 26 units of blood, 7 L of Gelofusine® , 4 L crystalloid, 12 units of FFP and 8 units of platelets. Her MAP had varied between 40 and 75 mmHg and her heart rate was 90–140/minute. Her oxygen saturation remained greater than 94% throughout. Despite measures to warm infused fluids and reduce heat loss, her core body temperature decreased and was 34.1°C [93.4°F] at the end of the procedure. Monitoring established intraoperatively included arterial and central venous lines. A pulmonary artery catheter introducer was placed in the right internal jugular vein and used for rapid blood transfusion. In addition to fluids, she received 10% mannitol 250 mL and an infusion of dopamine $3 \mu g\,kg^{-1}\,min^{-1}$. At the end of the procedure, she was transferred to the intensive care unit (ICU).

On admission to the ICU, she had a MAP of 62 mmHg, heart rate 127/minute and temperature 33.7°C [92.7°F]. She was sedated and controlled ventilation was continued. A warm-air warming blanket was put over her and blood transfusion continued while investigations were sent and monitoring established. Initial hematology results included hemoglobin $6.7\,g\,dL^{-1}$, platelet count $62 \times 10^9\,L^{-1}$, PT 37 s, APTT 68 s, fibrinogen $1.0\,g\,L^{-1}$, D-dimer $0.48\,mg\,L^{-1}$. Biochemical analysis was unremarkable except for a serum potassium of $5.9\,mmol\,L^{-1}$ and an $2.8\,mEq\,L^{-1}$ ionized calcium concentration of $0.72\,mmol\,L^{-1}$. Initial blood gas results on an F_IO_2 of 1.0 were: H^+ $49\,nmol\,L^{-1}$ [pH 7.31], P_aO_2 55.7 kPa [418 mmHg], P_aCO_2 4.2 kPa [31.5 mmHg], base excess $-6.8\,mmol\,L^{-1}$. Hemodynamic parameters were: HR 116/minute, MAP 69 mmHg, MPAP 17 mmHg, PAOP 7 mmHg, CI $5.4\,L\,min^{-1}\,m^{-2}$, SVR $929\,dyn\text{-}sec\,cm^{-5}$ and lactate $1.9\,mmol\,L^{-1}$. She received 4 units of blood, 4 units of FFP, 4 units of platelets and 8 units of cryoprecipitate because FFP contains little factor VIII. A 10 mg bolus of vitamin K was also given and calcium gluconate to maintain an ionized calcium above $0.85\,mmol\,L^{-1}$ [$3.39\,mEq\,L^{-1}$]. The dopamine infusion continued and her urine output was $40\,mL\,h^{-1}$.

Five hours later, she was cardiovascularly stable with: HR 102/minute, MAP 78 mmHg, PAOP 10 mmHg, CI 6.2 L min^{-1} m^{-2}, SVR 740 dyn-sec cm^{-5}. Her lactate was 1.8 mmol L^{-1}, urine output 40 mL h^{-1} and temperature 35.2°C [95.4°F]. Her coagulation had also improved to a platelet count 65 × 10^9 L^{-1}, PT 25 s, APTT 53 s; her Hb was 8.9 g dL^{-1}. Over the next hour, her MAP decreased to 58 mmHg despite blood transfusion, her HR was 132/minute, PAOP 4 mmHg, CI 6.1 L min^{-1} m^{-2}, SVR 987 dyn-sec cm^{-5} and lactate 2.7 mmol L^{-1}. Her temperature decreased to 34.9°C [94.8°F], her urine output to 20 mL h^{-1} and her abdomen was distended. She was transferred to the operating theater for laparotomy. At laparotomy, 4 L of blood was found in the abdominal cavity. Both sides of the pelvic wall were bleeding from multiple sites and the bleeding could not be controlled. Both internal iliac arteries were ligated and the bleeding was eventually controlled. During the procedure, the patient received 6 units of blood, 4 units of FFP and 4 units of platelets.

On return to the ICU, her temperature was 35.9°C, MAP 77 mmHg, HR 119/minute, PAOP 11 mmHg, CI 6.2 L min^{-1} m^{-2}, SVR 677 dyn-sec cm^{-5} and lactate 2.0 mmol L^{-1}. Her arterial blood gases on an F_IO_2 of 0.6 were: H$^+$ 48 nmol L^{-1} [pH 7.32], P_aO_2 97 mmHg [12.9 kPa], P_aCO_2 34.5 mmHg [4.6 kPa], base excess −4.2 mmol L^{-1}, and her coagulation status was: platelets 75 × 10^9 L^{-1}, PT 22 s, PTT 46 s, fibrinogen 1.2 g L^{-1}, D-dimer 0.41 mg L^{-1}. Her condition stabilized, her transfusion requirement decreased and by the next morning her temperature was 36.8°C [98.2°F], HR 89/minute, MAP 82 mmHg, PAOP 14 mmHg, CI 6.3 L min^{-1} m^{-2}, SVR 578 dyn-sec/cm^{-5}. Her lactate was 1.1 mmol L^{-1} and urine output 50 mL h^{-1}. Her Hb was 9.8 g dL^{-1}, platelets 69 × 10^9 L^{-1}, PT 20 s, APTT 48 s. Her arterial gases on an F_IO_2 of 0.4 were: H$^+$ 44 nmol L^{-1} [pH 7.36], P_aO_2 13.2 kPa [99 mmHg], P_aCO_2 5.1 kPa [38 mmHg] and base excess −1.6 mmol L^{-1}.

Trap 1

This patient had a massive blood transfusion to correct hemorrhage during her first operation. At this stage, it is important to watch for evidence of further blood loss in case hemorrhage persists. This may necesscitate re-exploration to control bleeding and if this is impossible to ligate the internal iliac arteries. Angiographic embolization of the internal iliac or its branches is also possible. It is also important to continue resuscitation and ensure that replacement of blood and blood products is adequate. This implies correction of any coagulopathy and ensuring the patient's body temperature returns to normal.

Trick 1

As well as control of bleeding, it is important to minimize the consequences of organ hypoperfusion which may have occurred during hemorrhage. Transfused blood may contain microaggregates and other substances not removed by even efficient filters. The lungs filter these out before they enter the systemic circulation. Because of this, the lungs may accumulate debris and massive transfusion is a risk factor for the development of ARDS. Other organs, predominantly the kidneys, gut and liver, suffer hypoperfusion as blood is diverted to other areas.

Vasoconstriction is a primary response to hemorrhage, so that the available blood is taken to important organs. The degree of vasoconstriction depends on the severity of hemorrhage but in hemorrhage of this magnitude some organs will suffer, particularly the kidneys, gut and liver. The degree of vasoconstriction to these organs can be minimized in two ways: first and most important, early and adequate fluid resuscitation to replace lost circulating volume; second and more controversial, the use of a dopaminergic agent such as dopamine or dopexamine to cause some renal and splanchnic vasodilation and maintain blood flow to these organs. A combination of these measures will reduce the consequences of hypoperfusion to these organs.

Trap 2

Hemorrhage is obvious when blood pours out of drains but intra-abdominal hemorrhage is often occult. A decreasing blood pressure or increasing heart rate are classic signs of hemorrhage but may be maintained by vasoconstriction and fluid infusion.

Trick 2

An early sign of hemorrhage is an increased SVR. Because vasoconstriction is part of the compensatory mechanism for hypovolemic shock, an increased SVR may occur before a decrease in blood pressure. The degree of vasoconstriction will depend on the compliance of the circulation. A decrease in hemoglobin is a late sign of hemorrhage and indicates the need for urgent management.

Trap 3

Blood is usually transfused to maintain a normal hemoglobin. The administration of blood products is usually governed by the results of PT, APTT and platelet count. Platelet transfusion is usually indicated if the patient had a count less than $50 \times 10^9 \, L^{-1}$ in the presence of bleeding.

Trick 3

Hemodilution is a physiological response to hemorrhage and appears to have a role in hemostasis. It is important not to overtransfuse the patient and some even advocate withholding blood during hemorrhage to allow the hemodilution mechanisms to produce hemostasis.

In the hypothermic patient, a low blood viscosity is important to allow flow through vasoconstricted vessels. As a result, coagulation is impaired in hypothermic patients. Measurement of PT and APTT is performed at 37°C [98.6°F]. Because of this, the PT and APTT may appear normal in a hypothermic patient and fail to reflect a profound clotting deficit. In this situation, it is vital to warm the patient: only then will hemostasis occur; the administration of clotting factors alone will not reverse the coagulopathy.

The time-honored definition of postpartum hemorrhage is more than 500 mL blood loss in the first 24 hours after delivery. This is now regarded as a normal blood loss following vaginal delivery and a practical definition of postpartum hemorrhage is blood loss which exceeds normal and has not responded to uterine massage and oxytocin. Since blood flow to the uterus and placenta can exceed $500 \, mL \, min^{-1}$ at term, significant blood loss can occur quickly. This usually occurs when the uterus fails to contract after the baby is delivered.

Initial management of postpartum bleeding is massage of the uterus and administration of oxytocin. Fluids should be given and blood obtained for transfusion. If these measures fail, ergometrine may be needed. Prostaglandins are used in some centers, given either intramyometrially, vaginally or intramuscularly. Failure of medical treatment dictates surgical management such as hysterectomy, ligation of vessels or angiographic embolization of vessels.

Follow-up

After the second operation the patient required 2 units of blood over the next 12 hours. At this stage, her sedation was stopped and her ventilatory support weaned. Her trachea was extubated and she remained cardiovascularly stable with a urine output of $50–60 \, mL \, h^{-1}$. She was discharged to the ward the next day and returned home with her baby a week later.

Bibliography

1 Zahn CM and Yeomans ER. Postpartum hemorrhage: placenta accreta, uterine inversion, and puerperal hematomas. *Clinical Obstetrics and Gynaecology* (1990) **33**: 473–481.
2 Cruikshank SH. Management of postpartum and pelvic hemorrhage. *Clinical Obstetrics and Gynaecology* (1986) **29**: 213–219.

11.4 Puerperal Sepsis
D.G. Greig and Maire P. Shelly

History

A 31-year-old woman was admitted to another hospital three weeks after a normal vaginal delivery of her second child at 39 weeks' gestation. She had been mildly but non-specifically unwell since delivery complaining of a yellow vaginal discharge which was treated with douches. The baby remained well. Three days before admission, she had developed 'flu-like symptoms with lethargy, rigors, sweating and right shoulder pain. On admission to hospital she was unwell, with a temperature of 38.2°C [100.8°F], a swollen, painful right shoulder and an erythematous rash which extended over her right axilla and right chest wall. No abnormality was found on vaginal examination. Blood cultures were taken and she was given intravenous flucloxacillin and a crystalloid infusion.

Her condition gradually deteriorated, despite aggressive fluid infusion. She became hypotensive, confused, oliguric, jaundiced and tachypneic, and she developed a coagulopathy. On the third day of admission a group A hemolytic streptococcus sensitive to penicillin was identified in her blood culture. Her antibiotic was changed to high-dose penicillin and she was transferred to the intensive care unit (ICU). sense

On admission to the ICU, she was sedated, paralyzed and ventilated. Her temperature was 35.6°C [96.1°F], heart rate 120/minute and arterial pressure 85/50 mmHg; her urine output was 25 mL in the first hour. The erythematous rash had become confluent and now covered her anterior chest and abdominal wall and extended laterally to both axillae and flanks (Figure 11.4.1). Blisters had developed down her right side. Chest examination revealed bilateral basal crackles and, on an F_IO_2 of 1.0, her pH was H^+ 56 nmol L^{-1} [7.25], P_aO_2 13.5 kPa [101 mmHg], P_aCO_2 6.7 kPa [49 mmHg] and base excess -5.4 mmol L^{-1}. Her abdomen was tense and distended. Hematological results were: hemoglobin 11.3 g dL^{-1}, white blood cell count 17.6 × 10^9 L^{-1} with a neutrophilia of 15.1 × 10^9 L^{-1}, platelet count 11 × 10^9 L^{-1}. Microscopy of a blood film revealed myelocytes, metamyelocytes, crenated red cells and toxic granulation. Her coagulation screen revealed PT 16 s, APTT 25.5 s, fibrinogen 2.6 mg mL^{-1}, and D-dimer 8 mg L^{-1}. Abnormal serum biochemistry included urea 139 mg dL^{-1} [23.1 mmol L^{-1}], creatinine 271 mmol L^{-1} [3.52 mg dL^{-1}], albumin 8 g L^{-1}, bilirubin 114 µmol L^{-1} [6.7 mg dL^{-1}], alkaline phosphatase 76 IU L^{-1}, alanine transferase 102 IU L^{-1}. Her first hemodynamic measurements revealed: MAP 55 mmHg, PAOP 6 mmHg, CI 6.6 L min^{-1} m^{-2}, SVR 321 dyn-sec cm^{-5}, PVR 109 dyn-sec cm^{-5}, D_{O_2I} 1042 mL min^{-1} m^{-2}, V_{O_2I} 66 mL min^{-1} m^{-2}, oxygen extraction ratio 6.3%, shunt fraction 65.7%, and blood lactate 2.0 mmol L^{-1}.

Vancomycin, imipenem, metranidazole and gentamicin were added to her penicillin chemotherapy to cover any additional organisms. Noradrenaline

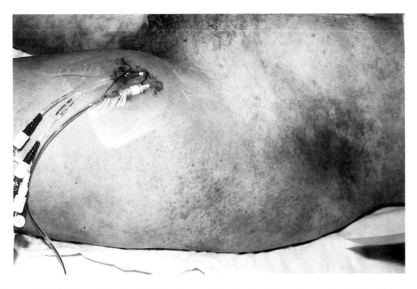

Figure 11.4.1. The patient with streptococcal toxic shock syndrome had this widespread rash with areas of incipient necrosis. The rash was confluent in both flanks and later blisters formed in the necrotic areas.

[norepinephrine] had no effect on her MAP or SVR, but phenylephrine in large doses (9.5 mg h^{-1}) maintained her MAP at 70 mmHg. Phenylephrine is a purer alpha agonist than norepinephrine and is an alternative in hypotension resistant to noradrenaline. In these cases, noradrenaline may have some beta activity and increase CI without an effect on SVR. It should be withdrawn with care if replaced by phenylephrine. The patient also received dopamine at 2.5 µg kg^{-1} min^{-1} to maintain renal and splanchnic perfusion. In spite of this her lactate increased to 2.8 mmol L^{-1} and her urine output remained around 20 mL h^{-1}. Dopexamine at up to 2.5 µg kg^{-1} min^{-1} was tried as an alternative dopaminergic agent but it had no effect on urine output or lactate. Her ventilatory support was pressure controlled ventilation with a pressure of 40 cmH$_2$O, 7.5 cmH$_2$O PEEP, I : E ratio 3 : 1 and F_1O_2 of 1.0. This produced a tidal volume of 0.7 L and arterial gases of H$^+$ 77 nmol L^{-1} [pH 7.11], P_aO_2 9.3 kPa [70 mmHg], P_aCO_2 7.2 kPa [54 mmHg], base excess -11.2 mmol L^{-1}. She also received vitamin C and N-acetyl cysteine as potential free radical scavengers. Ultrasound examination of her pelvis and abdomen revealed no abnormality but some ascites which, when tapped, revealed abundant white blood cells but no organisms. She had a yellowish vaginal discharge which was also sterile and no abnormality was found on vaginal examination.

The next day, she was bleeding from the sites of intravenous lines. Her clotting results were: platelets 8×10^9 L^{-1}, PT 30 s, APTT 50 s, fibrinogen 0.6 g L^{-1}, D-dimer 6 mg L^{-1} and she received 6 units each of FFP and platelets. By this time her WCC was 27.1×10^6 L^{-1} and her temperature was 39.3°C [102.7°F]. Hemodynamically she had deteriorated with HR 143/minute, MAP 55 mmHg,

PAOP 12 mmHg, MPAP 30 mmHg, CI 2.4 L min^{-1} m^{-2}, SVR 436 dyn-sec cm^{-5}, Do_{2I} 362 mL min^{-1} m^{-2}, Vo_{2I} 112 mL min^{-1} m^{-2} and lactate 2.1 mmol L^{-1}.

Dobutamine did not increase her CI but caused her HR to increase to 165/minute; the dobutamine was discontinued. This may occur if the patient is hypovolemic. Although her measured PAOP was 12 mmHg, her high intrathoracic pressures from controlled ventilation probably increased this value artificially. In this situation, measures of right ventricular ejection characteristics may provide a more accurate reflection of preload. Measurement of intrinsic PEEP may give some indication of the intrathoracic pressures. Her hypovolemia could be explained by continuous serous oozing from her skin. She had generalized edema and her rash was blistering on both sides. Despite continuous administration of colloids, her PAOP could only be maintained, not increased. A combination of adrenaline [epinephrine], dopexamine and milrinone eventually produced a MAP 74 mmHg, PAOP 13 mmHg, CI 3.6 L min^{-1} m^{-2}, SVR 672 dyn-sec cm^{-5}, Do_{2I} 478 mL min^{-1} m^{-2}, Vo_{2I} 126 mL min^{-1} m^{-2}, a lactate of 1.8 mmol L^{-1} and a urine output of 20 mL h^{-1}. Because of a deterioration in her respiratory function, her PEEP was increased in steps to 17 cmH$_2$O. This produced gases of H$^+$ 87 nmol L^{-1} [pH 7.06], P_aCO$_2$ 8.2 kPa [62 mmHg], P_aO$_2$ 7.3 kPa [55 mmHg], base excess -14 mmol L^{-1} still with an F_IO$_2$ of 1.0.

Trap 1

Because of the high mortality of septic shock and organ failure, the key to the management of septic patients is prompt recognition of the problem and aggressive early management. At this stage mediator release in response to the septic insult has begun but the downward spiral with activation of cascades and further mediator release may not have not become established. Several studies have investigated the effects of blocking mediators such as tumor necrosis factor, interleukin-1 and platelet activating factor, in the treatment of sepsis. To date these studies have not shown a benefit in reducing mortality.

Trick 1

The features of early sepsis are hypotension, tachycardia, tachypnea and pyrexia. This patient showed all these signs on admission to hospital and may have done so during the three days she was ill at home before admission. Treatment with antibiotics and fluids was started but she progressed to organ dysfunction as a result of hypoperfusion. Early invasive monitoring and optimization of oxygen delivery may have slowed the progress of her disease or avoided organ failure. Surgery to remove a septic focus was never performed, since a septic focus was not identified. A laparotomy may have been indicated but was not performed because of her poor condition and lack of evidence for a pelvic focus for her sepsis. Since she had a rapidly progressing disease mediated by toxins released by the group A hemolytic streptococcus, her ultimate death may have been inevitable.

Trap 2

Hypoperfusion and hypoxia lead to cellular ischemia and death and, ultimately, to organ ischemia and death. Optimizing oxygen delivery is one side of the equation which is often considered.

In sepsis, there is a fundamental problem with tissue oxygenation. The philosophy behind optimizing oxygen delivery is that sick tissues need more oxygen than usual and increasing oxygen delivery may increase oxygen consumption. Oxygen delivery depends on cardiac output, hemoglobin concentration and oxygenation. The balance needed is to increase oxygenation without impairing cardiac output, to increase cardiac output without myocardial ischemia and to increase hemoglobin without reducing blood flow. These are factors which need consideration on an individual patient basis.

Trick 2

The other side of the equation is to reduce tissue oxygen demand and to protect the tissues if possible from the adverse effects of ischemia and reperfusion. Oxygen demand can be reduced by limiting organ function. For example, sedation and anesthesia reduce cerebral oxygen demand and neuromuscular blockade reduces muscle oxygen demand. It may also be necessary to balance a proposed increase in oxygen demand against other factors, such as the use of diuretics to maintain urine flow.

Protection of tissues from ischemia and reperfusion is more difficult and more controversial. The generation of highly reactive free radicals is thought to contribute to tissue injury when tissues are reperfused after a period of hypoperfusion. Agents such as mannitol, vitamin C and N-acetylcysteine may scavenge free radicals before they can cause tissue damage and so protect the tissues. N-Acetylcysteine has been shown to reduce the incidence of multiple organ failure after late presentation of paracetamol overdose. The mechanism for this is thought to be free radical scavenging.

Sepsis is a state in which an infection results in impaired peripheral perfusion. When this state progresses so that the delivery of oxygen to the tissues does not meet their demands, it is known as 'septic shock'. The process ultimately leads to cell ischemia, dysfunction and death. The signs of sepsis include: fever or hypothermia, tachypnea, tachycardia and hypotension with clinical evidence of infection. Initially these may be mild but progression indicates the need for treatment. Evidence of end-organ dysfunction, such as altered conscious level, hypoxemia, raised lactate or acidemia, oliguria or coagulopathy, indicates a need for aggressive management. In the early stages mortality is about 20% but this increases rapidly as organ dysfunction becomes established.

Less than 1% of obstetric admissions have a documented bacteremia and only some 20% of these patients will become septic. However, because obstetric sepsis has a mortality of approximately 30%, it is an important cause of maternal mortality. Most obstetric sepsis is caused by Gram-negative organisms but the incidence of Gram-positive sepsis is increasing. The vagina has a mixed bacterial flora. Bacteria may enter the uterus through the cervix during labor and delivery and then enter the systemic circulation. Because pregnancy is a state of immunological compromise, there is a recognized risk of developing sepsis and an increased mortality. Endometritis is the most common cause of obstetric septic shock followed by septic abortion and intra-amniotic infections. Necrotizing fasciitis and toxic shock syndrome each cause less than 1% of cases with obstetric septic shock. Toxic shock syndrome is usually caused by *Staphylococcus aureus* and is diagnosed by the presence of pyrexia, a characteristic rash, hypotension, involvement of three or more organ systems and the ability to discount other causes of the infection. The same clinical features can be caused by a streptococcal infection and this is referred to as 'streptococcal toxic shock syndrome'. Both organisms produce potent toxins and the syndromes are thought to be caused by the toxins rather than the organisms themselves.

The isolation of a group A streptococcus from the patient's blood before transfer gave us the causative organism for the patient's sepsis but not its source. By the time of her ICU admission she had developed septic shock. Her cardiovascular system was hyperdynamic and vasodilated and she had a low oxygen consumption and oxygen extraction ratio, despite her increased global oxygen delivery. She also had evidence of inadequate tissue oxygenation with an increased lactate, increased base excess and acidemia. This patient had a calculated APACHE II score of 25 and evidence of impaired function of several organ systems: cardiovascular, respiratory, renal, hepatic, hematological, skin and probably gastrointestinal. A patient with this degree of illness has a mortality of over 70%.

Management of septic shock involves supporting the function of individual organs, optimizing delivery of oxygen to the tissues to reduce tissue ischemia and protecting organs from further injury. Identification and removal of the source of sepsis is important, as is antibiotic treatment of the causative organism. However, the toxin produced by the streptococcus is not inactivated by antibiotics and the disease may progress despite adequate antibiotic therapy. No antitoxin is currently available.

Follow-up

Over the next two days the patient's condition stabilized slightly but she then deteriorated further. Her hypotension became unresponsive to inotropes and vasopressors, her respiratory function worsened on significant ventilatory support, she became anuric, her lactate rose to $5.3 \, \text{mmol} \, \text{L}^{-1}$ and her coagulopathy worsened. As well as these factors, her extremities were starting to become gangrenous. In conjunction with the family, it was decided to withdraw treatment and she died 3 hours later. At post-mortem examination, she had evidence of multiple organ failure and sterile pus in both Fallopian tubes.

Bibliography

1 Pearlman M and Faro S. Obstetric septic shock: a pathophysiologic basis for management. *Clinical Obstetrics and Gynaecology* (1990) **33**: 482–492.
2 Fisher CJ and Panacek EA. Toxic shock syndrome. In: Shoemaker WC, Ayres S, Grenvik A, Holbrook PR and Thompson WL (eds) *Textbook of Critical Care* 2nd edn. Philadelphia, WB Saunders, pp 1002–1006, 1989.

Standard Abbreviations

Many abbreviations have been used in this book. The common ones used by the authors are shown below. Others, specific to certain chapters, are explained when they are used.

ABG	arterial blood gas
ACT	activated clotting time
ALT	alanine aminotransferase
APSAC	anisolated plasminogen-streptokinase activator complex
APTT	activated partial thromboplastin time
ARDS	acute respiratory distress syndrome
AST	aspartate aminotransferase
AIVR	accelerated idioventricular rhythm
BP	blood pressure
BUN	blood urea nitrogen
C_aO_2	arterial oxygen content
CI	cardiac index
CInt	confidence interval
cmH_2O	centimeters of water
CO	cardiac output
COAD	chronic obstructive airways disease
CPAP	constant positive airway pressure
CPR	cardiopulmonary resuscitation
CSF	cerebrospinal fluid
CSU	catheter specimen urine
CT	computed tomography
CVC	central venous catheter
CVP	central venous pressure
DIC	disseminated intravascular coagulopathy
ECG	electrocardiogram
EDTA	ethylenediaminetetraacetic acid
EEG	electroencephalogram
EMG	electromyogram
ESR	erythrocyte sedimentation rate
FBC	full blood count
FDP	fibrinogen degradation product
FEV_1	forced expiratory volume in one second
FFP	fresh frozen plasma

F_IO_2	fractional inspired oxygen concentration
FRC	functional residual capacity
FVC	forced vital capacity
h	hour
HR	heart rate
ICU	intensive care unit
IgG	immunoglobulin G
INR	interational normalised ratio
IPPV	intermittent positive-pressure ventilation
IU	international unit
IV	intravenous
JVP	jugular venous pressure
kPa	kilo Pascals
L	liters
LVSWI	left ventricular stroke work index
MABP	mean arterial blood pressure
MCV	mean corpuscular volume
MPAP	mean pulmonary artery pressure
min	minute
meq	milliequivalent
mL	milliliter
mmHg	millimeters of mercury
mmol	millimole
MRI	magnetic resonance image
MV	minute volume
P_aCo_2	partial pressure of carbon dioxide in arterial blood
P_aO_2	partial pressure of oxygen in arterial blood
PA	pulmonary artery
PAOP	pulmonary artery occlusion pressure
PEEP	positive end-expiratory pressure
PEFR	peak expiratory flow rate
PT	prothrombin time
PTT	partial thromboplastin time
PVRI	pulmonary vascular resistance index
RR	respiratory rate
rtPA	recombinant tissue plasminogen activator
RVSWI	right ventricular stroke work index
S_aO_2	oxygen saturation – arterial
S_pO_2	oxygen saturation – pulse oximeter
SIMV	synchronous intermittent mandatory ventilation
S_vO_2	mixed venous oxygen saturation
SVRI	systemic vascular resistance index
TV	tidal volume
WBC	white blood cell count

Normal Laboratory Values

Analyte	Conventional Units	SI Units	Fluid	Method or Instrument	Factor for Conversion to SI Units
General Chemistries					
Acetoacetate plus acetone	Negative	—	WB	—	—
Acid phosphatase, prostatic	0–0.8 U L^{-1}	0.0–13.0 nkat L^{-1}	S	Kinetic method	16.67
Alanineaminotransferase (ALT)					
Female	7–30 U L^{-1}	0.12–0.50 µkat L^{-1}			
Male	10–55 U L^{-1}	0.17–0.91 µkat L^{-1}			
Albumin	3.1–4.3 g dL^{-1}	31–43 g L^{-1}	S	Colorimetry (bromocresol purple)	10
Aldolase	0–7 U L^{-1}	0–117 nkat L^{-1}	S	Kinetic method	16.67
Alkaline phosphatase			S	Kinetic method	0.01667
Female	30–100 U L^{-1}	0.5–1.67 µkat L^{-1}			
Male	45–115 U L^{-1}	0.75–1.92 µkat L^{-1}			
Alkaline phosphatase leukocyte			WB	Histochemistry	
Female (not taking oral contraceptives)	30–160	None			None
Male	33–188	None			None
Alpha$_1$-antitrypsin	85–213 mg dL^{-1}	0.85–2.13 g L^{-1}	S	Nephelometry	0.01
Alpha fetoprotein (nonmaternal)	< 10 IU mL^{-1}	< 7.75 µg L^{-1}	S	Immunoassay	0.775
Ammonia	12–55 µmol L^{-1}	12–55 µmol L^{-1}	P	Enzymatic analysis	1
Amylase	53–123 U L^{-1}	0.88–2.05 nkat L^{-1}	S	Kinetic method	0.01667
	0–375 U L^{-1}	0–6.25 µkat L^{-1}	U	Kinetic method	
Angiotensin-converting enzyme (ACE)	10–50 U L^{-1}	167–834 nkat L^{-1}	S	Kinetic method	16.67
Ascorbic acid	0.4–1.5 mg dL^{-1}	23–85 µmol L^{-1}	WB	—	56.78
Aspartate aminotransferase (AST)			S	Kinetic method	0.01667
Female	9–25 U L^{-1}	0.15–0.42 µkat L^{-1}			
Male	10–40 U L^{-1}	0.17–0.67 µkat L^{-1}			
Bicarbonate (HCO$_3$)	22–26 mEq L^{-1}	22–26 mmol L^{-1}	WB,S	Calculation	1
Bilirubin	0.00	0.00	CSF	—	—
Bilirubin, direct	0.0–0.4 mg dL^{-1}	0–7 µmol L^{-1}	S	Colorimetry	17.1
Bilirubin, total	0.0–1.0 mg dL^{-1}	0–17 µmol L^{-1}	S	Colorimetry	17.1

Note: Values are also given in SI units (Systéme International d'Unitès).
Fluid abbreviations: S – serum; WB – whole blood; P – plasma; U – urine; CSF – cerebrospinal fluid; PRP – platelet-rich plasma.
Reprinted by permission of the publisher.

Analyte	Conventional Units	SI Units	Fluid	Method or Instrument	Factor for Conversion to SI Units
General Chemistries (*Continued*)					
CA-19-9 (cancer antigen)	< 37.0 U mL^{-1}	< 37.0 kU L^{-1}	S	Immunoassay	1
CA-125 (cancer antigen)	< 20.0 U mL^{-1}	< 20.0 kU L^{-1}	S	Immunoassay	1
Calcium	8.5–10.5 mg dL^{-1}	2.1–2.6 mmol L^{-1}	S	Colorimetry	0.25
	0.0–300 mg day^{-1}	0.0–7.5 mmol L^{-1}	U	Atomic absorption	0.025
Calcium, ionized	1.14–1.30 mmol L^{-1}	1.14–1.30 mmol L^{-1}	P	Ion-selective electrode	1
Carbon dioxide content, total	24.0–30.9 mmol L^{-1}	24.0–30.9 mmol L^{-1}	S	Carbon dioxide electrode	1
Carbon dioxide, partial pressure, arterial ($P_a\mathrm{CO}_2$)	35–45 mm Hg	4.7–6.0	WB	Carbon dioxide electrode	0.1333
Carbon monoxide	< 5% of total hemoglobin	Not applicable	WB	—	—
Carboxyhemoglobin	< 5% of total hemoglobin	< 0.05 fraction of total hemoglobin saturation	WB	Multiwavelength spectro- photometry	0.01
Carcinoembryonicantigen (CEA)	0.0–3.0 ng mL^{-1}	0.0–3.0 μg L^{-1}	P,S	Immunoassay	1
Carotenoids	0.8–4.0 μg mL^{-1}	1.5–7.4 μmol L^{-1}	S	—	—
Cerebrospinal fluid (adult)			CSF		
Albumin	11–48 mg dL^{-1}	0.11–0.48 g L^{-1}		Nephelometry	0.01
Cell count	0–5 mononuclear cells μL^{-1}	0–5 × 10^4 cells L^{-1}		Manual count	1 × 10^4
Chloride	120–130 mmol L^{-1}	120–130 mmol L^{-1}		Coulmetry	1
Glucose	50–75 mg dL^{-1}	2.8–4.2 mmol L^{-1}		Enzymatic analysis	0.05551
IgG	8.0–8.6 mg dL^{-1}	0.08–0.086 g L^{-1}		Nephelometry	0.01
Pressure	70–180 mm of water	70–180 arbitrary units		Manual measurement	1
Protein	15–45 mg dL^{-1}	0.15–0.45 g L^{-1}		Turbidometry	0.01
Ceruloplasmin	23–43 mg dL^{-1}	230–430 mg L^{-1}	S	Oxidose activity	10
Chloride	100–108 mmol L^{-1}	100–108 mmol L^{-1}	P,S	Coulometry	1
	10–200 mmol L^{-1}	10–200 mmol L^{-1}	U	Coulometry	1
Cholesterol			S	Colorimetry	0.02586
Desirable	< 200 mg dL^{-1}	< 5.18 mmol L^{-1}			
Borderline high	200–239 mg dL^{-1}	5.18–6.19 mmol L^{-1}			
High	⩽ 240 mg dL^{-1}	⩽ 6.20 mmol L^{-1}			
Copper	70–155 μg dL^{-1}	11.0–24.4 μmol L^{-1}	P	Atomic absorption	0.1574
	0–60 μg dL^{-1} day^{-1}	0.0–0.94 μmol day^{-1}	U	Atomic absorption	0.01574
Creatine	< 100 mg/24 hr or < 6% of creatinine; in pregnancy: up to 12% of creatinine; in children < 1 yr: may equal creatinine; in older children: up to 30% of creatinine	< 0.75 mmol 24 hr^{-1}	U	—	—
Creatine kinase (CK)			S	Kinetic method	0.01667
Female	40–150 U L^{-1}	0.67–2.50 μkat L^{-1}			
Male	60–100 U L^{-1}	1.00–6.67 μkat L^{-1}			

Analyte	Conventional Units	SI Units	Fluid	Method or Instrument	Factor for Conversion to SI Units
General Chemistries (*Continued*)					
Creatine kinase isoenzymes, MB fraction	0–7.5 ng mL^{-1}	0–7.5 µg L^{-1}	S	Immunoassay	1
Creatine kinase isoenzyme index	0.0%–3.0% relative index	None	S	$\dfrac{\text{ng/mL}}{\text{total CK (U/L)} \times 100}$	None
Creatinine	0.6–1.5 mg dL^{-1}	53–133 µmol L^{-1}	S	Colorimetry	88.4
	15–25 mg kg^{-1} day^{-1}	0.13–0.22 mmol kg^{-1} day^{-1}	U		0.0088
Cystine or cysteine	10–100 mg day^{-1}	40–420 µmol day^{-1}	U	—	4.161
Fecal fat (as stearic acid)	1–7 g day^{-1}	3.5–25 mmol day^{-1}	—	Gravimetry	3.515
Gamma-glutamyl transpeptidase (GGT)	1.0–60.0 U L^{-1}	0.02–1.00 µkat L^{-1}	S	Kinetic method	0.01667
Globulin	2.6–4.1 g dL^{-1}	26–41 g L^{-1}	S	Calculation: total protein – albumin	10
Glucose, fasting	70–110 mg dL^{-1}	3.9–6.1 mmol L^{-1}	P	Enzymatic analysis	0.05551
High-density lipoprotein, cholesterol, as major risk factor	< 35 mg dL^{-1}	< 0.91 mmol L^{-1}	S	Colorimetry	0.02586
Ketones	Negative	Negative	S,U	Colorimetry (nitroprusside)	—
Lactic acid	0.5–2.2 mmol L^{-1}	0.5–2.2 mmol L^{-1}	P	Enzymatic analysis	1
Lactic dehydrogenase (LDH)	110–210 U L^{-1}	1.83–3.50 µkat L^{-1}	S	Kinetic method	0.01667
Lactic dehydrogenase isoenzymes			S	Electrophoresis	0.01
LD$_1$	17%–27%	0.17–0.27			
LD$_2$	28%–38%	0.28–0.38			
LD$_3$	18%–28%	0.18–0.28			
LD$_4$	5%–15%	0.05–0.15			
LD$_5$	5%–15%	0.05–0.15			
Total LDH (when isoenzymes determined)	110–250 U L^{-1}	1.83–4.23 µkat L^{-1}			
Lead	⩽ 50 µg dL^{-1}	< 2.4 µmol L^{-1}	WB	—	0.04826
Lipase	4–24 u dL^{-1}	0.67–4.00 µkat L^{-1}	S	Kinetic method	0.1667
Low-density lipoprotein cholesterol					
Desirable	< 130 mg dL^{-1}	< 3.36 mmol L^{-1}			
Borderline high risk	130–159 mg dL^{-1}	3.36–4.11 mmol L^{-1}			
High risk	⩾ 160 mg dL^{-1}	⩾ 4.13 mmol L^{-1}			
Magnesium	1.5–2.0 mEq L^{-1}	0.8–1.0 mmol L^{-1}	S	Colorimetry	0.5
5′-Nucleotidase	1–11 U L^{-1}	0.02–0.18 µkat L^{-1}	S	Kinetic method	0.01667
Osmolality	280–296 mOsm kg^{-1} of water	280–296 mmol kg^{-1}	S	Freezing-point depression	1
Oxygen, partial pressure, arterial (P_aO_2), room air, age dependent	75–100 mm Hg	10.0–13.3 kPa	WB	Oxygen electrode	0.1333
Oxygen saturation, arterial	96%–100%	0.96%–1.00	WB	Pulse oximetry	0.01
pH, arterial	7.35–7.45 pH units	7.35–7.45 pH units	WB	pH electrode	1
Phospholipids	9–16 mg dL^{-1} as lipid phosphorus	2.9–5.2 mmol L^{-1}	S	—	—

Analyte	Conventional Units	SI Units	Fluid	Method or Instrument	Factor for Conversion to SI Units
General Chemistries (*Continued*)					
Phosphorus, inorganic	2.6–4.5 mg dL^{-1}	0.84–1.45 mmol L^{-1}	S	Spectrophotometry	0.3229
	average, 1 g day^{-1}	average, 32 mmol day^{-1}	U		32.29
Potassium	3.5–5.0 mmol L^{-1}	3.5–5.0 mmol L^{-1}	S	Ion-selective electrode	1
	Diet dependent	Diet dependent	U	Ion-selective electrode	1
Prostate-specific antigen			S	Immunoassay	1
Female	0.0–0.5 μg L^{-1}	0.0–0.5 μg L^{-1}			
Male < 40 yr	0.0–2.0 μg L^{-1}	0.0–2.0 μg L^{-1}			
Male ⩾ 40 yr	0.0–4.0 μg L^{-1}	0.0–4.0 μg L^{-1}			
Protein, total	6.0–8.0 g d L^{-1}	60–80 g L^{-1}	S	Colorimetry	10
	< 165 mg day^{-1}	< 0.165 g day^{-1}	U	Turbidometry	0.001
Pyruvic acid	0.0–0.11 mEq L^{-1}	0.0–0.11 mmol L^{-1}	WB	—	—
Sodium	135–145 mmol L^{-1}	135–145 mmol L^{-1}	S	Ion-selective electrode	1
	Diet dependent	Diet dependent	U	Ion-selective electrode	1
Stool nitrogen	< 2 g 24 hr^{-1} or 10% of urinary nitrogen	< 2 g 24 hr^{-1}	—		—
Total fatty acids	190–420 mg dL^{-1}	1.9–4.2 g L^{-1}	S	—	0.01
Total lipids	450–1,000 mg dL^{-1}	4.5–10.0 g L^{-1}	S	—	0.01
Triglycerides (fasting)	40–150 mg dL^{-1}	0.45–1.69 mmol L^{-1}	S	Spectrophotometry	0.01129
Urea nitrogen (BUN)	8–25 mg dL^{-1}	2.9–8.9 mmol L^{-1}	S	Conductivity	0.357
Uric acid					
Female	1.5–6.6 mg dL^{-1}	90–393 μmol L^{-1}			
Male	2.5–8.5 mg dL^{-1}	150–506 μmol L^{-1}			
Urobilinogen	⩽ 1.0 Ehrlich U	⩽ 1.0 arbitrary unit	U	—	—
Uroporphyrin	0–30 μg 24 hr^{-1}	< 36 nmol 24 hr^{-1}	U	—	—
Vitamin A	0.15–0.6 μg mL^{-1}	0.5–2.1 μmol L^{-1}	S	—	—
Endocrine Chemistry					
Aldosterone					
Standing (normal salt diet)	4–31 ng dL^{-1}	111–860 pmol L^{-1}	S,P	Immunoassay	27.74
Recumbent (normal salt diet)	< 16 ng dL^{-1}	< 444 pmol L^{-1}	S,P	Immunoassay	27.74
Normal salt diet (100–180 mEq of sodium)	6–25 μg day^{-1}	17–69 nmol day^{-1}	U	Immunoassay	2.774
Low salt diet (10 mEq of sodium)	17–44 μg day^{-1}	47–122 nmol day^{-1}	U	Immunoassay	2.774
High salt diet	0–6 μg day^{-1}	0–17 nmol day^{-1}	U	Immunoassay	2.774
Androstenedione	60–260 ng dL^{-1}	2.1–9.1 nmol L^{-1}	S	Immunoassay	0.0349
Antidiuretic hormone (arginine vasopressin)	1.0–13.3 pg mL^{-1}	1.0–13.3 ng L^{-1}	P	Immunoassay	1
C peptide	0.30–3.70 μg L^{-1}	0.10–1.22 nmol L^{-1}	S	Immunoassay	0.33
Calcitonin					
Female	0–20 μg mL^{-1}	0–20 ng L^{-1}			
Male	0–28 pg mL^{-1}	0–28 ng L^{-1}			

Analyte	Conventional Units	SI Units	Fluid	Method or Instrument	Factor for Conversion to SI Units
Endocrine Chemistry (*Contuinued*)					
Catecholamines					
Dopamine	65–400 µg day^{-1}	424–2,612 nmol day^{-1}	U	Liquid chromatography	6.53
	0–30 pg mL^{-1}	0–196 nmol L^{-1}	P	Liquid chromatography	6.53
Epinephrine	1.7–224 µg day^{-1}	9.3–122 nmol day^{-1}	U	Liquid chromatography	5.458
Supine	0–110 pg mL^{-1}	0–600 pmol L^{-1}	P	Liquid chromatography	5.458
Standing	0–140 pg mL^{-1}	0–764	P	Liquid chromatography	5.458
Norepinephrine	12.1–85.5 µg day^{-1}	72–505 mmol day^{-1}	U	Liquid chromatography	5.911
Supine	70–750 pg mL^{-1}	0.41–4.43 nmol L^{-1}	P	Liquid chromatography	0.005911
Standing	200–1,700 pg mL^{-1}	1.18–10.0 nmol L^{-1}	P	Liquid chromatography	0.005911
Chorionicgonadotrophin (hCG) (nonpregnant)	< 10 mIU mL^{-1}	< 10 IU L^{-1}	S	Immunoassay	1
Corticotrophin (ACTH)	6.0–76.0 pg mL^{-1}	1.3–16.7 pmol L^{-1}	P	Immunoassay	0.2202
Cortisol					
fasting, 8 A.M.–12 noon	5.0–25.0 µg dL^{-1}	138–690 nmol L^{-1}			
12 noon–8 P.M.	5.0–15.0 µg dL^{-1}	138–410 nmol L^{-1}			
8 P.M.–8 A.M.	0.0–10.0 µg dL^{-1}	0–276 nmol L^{-1}			
Cortisol free	20–70 µg day^{-1}	55–193 nmol day^{-1}	U	Immunoassay	2.759
11-Deoxycortisol (after metyrapone)	> 75 µg dL^{-1}	> 216 nmol L^{-1}	P	Immunoassay	28.86
1,25-Dihydroxyvitamin D	16–42 pg mL^{-1}	38–101 pmol L^{-1}	S	Immunoassay	2.4
Erythropoietin	< 19 mU mL^{-1}	⩽ 19 U L^{-1}	S	Immunoassay	1
Estradiol			S,P	Immunoassay	3.671
Female					
Premenopausal adult	23–361 pg mL^{-1}	84–1,325 pmol L^{-1}			
Postmenopausal	< 30 pg mL^{-1}	< 110 pmol L^{-1}			
Prepubertal	< 20 pg mL^{-1}	< 73 pmol L^{-1}			
Male	< 30 pg mL^{-1}	< 184 pmol L^{-1}			
Follicle-stimulating hormone (FSH)			S,P	—	1
Female					
Preovulatory or postovulatory	4.6–22.4 mU mL^{-1}	4.6–22.4 arbitrary units			
Midcycle peak	13–41 mU mL^{-1}	13–41 arbitrary units			
Postmenopausal	30–170 mU mL^{-1}	3—170 arbitrary units			
Male	3–18 mU mL^{-1}	3–18 arbitrary units			
Gastrin	0–200 pg mL^{-1}	0–200 ng L^{-1}	P	Immunoassay	1
Growth hormone	2.0–6.0 ng mL^{-1}	2.0–6.0 µg L^{-1}	P	Immunoassay	1
Hemoglobin A$_{10}$	3.8%–6.4%	0.038–0.064	P	Liquid chromatography	0.01
Homovanillicacid	0.0–15.0 mg day^{-1}	0–82 µmol day^{-1}	U	Liquid chromatography	5.489

Endocrine Chemistry (*Contuinued*)

Analyte	Conventional Units	SI Units	Fluid	Method or Instrument	Factor for Conversion to SI Units
17-Hydroxycorticosteroids			U	Colorimetry	2.759
Female	2.0–6.0 mg day^{-1}	5.5–17.0 μmol day^{-1}			
Male	3.0–10.0 mg day^{-1}	8–28 μmol day^{-1}			
5-Hydroxyindoleacetic acid (lower in women than in men)	2–9 mg day^{-1}	10–47 μmol day^{-1}	U	Colorimetry	5.23
17-Hydroxyprogesterone			S	Immunoassay	3.026
Female					
Prepubertal	0.20–0.54 μg L^{-1}	0.61–1.63 nmol L^{-1}			
Follicular	0.02–0.80 μg L^{-1}	0.61–2.42 nmol L^{-1}			
Luteal	0.90–3.04 μg L^{-1}	2.72–9.20 nmol L^{-1}			
Postmenopausal	< 0.45 μg L^{-1}	< 1.36 nmol L^{-1}			
Male					
Prepubertal	0.12–0.30 μg L^{-1}	0.36–0.91 nmol L^{-1}			
Adult	0.20–1.80μg L^{-1}	0.61–5.45 nmol L^{-1}			
25-Hydroxyvitamin D	8–55 ng mL^{-1}	20–137 nmol L^{-1}	S	Immunoassay	2.496
Insulin	0–29 μU mL^{-1}	0–208 pmol L^{-1}	S	Immunoassay	7.175
17-Ketogenic steroids			U	Colorimetry	3.467
Female	3.0–15.0 mg day^{-1}	10–52 μmol day^{-1}			
Male	5.0–23.0 mg day^{-1}	17–80 μmol day^{-1}			
17-Ketosteroids			U	Colorimetry	3.467
Female and male ⩽ 10 yr	0.1–3.0 mg day^{-1}	0.4–10.4 μmol day^{-1}			
Female and male 11–14 yr	2.0–7.0 mg day^{-1}	6.9–24.2 μmol day^{-1}			
Female ⩾ 15 yr	5.0–15.0 mg day^{-1}	17.3–52.0 μmol day^{-1}			
Male ⩾ 15 yr	9.0–22.0 mg day^{-1}	31.2–76.3 μmol day^{-1}			
Luteinizing hormone (LH)			S,P	—	1
Female					
Preovulatory or postovulatory	2.4–34.5 mU mL^{-1}	2.4–34.5 arbitrary units			
Midcycle peak	43–187 mU mL^{-1}	43–187 arbitrary units			
Postmenopausal	30–150 mU mL^{-1}	30–150 arbitrary units			
Male	3–18 mU mL^{-1}	3–18 arbitrary units			
Metanephrines, total	0.0–0.90 mg day^{-1}	0.0–4.9 μmol day^{-1}	U	Spectrophotometry	5.458
Parathyroid hormone	10–60 pg mL^{-1}	10–60 ng L^{-1}	P	Immunoassay	1
Parathyroid-related potein	< 1.5 pmol L^{-1}	< 1.5 pmol L^{-1}	P	Immunoassay	1
Pregnanediol			U	Gas chromatography	3.12
Female	0.2–6.0 mg day^{-1}	0.6–18.7 μmol day^{-1}			
Follicular phase	0.1–1.3 mg day^{-1}	0.3–5.3 μmol day^{-1}			
Luteal phase	1.2–9.5 mg day^{-1}	3.7–29.6 μmol day^{-1}			
Pregnancy	Gestation-period dependent	Gestation-period dependent			
Male	0.2–1.2 mg day^{-1}	0.6–3.7 μmol day^{-1}			
Pregnanetriol	0.5–2.0 mg day^{-1}	1.5–6.0 μmol day^{-1}	U	Gas chromatography	2.972
Progesterone			S,P	—	3.180
Female					
Follicular phase	0.2–0.6 ng mL^{-1}	0.6–1.9 nmol day^{-1}			
Midcycle peak	0.3–3.5 mg mL^{-1}	0.95–11 nmol L^{-1}			
Postovulatory	6.5–32.2 ng mL^{-1}	21–102 nmol L^{-1}			
Male	< 1.0 ng mL^{-1}	< 3.2 nmol L^{-1}			

Analyte	Conventional Units	SI Units	Fluid	Method or Instrument	Factor for Conversion to SI Units
Endocrine Chemistry (*Contuinued*)					
Prolactin					
Female	0–15 ng mL^{-1}	0.15 µg L^{-1}			
Male	0–10 ng mL^{-1}	0–10 µg L^{-1}			
Renin activity			P	Immunoassay	0.2778
Normal salt intake					
Recumbent 6 hr	0.5–1.6 ng mL^{-1} hr^{-1}	0.14–0.44 ng (liter sec)$^{-1}$			
Upright 4 hr	1.9–3.6 ng mL^{-1} hr^{-1}	0.53–1.00 ng (liter sec)$^{-1}$			
Low salt intake					
Recumbent 6 hr	2.2–4.4 ng mL^{-1} hr^{-1}	0.61–1.22 ng (liter sec)$^{-1}$			
Upright 4 hr	4.0–8.1 ng mL^{-1} hr^{-1}	1.11–2.25 ng (liter sec)$^{-1}$			
Upright 4 hr, with diuretic	6.8–15.0 ng mL^{-1} hr^{-1}	1.89–4.17 ng (liter sec)$^{-1}$			
Resin triiodothyronine uptake	25%–35%	0.25–0.35	S	—	0.01
Reverse triiodothyronine	13–53 ng mL^{-1}	0.2–0.3 nmol L^{-1}	S	—	—
Somatomedin C (Sm-C, IGF-1)			P	Immunoassay	1
Female					
Preadolescent	60.8–724.5 ng mL^{-1}	60.8–724.5 µg L^{-1}			
Adolescent	112.5–450.0 ng mL^{-1}	112.5–450.0 µg L^{-1}			
Adult	141.8–389.3 ng mL^{-1}	141.8–389.3 µg L^{-1}			
Male					
Preadolescent	65.5–843.5 ng mL^{-1}	65.5–841.5 µg L^{-1}			
Adolescent	83.3–378.0 ng mL^{-1}	83.3–378.0 µg L^{-1}			
Adult	54.0–328.5 ng mL^{-1}	54.0–328.5 µg L^{-1}			
Testosterone: total, morning sample			P	Immunoassay	0.03467
Female	20–90 ng dL^{-1}	0.7–3.1 nmol L^{-1}			
Male, adult	300–1,100 ng dL^{-1}	10.4–38.1 nmol L^{-1}			
Testosterone, unbound, morning sample					
Female, adult	0.09–1.29 ng dL^{-1}	3–45 pmol L^{-1}			
Male, adult	3.06–24.0 ng dL^{-1}	106–832 pmol L^{-1}			
Thyroglobulin	0.60 ng mL^{-1}	0–60 µg L^{-1}	S	Immunoassay	1
Thyroid hormone-binding index	0.83–1.17	0.83–1.17	—	Charcoal resin	1
Thyroid-stimulating hormone (TSH)	0.5–5.0 µU mL^{-1}	0.5–5.0 m UL^{-1}	S	Immunoassay	1
Thyroxine, free (FT$_4$)	0.8–2.7 ng dL^{-1}	10–35 pmol L^{-1}	S	Direct equilibrium dialysis	12.87
Thyroxine-binding globulin	Age and sex dependent	Age and sex dependent	S	Immunoassay	—
Thyroxine, free, index	4.6–11.2	4.6–11.2	—	Calculation	1
Thyroxine, total (T$_4$)	4–12 µg dL^{-1}	51–154 nmol L^{-1}	S	Immunoassay	12.87
Triiodothyronine, total (T$_3$)	75–195 ng dL^{-1}	1.2–3.0 nmol L^{-1}	S	Immunoassay	0.01536
Vanillymandelic acid (VMA)	1.4–6.5 mg day^{-1}	7.1–32.7 µmol day^{-1}	L	Liquid chromatography	5.046

Analyte	Conventional Units	SI Units	Fluid	Method or Instrument	Factor for Conversion to SI Units
Immunology					
Autoantibodies					
Adrenal gland	Negative 1:10 dilution	Not applicable	S	Indirect immuno-fluorescence	—
Anticentromere antibodies	Negative at 1:40 dilution	Not applicable	S	Indirect immuno-fluorescence	—
Anti-native DNA antibodies	Negative at 1:10 dilution	Not applicable	S	Indirect immuno-fluorescence	—
Antineutrophil antibodies, direct	Negative	Not applicable	WB	Autologous immunologic assay	—
Antientrophil antibodies, indirect	Negative	Not applicable	S	Staphylococcal conjugated immunologic assay	—
Antinuclear antibodies	Negative at 1:8 dilution	Not applicable	S	Indirect immuno-fluorescence	—
Gastric parietal cells	Negative at 1:20 dilution of serum	Not applicable	S	—	—
Interstitial cells of the testes	Negative at 1:10 dilution of serum	Not applicable	S		—
La	None detected	Not applicable	S	Indirect immuno-fluorescence	—
Mitochondrial	Negative at 1:20 dilution	Not applicable	S	Indirect immuno-fluorescence	—
RNP	None detected	Not applicable	S	Indirect immuno-fluorescence	—
Ro	None detected	Not applicable	S	Indirect immuno-fluorescence	—
Skeletal muscle	Negative at 1:60 dilution of serum	Not applicable	S	—	—
Sm	None detected	Not applicable	S	Indirect immuno-fluorescence	—
Smooth muscle	Negative at 1:20 dilution	Not applicable	S	Indirect immuno-fluorescence	—
Thyroid colloid and microsomal antigens	Negative at 1:10 dilution	Not applicable	S	Indirect immuno-fluorescence or hemagglutination	—
Bence Jones protein	No Bence Jones protein detected in a 50-fold concentrate of urine	Not applicable	S	—	—
C1 esterase inhibitor protein	12.6–24.6 mg dL^{-1}	0.13–0.25 g L^{-1}	S	Nephelometry	0.01
Complement					
C3	83–177 mg dL^{-1}	0.83–1.77 g L^{-1}	S	Nephelometry	0.01
C4	15–45 mg dL^{-1}	0.15–0.45 g L^{-1}	S	Nephelometry	0.01
Total hemolytic (CH$_{50}$)	150–250 U mL^{-1}	150–250 U L^{-1}	S	Sheep red cell hemolysis	1
Factor B	17–42 mg dL^{-1}	0.17–0.42 g L^{-1}	S	Nephelometry	0.01

Analyte	Conventional Units	SI Units	Fluid	Method or Instrument	Factor for Conversion to SI Units
Immunology (*Contuinued*)					
Cryoprecipitable proteins	None detected	Not applicable	S	—	—
DNA binding[a]	Significant if > 25 units	Not applicable	S	—	—
Extractable nuclear antigen[a]	Abnormal if present	Not applicable	S	—	—
Immunoglobulin, quantitation			S	Nephelometry	
IgA	70–312 mg dL^{-1}	0.70–3.12 g L^{-1}			0.01
IgC	639–1,349 mg dL^{-1}	6.39–13.49 g L^{-1}			0.01
IgM	56–352 mg dL^{-1}	0.56–3.52 g L^{-1}			0.01
IgE	< 103 IU mL^{-1}	< 247 μg L^{-1}			2.4
Rheumatoid factor (fasting sample)	< 30 IU L^{-1}	< 30 kIU L^{-1}	S	Nephelmoetry	1
Viscosity	1.4–1.8 relative viscosity units, as compared with water	1.4–1.8 relative viscosity units, as compared with water	S	Ostwald viscosimetry	1
Hematology and Coagulation					
Alpha$_2$-antiplasmin, functional	80%–130%	0.80–1.30	P	Chromogenic assay	0.01
Anti-factor VIIIC titer	0 Bethesda units	0 Betheseda units	P	Automated clothing assay	1
Antiplatelet antibodies	Negative	Negative	P	Serotonin release	1
Antithrombin III			P		
Immunologic	22–39 mg dL^{-1}	220–390 mg L^{-1}		Immunoassay	10
Functional	80%–120%	0.80–1.20		Chromogenic assay	0.01
Bleeding time	2.0–9.5 ming	2.0–9.5 min	—	Surgicutt	1
Clot retraction	50%–100%/2 hr	0.50–1.00/2 hr	—	Manual	0.01
p-Dimer screen	< 0.5 μg mL^{-1}	< 0.5 mg L^{-1}	P	Latex agglutination	1
Differential bone marrow count	Observed range (mean)	Observed range (mean)	—	—	—
Neutrophilic series (total)	49.2%–65.0% (53.6%)	0.492–0.650 (0.536)			
Myeloblasts	0.2%–1.5% (0.9%)	0.002–0.015 (0.009)			
Promyelocytes	2.1%–4.1% (3.3%)	0.021–0.041 (0.033)			
Myelocytes	8.2%–15.7% (12.7%)	0.082–0.157 (0.127)			
Metamyelocytes	9.6%–24.6% (15.9%)	0.096–0.246 (0.159)			
Band	9.5%–15.3% (12.4%)	0.095–0.153 (0.124)			
Segmented	6.0%–12.0% (7.4%)	0.060–0.120 (0.074)			
Eosinophilic series (total)	1.2%–5.3% (3.1%)	0.012–0.053 (0.031)			
Myelocytes	0.2%–1.3% (0.8%)	0.002–0.013 (0.008)			
Metamyelocytes	0.4%–2.2% (1.2%)	0.004–0.022 (0.012)			
Band	0.2%–2.4% (0.9%)	0.002–0.24 (0.009)			
Segmented	0%–1.3% (0.5%)	0–0.013 (0.005)			
Basophilic and mast cells	0%–0.2% (0.1%)	0–0.002 (0.001)			

[a]Laboratory test value is that used by the Stanford University Hospital.

Hematology and Coagulation (*Contuinued*)

Analyte	Conventional Units	SI Units	Fluid	Method or Instrument	Factor for Conversion to SI Units
Erythrocytic series (total)	18.4%–33.8% (25.6%)	0.184–0.338 (0.236)			
Pronormoblasts	0.2%–1.3% (0.6%)	0.002–0.013 (0.006)			
Basophilic	0.5%–2.4% (1.4%)	0.005–0.024 (0.014)			
Polychromatophilic	17.9%–29.2% (21.6%)	0.179–0.292 (0.216)			
Orthochromatic	0.4%–4.6% (2.0%)	0.004–0.046 (0.020)			
Lymphocytes	11.1%–23.2% (16.2%)	0.111–0.232 (0.162)			
Plasma cells	0.4%–3.9% (1.3%)	0.004–0.039 (0.013)			
Monocytes	0%–0.8% (0.3%)	0–0.008 (0.003)			
Megakaryocytes	0%–0.4% (0.1%)	0–0.004 (0.001)			
Reticular cells	0%–0.9% (0.3%)	0–0.009 (0.003)			
M:E ratio	1.5–3.3 (2.3)	1.5–3.3 (2.3)			
Differential blood count			WB	Automated cell counter	0.01
Neutrophils	45%–74%	0.45–0.74			
Bands	0%–4%	0–0.04			
Lymphocytes	16%–45%	0.36–0.45			
Monocytes	4%–10%	0.04–0.10			
Eosinophils	0%–7%	0–0.07			
Basophils	0%–2%	0–0.02			
Erythrocyte count	$4.15–4.90 \times 10^6\,\text{mm}^{-3}$	$4.15–4.90 \times 10^{12}\,\text{L}^{-1}$	WB	Automated cell counter	1
Erythrocyte sedimentation rate			WB	Manual (modified Westergren method)	1
Female	$1–30\ \text{mm hr}^{-1}$	$1–30\ \text{mm hr}^{-1}$			
Male	$1–13\ \text{mm hr}^{-1}$	$1–13\ \text{mm hr}^{-1}$			
Euglobulin lysis time	No lysis in 2 hr	0 (in 2 hr)	P	—	—
Factor I, fibrinogen	$0.15–0.35\ \text{g dL}^{-1}$	$4.0–10.0\ \mu\text{mol L}^{-1}$	P	Automated clotting assay	29.41
Factor II, prothrombin	60%–140%	0.60–1.40	P	Automated clotting assay	0.01
Factor V	60%–140%	0.60–1.40	P	Automated clotting assay	0.01
Factor VII	60%–140%	0.60–1.40	P	Automated cloting assay	0.01
Factor VIII	50%–200%	0.50–2.00	P	Automated clotting assay	0.01
Factor IX	60%–140%	0.60–1.40	P	Automated clotting assay	0.01
Factor X	60%–140%	0.60–1.40	P	Automated clotting assay	0.01
Factor XI	60%–140%	0.60–1.40	P	Automated clotting assay	0.01
Factor XII	60%–140%	0.60–1.40	P	Automated clotting assay	0.01
Factor XIII screen	Negative	Negative	P	Urea clot dissolution	1
Ferritin			S	Immunoassay	1
Normal	$> 20\ \text{ng mL}^{-1}$	$> 20\ \mu\text{g L}^{-1}$			

Analyte	Conventional Units	SI Units	Fluid	Method or Instrument	Factor for Conversion to SI Units
Hematology and Coagulation (*Contiuined*)					
Borderline deficient	13–20 ng mL^{-1}	13-20 µg L^{-1}			
Deficient	0–12 ng mL^{-1}	0–12 µg L^{-1}			
Excessive	> 400 ng mL^{-1}	> 400 µg L^{-1}			
Fibrin(ogen) degradation products	< 10µg mL^{-1}	< 100 mg L^{-1}	S	Latex agglutination	10
Fletcher factor screen	Negative	Negative	P	Automated cloting assay	1
Folate (folic acid)			S	Immunoassay	2.266
Normal	⩾ 3.3 ng mL^{-1}	> 7.3 nmol L^{-1}			
Borderline deficient	2.5–3.2 ng mL^{-1}	5.7–7.3 nmol L^{-1}			
Deficient	< 2.5 ng mL^{-1}	< 5.7 nmol L^{-1}			
Glucose-6-phosphate dehydrogenase (erythrocyte enzyme)	5–15 U/g of hemoglobin	5–15 u/g of hemoglobin	WB	Colorimetry	1
Haptoglobin	13–163 mg dL^{-1}	0.13–1.63 g L^{-1}	S	Nephelometry	0.01
Hematocrit			WB	Automated cell counter	0.01
Female	37%–48%	0.37–0.48			
Male	42%–52%	0.42–0.52			
Hemoglobin			WB	Automated cell counter	—
Female	12–16 g dL^{-1}	7.4–9.9 mmol L^{-1}	WB	Automated cell counter	—
Male	13–18 g dL^{-1}	8.1–11.2 mmol L^{-1}			
Hemoglobin and myoglobin	0	0	U	—	—
Hemoglobin studies					
Elecrophoresis for abnormal hemoglobin	3.0%	0.030	WB	—	—
Elecrophoresis for hemoglobin A$_2$	3.0%–3.5% (borderline)	0.030–0.035 (borderline)	WB	—	—
Hemoglobin F (fetal hemoglobin)	< 2%	< 0.02	WB	—	—
Hemoglobin met- and sulf-	0	0	WB	—	—
Serum hemoglobin	2–3 mg dL^{-1}	1.2–1.9 µmol L^{-1}	S	—	—
Thermolabile hemoglobin	0	0	WB	—	—
Iron	50–150 µg dL^{-1}	9.0–26.9 µmol L^{-1}	S	Colorimetry	0.1791
Iron-binding capacity	250–410 µg dL^{-1}	45–73 µmol L^{-1}	S	Colorimetry	0.1791
Leukocyte count	4.3–10.8 × 10^3	4.3–10.8 × 10^{9}L^{-1}	WB	Automated cell counter	1
Lupus inhibitor tests				Automated clotting assay	1
Tissue thromboplastin inhibition test	Negative	Negative	P		
Dilute Russell's viper venom test	Negative	Negative	P		
Platelet neutralization procedure	Negative	Negative	P		
Anticardiolipin antibody			S	Immunoassay	1
IgG	0–23 anti-IgG units	0–23 arbitrary units			
IgM	0–11 anti-IgM units	0–11 arbitrary units			

Hematology and Coagulation (*Contiuued*)

Analyte	Conventional Units	SI Units	Fluid	Method or Instrument	Factor for Conversion to SI Units
Mean corpuscular hemoglobin (MCH)	28–33 pg cell^{-1}	28–33 pg cell^{-1}	WB	Automated cell counter	1
Mean corpuscular hemoglobin	32–36 g dL^{-1}	320–360 g L^{-1}	WB	Automated cell counter	10
Mean corpuscular volume (MCV)	86–98 μm^3	86–98 fl	WB	Automated cell counter	1
50:50 Mixing studies	Correction = factor deficiency		P	Automated clotting assay	1
Muramidase (lysozyme)	3–7 μg mL^{-1}	3–7 mg L^{-1}	S	—	—
	0–2 μg mL^{-1}	0–2 mg L^{-1}	U	—	—
Osmatic fragility of erythrocytes	Increased if hemolysis occurs at > 0.5% sodium chloride	Not applicable	WB	Spectrophotometry	1
Partial thromboplastin time, activated	24–37 sec	24–37 sec	P	Automated clotting assay	1
Peroxide hemolysis	< 10%	< 0.10	WB	Manual	0.01
Plasminogen, functional	80–130%	0.80–1.30	P	Chromogenic assay	0.01
Platelet aggregation	> 65% aggregation in response to adenosine diphosphate, epinephrine, collagen, ristocetin and arachidonic acid	Not applicable	PRP	Platelet aggregometry	Not applicable
Platelet count	150–350 × 10^3 mm^{-3}	150–350 × 10^9 L^{-1}	WB	Automated cell counter	1
Platelet, mean volume	6.6–11.0 μm^3	6.6–11.0 n	WB	Automated cell counter	1
Protein C					0.01
Immunologic	70%–140%	0.70–1.40		Immunoassay	
Functional	70%–140%	0.70–1.40		Automated clotting assay	
Protein S			P		0.01
Total antigen	70%–140%	0.70–1.40		Immunoassay	
Functional	70%–140%	0.70–1.40		Automated clotting assay	
Prothrombin time	8.8–11.6 sec	8.8–11.6 sec	P	Automated clotting assay	1
Pyruvate kinase (erythrocyte enzyme)	13–17 U gHb^{-1}	13–17 U g^{-1}	WB	—	—
Red cell distribution width	11.5%–14.5%	0.115–0.145	WB	Automated clotting assay	0.01
Reptilase time	Within 5 sec of control	Within 5 sec of control	P	Automated clotting assay	1
Reticulocyte count	0.5%–2.5% red cells	0.005–0.025 red cells	WB	Manual	0.01
Ristocetin cofactor (functional von Willebrand factor)	50%–150%	0.50–1.50	P	Platelet agglutination	0.01

Analyte	Conventional Units	SI Units	Fluid	Method or Instrument	Factor for Conversion to SI Units
Hematology and Coagulation (*Contuinued*)					
Thrombin time	Within 5 sec of control	Within 5 sec of control	P	Automated clotting assay	1
Vitamin B_{12}					
Normal	205–876 pg mL^{-1}	151–646 pmol L^{-1}			
Borderline	140–204 pg mL^{-1}	103–150 pmol L^{-1}			
Deficient	< 140 pg mL^{-1}	< 103 pmol L^{-1}			
von Willebrand factor (vWF) antigen (factor VIII:R antigen)	50%–150%	0.50–1.50	P	Immunoassay	0.01
Von Willebrand factor multimers	Normal distribution	Normal distribution	P	Western blotting	1
Whole blood clot lysis time	No clot lysis in 24 hr	0 (in 24 hr)	WB	—	—

Index